DID YOU KNOW?

- No-fat foods can cause you to gain weight.

- A single natural supplement can help people who have age-related memory problems regain twelve years of brain power.

- Essential fatty acids can keep your skin moist and healthy.

- Low potassium levels can cause caffeine cravings and a "sweet tooth."

- Men who eat three servings a week of cruciferous vegetables reduce the risk of prostate cancer by 41 percent.

- Magnesium is an aid in fighting depression and preventing heart attacks.

- Antioxidants can lower cholesterol, protect you from environmental pollution, and even help detoxify carcinogens.

- Onions, garlic, radishes, and leeks contain a natural antibiotic that can destroy disease-causing germs without harming good bacteria.

- Vitamin B6, folic acid, and vitamin B12 can save your life.

- Vitamin D deficiency weakens your immune system and could lead to an increased risk of complications to infections.

- More than 23 million Americans, including millions of children, live in food deserts—areas that are more than one mile from a supermarket at which they can buy fresh fruits and vegetables.

- 95 percent of Americans and 98 percent of teens do not have an adequate vitamin D intake.
- 61 percent of adults and 90 percent of teens do not get enough magnesium daily.
- 31 percent of the US population is at risk for at least one vitamin deficiency or anemia.
- Gummies warning: They have a shorter shelf life (they lose potency more quickly than other vitamins). There are non-uniform amounts of vitamins in gummies; they may contain more or less than the listed ingredient amounts. There is 1 gram of sugar per gummy. It's like eating a Halloween candy 365 days a year.

**UP-TO-DATE AND COMPREHENSIVE
EVERYTHING YOU'VE EVER WANTED
TO KNOW
ABOUT VITAMINS AND SUPPLEMENTS**

DR. EARL MINDELL'S

VITAMIN BIBLE

REVISED AND UPDATED

Over 200 Vitamins and
Supplements for Improving
Health, Wellness, and Longevity

Earl Mindell, RPh, PhD with
Hester Mundis

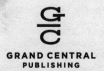

GRAND CENTRAL
PUBLISHING

NEW YORK BOSTON

The regimens throughout this book are recommendations, not prescriptions, and are not intended as medical advice. Before starting any new program, check with your physician or a nutritionally oriented doctor (see section 462), especially if you have a specific physical problem or are taking any medication.

Grand Central Publishing
Hachette Book Group
1290 Avenue of the Americas, New York, NY 10104
grandcentralpublishing.com
twitter.com/grandcentralpub

First premium mass market edition: August 2021

Grand Central Publishing is a division of Hachette Book Group, Inc. The Grand Central Publishing name and logo is a trademark of Hachette Book Group, Inc.

The publisher is not responsible for websites (or their content) that are not owned by the publisher.

The Hachette Speakers Bureau provides a wide range of authors for speaking events. To find out more, go to www.hachettespeakersbureau.com or call (866) 376-6591.

Print book interior design by Charles A. Sutherland

ISBN: 978-1-5387-3726-2 (mass market); 978-1-4555-0913-3 (ebook)

Printed in the United States of America

OPM

10 9 8 7 6 5 4 3 2 1

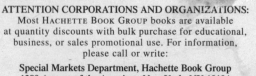

This book is dedicated to
GAIL, ALANNA, EVAN, LILY, RYAN
and our parents, families, and friends
and to
the future

Acknowledgments

I wish to express my deep and lasting appreciation to my friends and associates who have assisted me in the preparation of this book since its first publication, especially Linus Pauling, PhD; Harold Segal, PhD; Bernard Bubman, RPh; Sal Messineo, PharmD; Robert Mendelson, MD; Donald Cruden, OD; Robert Kotler, MD; Alan Needleman, RPh; Peter Mallory; Teri Cox; Carol Coleman Gerber; Hester Mundis; and Haley Weaver.

I would also like to thank the Nutrition Foundation; the International College of Applied Nutrition; the American Medical Association; the American Pharmacists Association; the New York Blood Center; the American Academy of Pediatrics; the American Dietetic Association; the National Academy of Sciences; the National Dairy Council; the Society for Nutrition Education; the United Fresh Fruit and Vegetable Association; Chapman University College of Pharmacy, Ronald Jordan, Dean; the Albany College of Pharmacy; Edward Leavitt, DVM; Jane Bicks, DVM; Betty Haskins; Shelby Zoad; Jim Zeeperman; Stephanie Marco; Susan Towlson; Sandra Scheur; Ronald Borenstein; Laura Borenstein; Glenn Williams; and Richard Curtis, without whom a project of this scope could never have been completed.

The first wealth is health.

—*Ralph Waldo Emerson,*
The Conduct of Life

Contents

IX. How to Find Out What Vitamins You Really Need

XVII. So You Think You Don't Eat Much Sugar and Salt

XVIII. Staying Beautiful—Staying Handsome

A Note to the Reader About This Revised and Updated 40th Anniversary Edition

Widely expanded and thoroughly revised, this new edition of the *Vitamin Bible* marks its 40th anniversary in print. Since the book's publication, this is the FIFTH time it has been updated to ensure it continues to be the trusted, reliable source of current nutritional information that it has been for more than two decades for millions of people around the world. My hope is that this latest iteration is the most comprehensive ever, providing the essential information and explicit guidance you need to safely pursue and successfully achieve optimal health for yourself and your family.

Although there is an abundance of nutritional information on the internet, there is an equal abundance of misinformation—about supplements, potential food and drug interactions, toxicity levels, and more. Not knowing what or what not to believe, what to look and look out for, can seriously jeopardize your health. The *Vitamin Bible* was designed to prevent that from happening by becoming the ultimate go-to nutritional reference guide, furnishing facts that you need when you want them—and right at your fingertips.

Along with more than thirty-five new sections in this edition and updated supplement regimens that include superfruits, herbal alternatives to drugs, and the latest nutraceuticals for everything from increasing fertility and dealing with postpartum depression to regaining memory brain power and sidestepping swine flu; from coping with COPD (chronic obstructive pulmonary disease) and dealing with RLS (restless legs syndrome) to protecting the prostate from BPH (benign prostatic hyperplasia) and boosting the immune system to new heights (*and much more*), the vitamin and mineral listings have all been expanded to include new FDA dosage recommendations and interactions with drugs. Also included are eye-opening sections on phytoestrogens (chemicals in plants that can act like the hormone estrogen in the body), prebiotics (nutrients for probiotics), cortisol (the stress or death hormone), fake-fat falsehoods, and, with heart disease now the leading killer among women, the top heart-protecting supplements every woman needs to know about.

The *Vitamin Bible*'s user-friendly sections are still cross-referenced in the text so you can easily find out more about what you want to know without having to refer to the index. Remember this: The more you know about how vitamins and supplements work, and how they can work for you, the more empowered you are and the more proactive you can be on your journey to optimal health.

ONE IMPORTANT REMINDER

The regimens throughout this book are recommendations, not prescriptions, and are not intended as medical advice. Before starting any new program, check with your physician or a nutritionally oriented doctor (see section 462), especially if you have a specific physical problem or are taking any medication.

Preface

This book is written for *you*—the untold legions of men and women who are forever trying to fit yourselves into statistical norms only to find that the charts are designed for some mythical average person who is taller, shorter, fatter, skinnier, less or more active than you'll ever be. It is a guide to healthy living for individuals, not statistics. Wherever feasible I have given personal advice. For this, I believe, is the only way to lead anyone to optimal health, which is the purpose of this book.

In these pages I have combined my knowledge of pharmacy with that of nutrition to best explain the confusing, often dangerous, interrelation of drugs and vitamins. I've attempted to personalize and be specific so as to eliminate much of the confusion about vitamins that has arisen with generalizations.

In using the book you will occasionally find that your vitamin needs fall into several different categories. In this case, let common sense dictate the necessary adjustment. (If you are already taking B6, for example, there's no need to double up on it unless a higher dosage is called for.)

The recommendations I've made are not meant to be prescriptive but can easily be used as flexible programs when working with your doctor. No book can substitute for professional care.

It is my sincere hope that I have provided you with information that will help you attain the longest, happiest, and healthiest of lives.

EARL L. MINDELL, RPh, PhD
WWW.DREARLMINDELL.COM

I

GETTING INTO VITAMINS

1. Why I Did

Starting out, my professional education was strictly establishment when it came to vitamins. My courses in pharmacology, biochemistry, organic and inorganic chemistry, and public health hardly dealt with vitamins at all—except in relation to deficiency diseases. (Lack of C? Scurvy. Out of B1? Beriberi. Insufficient vitamin D? Rickets.)

There were no references to vitamins being used for disease prevention or as ways to optimum health.

In 1965 I opened my first pharmacy. Until then I had never realized just how many drugs people were taking, not for illness but simply to get through the day. My partner at the time was very vitamin-oriented. Both of us were working fifteen hours a day, but only *I* looked and felt it. When I asked him what his secret was, he said it was not a secret at all. It was vitamins. I realized what he was talking about had very little to do with scurvy and beriberi and a lot to do with me. I instantly became an eager pupil, and have never since regretted it. After embarking on the most elementary vitamin regimens, I was not only convinced, I was converted.

Suddenly nutrition became the most important thing in my life. I read every book I could find on the subject, clipped articles and tracked down their sources, dug out my pharmacy school texts and discovered the amazingly close relationship that did indeed exist between biochemistry and nutrition. I attended any health lecture I could. In fact, it was at one such lecture that I learned of antioxidants and their age-reversing properties. (I have been taking antioxidant supplements since then, as well as SOD—superoxide dismutase, an enzyme present in green and white tea extracts. Today, because of these, most people guess me to be five to ten years younger than I am.) I was excited about each new discovery in the field, and it showed.

A whole new world had opened up for me, and I wanted others to share it.

By 1970 I was totally committed to nutrition and preventive medicine. Today, as a nutritionist, lecturer, and author, I'm still excited about the world that opened up to me more than forty years ago—a world that continues to grow with each new discovery that is made.

2. What Vitamins Are

When I mention the word *vitamin*, most people think *pill*. Thinking *pill* brings to mind confusing images of medicine and drugs. Though vitamins can and certainly often do the work of both medicine and drugs, they are neither.

• Quite simply, vitamins are organic substances necessary for life. Vitamins are essential to the normal functioning of our bodies and, save for a few exceptions, cannot be manufactured or synthesized internally. Necessary for our growth, vitality, and general well-being, they are found in minute quantities in all natural food. We must obtain vitamins from these foods or from dietary supplements.

What you have to keep in mind is that supplements, which are available in tablet, capsule, liquid, powder, spray, patch, and injection forms, are still just food substances, and, unless synthetic, are also derived from living plants and animals.

- It is impossible to sustain life without *all* the essential vitamins.

3. What Vitamins Are Not

A lot of people think vitamins can replace food. They cannot. In fact, vitamins cannot be assimilated without ingesting food. There are a lot of erroneous beliefs about vitamins, and I hope this book will clear up most of them.

- Vitamins are not pep pills and have no caloric or energy value of their own.
- Vitamins are not substitutes for protein or for any other nutrients, such as minerals, fats, carbohydrates, water—or even for one another!
- Vitamins themselves are not the components of our body structures.
- You cannot take vitamins, stop eating, and expect to be healthy.

4. How They Work

If you think of the body as an automobile's combustion engine and vitamins as spark plugs, you have a fairly good idea of how these amazing substances work for us.

Vitamins are components of our enzyme systems that, acting like spark plugs, energize and regulate our metabolism, keeping us tuned up and functioning at high performance.

Compared with our intake of other nutrients like proteins, fats, and carbohydrates, our vitamin intake (even on some megadose regimens) is minuscule. But a deficiency in even one vitamin can endanger the whole human body.

5. Should You Take Supplements?

Since vitamins occur in all organic material, some containing more of one vitamin than another and in greater or lesser amounts, you could say that if you ate the "right" foods in a well-balanced diet, you would get all the vitamins you need. And you would probably be right. The problem is, very few of us are able to arrange this mythical diet. According to Dr. Daniel T. Quigley, author of *The National Malnutrition,* "Everyone who has in the past eaten processed sugar, white flour, or canned food has some deficiency disease, the extent of the disease depending on the percentage of such deficient food in the diet." Additionally, the October 2002 *Journal of the American Medical Association* reported a research study stating categorically that "every adult should take a multiple vitamin since it is impossible to obtain all the nutrients needed in our daily food intake today."

Because most restaurants tend to reheat food or keep it warm under heat lamps, if you frequently eat out or take out you run the risk of vitamin A, B1, and C deficiencies. Also, since so many of our foods are processed or genetically modified (75 percent of the food in grocery stores has been genetically modified), lack of calcium, folic acid, and magnesium is epidemic. (And if you're a woman between the ages of thirteen and forty, this sort of work-saving dining is likely to cost you invaluable bone-building calcium and iron.)

Processed foods have been depleted in nutrients. Take breads and cereals, for example. Practically all of them you find in today's supermarkets are high in nothing but carbohydrates. "But they are enriched!" you say. It's written right on the label: *enriched.*

Enriched? Enrichment means replacing nutrients in foods that once contained them but because of heat, storage, and so forth no longer do. Foods, therefore, are "enriched" to the levels found in the natural product before processing. Unfortunately, standards of enrichment leave much to be desired nutritionally. For example, the standard of enrichment for white flour is to replace the twenty-two natural nutrients that are removed with three B vitamins, vitamin D, calcium, and iron salts. Now really, for the staff of life, that seems a pretty flimsy stick.

I think you can see why my feeling about taking supplements is clear.

6. What Are Nutrients?

They're more than vitamins, though people often think they are the same thing. Carbohydrates, proteins (which are made up of amino acids), fats, minerals, vitamins, and water are all nutrients—absorbable components of foods— and necessary for good health. Nutrients are necessary for energy, organ function, food utilization, and cell growth.

7. The Difference Between Micronutrients and Macronutrients

Micronutrients, like vitamins and minerals, do not themselves provide energy. The macronutrients—carbohydrates, fat, and protein—do that, but only when there are sufficient micronutrients to release them.

The amount of micronutrients and macronutrients you need for proper health is vastly different—but each is important. (See section 75 for the protein–amino acid connection.)

8. How Nutrients Get to Work

Nutrients basically work through digestion. Digestion is a process of continuous chemical simplification of materials that enter the body through the mouth. Materials are split by enzymatic action into smaller and simpler chemical fragments, which can then be absorbed through walls of the digestive tract—an open-ended muscular tube, more than thirty feet long, which passes through the body—and finally enter the bloodstream.

9. Understanding Your Digestive System

Knowing how your digestive system works will clear up some of the more common confusions about how, when, and where nutrients operate.

Mouth and Esophagus

Digestion begins in the mouth with the grinding of food and a mixture of saliva. An enzyme called ptyalin in the saliva begins to split starches into simple sugars. The food is then forced to the back of the mouth and into the esophagus, or gullet. Here is where peristalsis begins. This is a kneading, "milking" constriction and relaxation of muscles that propels material through the digestive system. To prevent backflow of materials, and to time the release of proper enzymes—since one enzyme cannot do another enzyme's work—the digestive tract is equipped with valves at important junctions.

The tiny valve at the end of your esophagus opens long enough for chewed-up particles to enter the stomach. Occasionally, especially after eating, this valve relaxes—which is what enables you to belch. But a relaxed valve can also allow the acid from your stomach to be pushed back up into the esophagus, causing what's known as gastroesophageal reflux disease (GERD)—better known to those who experience it as heartburn (see section 305).

Stomach

This is the biggest bulge in the digestive tract, as most of us are well aware. But it is located higher than you might think, lying mainly behind the lower ribs, not under the navel, and it does not occupy the belly. It is a flexible bag enclosed by restless muscles, constantly changing form.

Virtually nothing is absorbed through the stomach walls except alcohol.

Watery substances, such as soup, leave the stomach quite rapidly. Fats remain considerably longer. An ordinary meal of carbohydrates, proteins, and fats is emptied from the average stomach in *three* to *five* hours. Stomach glands and specialized cells produce mucus, enzymes, hydrochloric acid, and a factor that enables vitamin B12 to be dissolved through intestinal walls into the circulation. A normal stomach is definitely on the acid side, and gastric juice, the stomach's special blend, consists of many substances:

Pepsin The predominant stomach enzyme, a potent digester of meats and other proteins. It is active only in an acid medium.

Rennin Curdles milk.

HCl (hydrochloric acid) Produced by stomach cells and creates an acidic state.

The stomach is not absolutely indispensable to digestion. Most of the process of digestion occurs beyond it.

Small Intestine

Twenty-two feet long, this is where digestion is completed and virtually all absorption of nutrients occurs. It has an alkaline environment, brought about by highly alkaline bile, pancreatic juice, and secretions of the intestinal walls. The alkaline environment is necessary for the most important work of digestion and absorption. The *duodenum,* which begins at the stomach outlet, is the first part of the small intestine. This joins with the *jejunum* (about ten feet long), which joins with the *ileum* (ten to twelve feet long). When semiliquid contents of the small intestine are moved along by peristaltic action, we often say we hear our stomachs "growling." Actually the stomach lies above these rumblings (called *borborygmi*), but even with the truth known it's doubtful the phrase will change.

Large Intestine (Colon)

Any material leaving the ileum and entering the *cecum* (where the small and large intestine join) is quite watery. Backflow is prevented at this junction by a muscular valve.

Very little is absorbed from the large intestine except water.

The colon is primarily a storage and dehydrating organ. Substances entering in a liquid state become semisolid as water is absorbed. It takes twelve to fourteen hours for contents to make the circuit of the intestine.

The colon, in contrast to a germ-free stomach, is lavishly populated with bacteria, normal intestinal flora. A large part of the feces is composed of bacteria, along with indigestible material, chiefly cellulose, and substances eliminated from the blood and shed from the intestinal walls.

Liver

The liver is the largest solid organ of the body and weighs about four pounds. It is an incomparable chemical plant. It can modify almost any chemical structure. It is a powerful detoxifying organ, breaking down a variety of toxic molecules and rendering them harmless. It is also a blood reservoir and a storage organ for vitamins such as A and D and for digested carbohydrate (glycogen), which is released to sustain blood sugar levels. It manufactures enzymes, cholesterol, proteins, vitamin A (from carotene), and blood coagulation factors.

One of the prime functions of the liver is to produce bile. Bile contains salts that promote efficient digestion of fats by detergent action, emulsifying fatty materials.

Gallbladder

This is a saclike storage organ about three inches long. It holds bile, modifies it chemically, and concentrates it tenfold. The taste or sometimes even the sight of food may be sufficient to empty it out. Constituents of gallbladder fluids sometimes crystallize and form gallstones.

Pancreas

This gland is about six inches long and is nestled into the curve of the duodenum. Its cell clusters secrete insulin, which accelerates the burning of sugar in the body. Insulin is secreted into the blood, not the digestive tract. The larger part of the pancreas manufactures and secretes pancreatic juice, which contains some of the body's most important digestive enzymes—*lipases,* which split fats; *proteases,* which split protein; and *amylases,* which split starches.

10. The Importance of Enzymes

Enzymes are necessary for the digestion of food, releasing valuable vitamins, minerals, and amino acids that keep us alive and healthy.

Enzymes are catalysts, meaning they have the power to cause an internal action without themselves being changed or destroyed in the process.

Enzymes are destroyed under certain heat conditions.

Enzymes are best obtained from uncooked or unprocessed fruits, vegetables, eggs, meats, and fish.

Each enzyme acts upon a specific food; one cannot substitute for the other. A deficiency, shortage, or even the absence of one single enzyme can mean the difference between sickness and health.

Enzymes that end in *-ase* are named by the food substance they act upon. For example, with phosphorus the enzyme is called phosphatase; with sugar (sucrose) it is known as sucrase.

Pepsin is a vital digestive enzyme that breaks up the proteins of ingested food, splitting them into usable amino acids. Without pepsin, protein could not be used to build healthy skin, strong skeletal structure, rich blood supply, and strong muscles.

Rennin is a digestive enzyme that causes coagulation of milk, changing its protein, casein, into a usable form in the body. Rennin releases the valuable minerals from milk, calcium, phosphorus, potassium, and iron, which are used by the body to stabilize the water balance, strengthen the nervous system, and produce strong teeth and bones.

Lipase splits fat, which is then utilized to nourish the skin cells, protect the body against bruises and blows, and ward off the entrance of infectious virus cells and allergic conditions.

Hydrochloric acid in the stomach works on tough foods such as fibrous meats, vegetables, and poultry. It digests protein, calcium, and iron. Without HCl, problems such as pernicious anemia, gastric carcinoma, congenital achlorhydria, and allergies can develop. Because stress, tension, anger, and anxiety before eating, as well as deficiencies of some vitamins (B complex primarily) and minerals, can all cause a lack of HCl, more of us are short of it than we realize. If you think that you have an overacid problem or heartburn, for which you are dosing yourself with an antacid such as Pepsid Complete, Tums, Rolaids, or Alka-Seltzer, you are probably unaware that *the symptoms of having too little acid are exactly the same as having too much,* in which case the taking of antacids could be the worst possible thing for you to do.

Dr. Alan Nittler, author of *A New Breed of Doctor*, has stated emphatically that everyone over the age of forty should be using an HCl supplement.

Betaine HCl and glutamic acid HCl are the best forms of commercially available hydrochloric acid.

CAUTION: *If you have an ulcer condition, consult your doctor before using these supplements.*

11. Why You Need Carbohydrates

Carbohydrates, the scourge of misinformed dieters, are the main suppliers of the body's energy. During digestion, starches and sugars, the principal kinds of carbohydrates, are broken down into glucose, better known as blood sugar. This blood sugar provides the essential energy for the brain and central nervous system.

You need carbohydrates in your daily diet so that vital tissue-building protein is not wasted for energy when it might be needed for repair. If you eat too many carbohydrates, more than can be converted into glucose or glycogen (which is stored in liver and muscles), the result, as we know all too well, is fat. When the body needs more fuel, the fat is converted back to glucose and you lose weight.

Don't be too down on carbohydrates. They're as important for good health as other nutrients—and gram for gram they have the same 4 calories as protein. Though no official requirement exists, a minimum of 50 g. daily is recommended to avoid ketosis, an acid condition of the blood that can happen when your own fat is used primarily for energy.

12. Name That Vitamin

Because at one time no one knew the chemical structure of vitamins and therefore could not give them a proper scientific name, most are designated by a letter of the alphabet. The following vitamins are known today; many more may yet be discovered: vitamin A (retinol, carotene); vitamin B-complex group: B1 (thiamin), B2 (riboflavin), B3 (niacin, niacinamide), B4 (adenine), B5 (pantothenic acid), B6 (pyridoxine), B10, B11 (growth factors), B12 (cobalamin, cyanocobalamin), B13 (orotic acid), B15 (pangamic acid), B1, Bc (folic acid), Bt (carnitine), Bx or PABA (para-aminobenzoic acid); choline; inositol; C (ascorbic acid); D (calciferol, viosterol, ergosterol); E (tocopherol); F (fatty acids); G (riboflavin); H (biotin); K (menadione); L (necessary for lactation); M (folic acid); P (bioflavonoids); Pp (nicotinamide); P4 (troxerutin); T (growth-promoting substances); U (extracted from cabbage juice).

Japanese scientists at the Tokyo-based Institute of Physical and Chemical Research say that PQQ (pyrroloquinoline quinone), a substance discovered in 1979 and subsequently shown to play an important role in fertility in mice and possibly in humans, could be categorized as a vitamin. If so, it would be the first new vitamin identified in fifty-five years.

What is known about PQQ: It is an antioxidant and believed to belong to the B-complex family. The best natural source is natto, a pungent Japanese dish of fermented soybeans. It is also found in parsley, green tea, green peppers, kiwi fruit, and papaya. (Personal advice: If you want to add some PQQ to your diet naturally, I'd suggest you go the parsley, green tea, peppers, papaya, and kiwi route. Having tasted natto, it's not something I'd recommend, unless you really enjoy a flavor with the pungency of well-worn socks.)

13. Name That Mineral

Although about eighteen known minerals are required for body maintenance and regulatory functions, recommended dietary intake (RDI) has been established for only seven—calcium, iodine, iron, magnesium, phosphorus, selenium, and zinc.

The active minerals in your body are calcium, chlorine, chromium, cobalt, copper, fluorine, iodine, iron, magnesium, manganese, molybdenum, phosphorus, potassium, selenium, sodium, sulfur, vanadium, and zinc. Trace minerals such as boron, silicon, nickel, and arsenic are also necessary for optimal growth and membrane function.

14. Your Body Needs Togetherness

As important as vitamins are, they can do nothing for you without minerals. I like to call minerals the Cinderellas of the nutrition world because, though very few people are aware of it, vitamins cannot function and cannot be assimilated without the aid of minerals. And though the body can synthesize some vitamins, it cannot manufacture a *single* mineral.

15. Name That Antioxidant

Antioxidants (good guys) are those enzymes, amino acids, supplements, vitamins, and minerals that protect our bodies from *free radicals* (bad guys), uncontrolled oxidations that damage cells and weaken the immune system. The body generates free radicals daily simply by burning fuel for energy. In other words, they're a necessary but unwanted by-product. Various environmental and physical stresses—from air pollution, smoking, drinking alcohol, and disease to charcoal-broiled food, old age, and vigorous exercise—generate extra free radicals. To keep free radicals in check, our bodies produce different types of natural antioxidants. The best way to understand how antioxidants work is to take an apple, slice it in half, and put the two halves on a countertop. What happens to the exposed apple after a while? It turns brown, it oxidizes, it rusts. The same thing happens in your body. If you squeeze some lemon juice on one-half of the exposed apple before it turns brown, it prevents this rusting from occurring, because the vitamin C in the lemon juice is an antioxidant. The most notable antioxidants are catalase, coenzyme-Q10, glutathione, melatonin, vitamin A, alpha- and beta-carotene, vitamin C, vitamin E, lipoic acid, selenium, superoxide dismutase (SOD), grape-seed and grape-skin extract, green and white tea extract, resveratrol, and zinc. Unfortunately, as we age, more free radicals accumulate and less natural antioxidants are produced, significantly increasing the risk of cancer and heart disease. Because of this, antioxidant-rich foods and supplements such as ginkgo biloba, grape-seed extract, green tea extract, isoflavones, lutein, and lycopene are needed in our diets, and the sooner they are included the greater the long-term benefits. (See chapter VII.)

16. Name That Nutraceutical

Nutraceuticals are possibly the most exciting break-through in preventive medicine in decades. They are derived from natural products (food substances or parts of a food) that have proven therapeutic benefits similar to pharmaceuticals—such as isoflavones from soy, which have anticancerous properties; and hypericum and polyphenols in St. John's wort, which have antidepressant properties. These naturally occurring compounds extracted from plants, algae, and other biological sources are concentrated into pills, powders, and capsules and are now being used to prevent numerous diseases as well as to treat common ailments—an area formerly ruled by prescription drugs. For example, antidepressants such as Paxil and Prozac, selective serotonin reuptake inhibitors (SSRIs), have been found to be matched in effectiveness by nutraceuticals such as 5-HTP (see section 81), which is made from a natural extract from the seeds of the Griffonia simplicifolia tree.

Nutraceuticals can also concentrate the best of food chemicals for daily consumption. Since only 9 percent of Americans eat five servings of fruits and vegetables a day, these supplements are playing an increasingly important role in our nation's health. There are phytochemical-enriched foods, for example, snack bars fortified with soy phytochemicals (phytoestrogens), to alleviate symptoms such as hot flashes in menopausal women and to prevent prostate problems in men, nutraceutical-enriched margarine to lower blood serum cholesterol, as well as phytochemical-enriched candy for children who don't care for vegetables. There are a lot more ways, these days, to get what's good for you into you.

17. Name That Alternative Therapy

Just as no one supplement fits all, no one alternative therapy is suited to everyone. Today, dozens of alternatives to conventional medicine are available, gaining in acceptance and evidencing remarkable results. (To locate a nutritionally oriented doctor or alternative practitioner, see section 462.) Among the better known alternative therapies are:

Ayurveda One of the oldest recorded medical systems in the world, India's ayurvedic medicine is still practiced in that country today. It has been dubbed the "mother of all healing" because of its profound influence on nearly all other medical systems. Ayurveda does not just treat the symptoms of a disease: The treatment must encompass the entire body—as well as mind, spirit, and lifestyle. The belief is that it's as important to keep healthy people healthy as it is to cure the sick, and that early intervention— before symptoms appear—is essential to well-being.

More than two thousand different preparations are used in ayurvedic medicine. Herbs are generally used only in combination with other herbs. In fact, ayurvedic healers use the whole plant, as opposed to the Western concept of extracting the one or two active ingredients, because they believe that every chemical in a plant is designed to work in harmony with the body. Ayurvedic medicine is designed to bolster and support all body systems.

Acupuncture An ancient Chinese healing medicine based on the belief that a life force, *qi* (pronounced *chee*) flows through fourteen channels in the body and can be stimulated by the insertion of needles into some of the body's 360 acupuncture points to restore its energy balance. Acupuncture has been shown to have the ability in many instances to reverse temporary discomforts as well as organic disease. Acupuncturists also use herbs in healing therapies. In most states in the US, completion of a recognized program of study and a license to practice is required to become a doctor of acupuncture or a doctor of Oriental medicine. Naturopathic doctors (NDs) are also licensed to practice acupuncture.

Chiropractic Chiropractic medicine focuses on spinal manipulations to achieve health. Many chiropractors (DCs) also practice nutritional medicine. They have had four to five years of study in an accredited chiropractic school after a minimum of two years of undergraduate school and are licensed to work in all fifty states, Australia, New Zealand, Canada, most of Europe, Africa, and the Middle East. They cannot prescribe drugs or do surgery.

Herbal medicine The most widely used form of medicine for thousands of years and recognized as today's leading trend in self-care. Herbal medicine is rooted in the same theory as establishment pharmacology. In fact, nearly 50 percent of all drugs commonly used and prescribed either are derived from a plant source or contain chemical imitations of a plant compound. Today, the efficacy of many herbal remedies is undisputed and well documented. (See chapter VIII.)

Homeopathy Based on the findings of Samuel Hahnemann, homeopathy uses medicines to stimulate the body's natural defense mechanisms and is based on the premise that "like cures like." For instance, a substance that can trigger symptoms in a healthy individual when taken in large doses can cure similar symptoms in a sick person when taken in extremely small doses. The homeopathic approach to treating illness—viewing the individual (mentally, physically, emotionally) as a whole—is founded on the understanding that symptoms are an expression of the body's attempt to correct an imbalance and restore health. Rather than suppressing these symptoms, homeopathic medicines (which come from naturally occurring plant, mineral, or animal substances and are nontoxic) act quickly to stimulate and regulate the body's defenses—*with no side effects when used as directed* (see section 230). There is no licensing at this writing for the practice of homeopathic medicine. A physician (MD, DO, ND, or DC) can become a doctor of homeopathy (DHt) after six weeks of study.

Naturopathic Naturopathic medicine encompasses herbal medicine, massage, acupuncture, and a broad spectrum of other alternative treatments. Naturopathic doctors (NDs) are required to pass a national licensing exam after completing four years in a naturopathic medical college.

Orthomolecular medicine An alternative therapy that aims to provide optimal levels of substances normally found in the body through nutrients. Aside from using various supplements to allow the body to produce the biochemicals necessary for health, orthomolecular medicine also involves the removal of harmful substances such as drugs, pollutants, and allergens from the body. The majority, though not all, of orthomolecular practitioners are MDs.

Osteopathy Osteopathic physicians (DOs) have the same medical education as an MD and are licensed to do everything an MD can do, including surgery. The *big* difference is that unlike traditional (allopathic) MDs, who tend to specialize in certain diseases or organs, osteopaths are holistic in their approach to healing and, as a rule, are far better versed in preventive nutrition.

DID YOU KNOW?

- It is impossible to sustain life without *all* the essential vitamins.
- The body can synthesize some vitamins but cannot manufacture a *single* mineral.
- A deficiency in even one vitamin can endanger the whole human body.

---

18. Any Questions About Chapter I?

I've seen quite a few amino acid supplements in natural food stores. Are these considered nutrients? Are they as important as vitamins?

Emphatically yes, and yes again! Amino acids (see section 75) are the building blocks of one of our most important nutrients—protein.

Every cell in your body contains (and needs) protein. It's used to build new tissue and repair damaged cells, as well as to make hormones and enzymes, keep the acid-alkaline blood content balanced, and eliminate the unwanted garbage, among other things. As protein is digested, it's broken down into smaller compounds called amino acids. When these amino acids reach the cells in your body, they're formed into protein again. It's a wonderful cycle.

The importance of vitamins and amino acids in nutrition is equal, because you'll get no value from one without the proper amount of the other. As for amino acid supplements and their value to you as an individual, I'd suggest looking over sections 75 and 80, which discuss some of the remarkable benefits supplementation has been shown to provide.

I know that vitamins can't work properly without minerals, but do some minerals make them work more effectively than others?

Absolutely. Vitamin A, for instance, works best with the minerals calcium, magnesium, phosphorus, selenium, and zinc. The B vitamins are also potentiated by these minerals, along with cobalt, copper, iron, manganese, potassium, and sodium. For vitamin C, the five minerals found to promote the most effectiveness are calcium, cobalt, copper, iron, and sodium; for vitamin D, they are calcium, copper, magnesium, selenium, and sodium; and for vitamin E, they are calcium, iron, manganese, phosphorus, potassium, selenium, sodium, and zinc. To find out what minerals—and other vitamins—can increase the effectiveness of individual vitamins, see sections 30–53.

What is boron?

Underappreciated! It's a trace mineral needed by the body in only minuscule amounts, which is why there's no official recommended daily allowance. But this does not diminish its importance in working with calcium, magnesium, and vitamin D to help prevent osteoporosis. And it may even help your brain to work better. It's found in most fruits and vegetables; however, dried fruits such as prunes and apricots are the best source. As a supplement, I recommend 3 mg. daily. (Do not exceed 10 mg. daily.)

What's the difference between nutraceuticals and functional foods?

Nutraceuticals and functional foods (often referred to interchangeably) are food components that have health-promoting, disease-preventing, or medicinal properties above and beyond their basic nutritional functions. But while a functional food is similar to a conventional food, a nutraceutical is isolated from a food and can be sold in dosage form.

What are phytochemicals?

Phytochemicals are chemicals found in plants; health-promoting nutrients that give fruits, vegetables, grains, and legumes their color, flavor, and natural protection against disease. They are, essentially, the plants' immune system. They are potent antioxidants and can provide protection against free radical damage, helping the body ward off a variety of ailments, including heart disease and cancer.

I have a mitral valve prolapse and take antibiotics often. I've heard about probiotics, but don't know what they are. Should I be taking them?

You sure should! *Probiotic,* which means "for life," is a general term for microorganisms known as friendly bacteria, which support the body's own defenses against infection and disease. There are billions of friendly bacteria in our bodies, and they do some wonderful things, such as aid in digestion, improve immune function, help keep hormone levels normal, protect against overgrowth infection from fungi and yeasts (which may be absorbed into the bloodstream and contribute to other serious diseases), manufacture some B vitamins, and more.

Unfortunately, antibiotics can't distinguish between good and bad bacteria. Overuse can lead to an increase in drug-resistant strains and, therefore, make you more susceptible to illness. You can increase your good bacteria levels by adding more fiber to your diet (intestinal bacteria consume dietary fiber and metabolize it into acids that inhibit the growth of bad bacteria) and eating yogurt— preferably nonfat or low-fat—made with live, active cultures. (Dairy-free probiotics are also available.) But the easiest way would be to take a daily probiotic supplement during the time you're taking the antibiotics—and for about a month afterward to replenish your good bacteria. I'd suggest 1 capsule (or 1 tbsp. liquid) three times a day, half an hour before meals. *NOTE*: You may experience gas or bloating when you first start taking probiotics. This is an indication that the good bacteria are fermenting and the problem should disappear in a week or so when your body adjusts to the change. (See section 131.)

What are carotenoids?

The most important thing to know about carotenoids is that they're good for you (see section 107). They're a class of compounds related to vitamin A, the best-known being beta-carotene (others include alpha-carotene, gamma-carotene, lutein, and lycopene), which has long been shown to be helpful in preventing many types of cancer. The beta-carotene in foods is converted into vitamin A, but, unlike vitamin A, large amounts are not toxic. (Too much beta-carotene could, though, make you look as if you've been overdoing it on bronzers by turning your skin an orangey yellow.)

Lycopene, the substance that gives tomatoes,

watermelon, pink grapefruit, and other fruits and vegetables their distinctive red color, is the new popular carotenoid on the nutritional block. Findings from Harvard University, the U.S. Department of Agriculture, and the Dana-Farber Cancer Institute indicate that tomato consumption reduces the risk of cancer in general and prostate cancer in particular. In fact, the study showed that men who consumed large amounts of tomatoes had only about half the risk of prostate cancer as did men who consumed small amounts of tomato products. Because fat helps move lycopene into the bloodstream, pizza might finally have a redeeming nutritional feature. Just don't cancel it out with pepperoni and extra cheese!

I know that antioxidants fight oxidation in the body, but what exactly is oxidation and what causes it?

Oxidation is what happens to metal when it rusts or an apple when it turns brown. Unstable oxygen molecules called free radicals steal electrons from other molecules in an attempt to become stable. In the process, the free radicals damage cells, shortening their life span and speeding up the aging process. Once oxidation begins it can be hard to stop. The consequences range from infections to various degenerative conditions including heart disease, arthritis, and cancer.

What causes oxidation? Dozens of things, but the most common culprits are pollutants, chemicals, and toxins, such as cigarette smoke. (See section 104.)

What are "smart nutrients" and do they really make you smart?

Well, you're smart if you're getting them. They're the nutrients that have been shown to protect and enhance brain function. Our levels of naturally produced antioxidants, which protect the brain from destructive free radicals, decline with age. Because of this, antioxidant supplements—which include vitamins, minerals, amino acids, and herbs—have been deemed smart nutrients. (See chapter VII.)

Some smart nutrients you'd be wise to look into and look for, especially in combination supplements, are: vitamin E, gamma tocotrienol, sage extract, wild green oats, spearmint tea, lithium orotate, ashwagandha extract, grape-seed extract, lipoic acid, NADH (coenzyme I), vitamin B1 (thiamin), vitamin B3 (niacin), vitamin B6 (pyridoxine), vitamin B12, folic acid, choline, L-carnitine, phenylalanine, DHA (docosahexaenoic acid), DMAE (dimethylamino-ethanol), phosphatidylethanolamine, phosphatidylcephalin, fo-ti root, schizandra berry, l-glutamine, vinpocetine, ginkgo biloba, gotu kola, blueberry (*brain berries*) extract, hupA (huperzine A), magnesium, pregnenolone, phosphatidylserine, phosphatidylcholine, inositol, and zinc. None of these brain-boosters will make you an Einstein, but they can help you remember where you put your car keys.

Are genetically engineered foods safe to eat? And how do we know if the food we're eating has been genetically altered?

If you can avoid eating them, you're better off. Unfortunately, at this point in time it's nearly impossible. Virtually all of our processed food contains genetically modified ingredients somewhere in their production—the wheat used for wheat flour has been genetically modified, as has the corn in cornstarch, and so on. Products can even be labeled "all natural" and "organic" (see section 243) and still contain GM foods. As for the safety, the FDA has green-lighted them, but the long-term effects are still unknown. My advice is to at least minimize your GM intake by limiting the processed foods you eat, cutting back on visits to fast-food restaurants, and, whenever possible, shop organic.

To tell if your tomatoes are genetically modified, throw one against a wall. If it bounces back unbruised, you know it has been genetically modified. Genetically modified tomatoes have thicker skins so that they do not bruise as easily. They are also making tomatoes grow squarer so that they can be shipped in boxes more efficiently.

II

A Vitamin Pill Is a Vitamin Pill Is a...

19. Where Vitamins Come From

Because vitamins are natural substances found in foods, the supplements you take—be they capsules, tablets, powders, or liquids—also come from foods. Though many of the vitamins can be synthesized, most are extracted from basic natural sources.

For example: Vitamin A usually comes from fish liver oil. Vitamin B complex comes from yeast or liver. Vitamin C is best when derived from rose hips, the berries found on the fruit of the rose after the petals have fallen off—or from tapioca. And vitamin E is generally extracted from soybeans, wheat germ, or corn.

20. Why Vitamins Come in Different Forms

Everyone's needs are different, and for this reason manufacturers have provided many vitamins in a variety of forms.

Tablets are the most common and convenient form.

They're easier to store, carry, and have a longer shelf life than powders or liquids—and they cannot be adulterated.

Caplets are capsule-shaped tablets. These can be enteric coated so that they dissolve in the intestine, not in the stomach (which is acid).

Capsules, like tablets, are convenient and easy to store, and are the usual supplement for oil-soluble vitamins such as A, D, and E. They contain fewer excipients than do tablets.

Gelatin capsules are made with gelatin, an animal product. They should be stored away from light in a cool, dry area to prevent oxidation.

Vegetable capsules are free of any animal products, starches, sugars, and other allergens. They're made from cellulose and plant fiber from trees, which is resistant to fungal and bacterial problems. They can withstand storage in a high-temperature environment without melting or sticking together. They're not affected by cold, dry climates that may cause gelatin caps to become brittle. Unfortunately, they can react with the ingredients in them and are therefore not used as much as gelatin capsules. They are also more expensive.

Softgels (or *gelcaps*) are soft gelatin capsules that many people find easier to swallow than regular capsules. Like tablets and capsules, softgels must be processed through the digestive system, so they're slower acting than their liquid and powder counterparts.

Powders have the advantages of extra potency (1 tsp. of many vitamin C powders can give you as much as 4,000 mg.) and the added benefit of no fillers, binders, or additives for anyone with allergies.

Liquids are available for easy mixing with beverages and for people unable to swallow capsules or tablets.

Intraoral sprays deliver *low-dose* concentrations of

nutrients directly into the mouth, under the tongue. They are absorbed into the bloodstream through the mucous membranes and bypass the gastrointestinal tract, generally within fifteen minutes.

Sublinguals are tablets that dissolve under the tongue. (For vitamin B12, this is my recommended form of supplement because it is better absorbed by the body.)

Patches and implants supply continuous, measured amounts of nutrients, though at this writing they are available only for a limited number of nutritional supplements and are considered drug-delivery systems in the United States.

Gummies are often "chewable candy." Look for gummies that contain no sugar, unless you enjoy dental visits.

21. Oil vs. Dry or Water Soluble

The oil-soluble vitamins, such as A, D, E, and K, are available and advisable in "dry" or water-soluble form for people who tend to get upset stomachs from oil, for acne sufferers or anyone with a skin condition where oil ingestion is not advised, and for dieters who have cut most of the fat from their meals. (Fat-soluble vitamins need fat for proper assimilation. If you're on a low-fat diet and taking A, D, E, or supplements, I suggest you use the dry form.)

22. Synthetic vs. Natural and Inorganic vs. Organic

When I'm asked if there's a difference between synthetic and natural vitamins, I usually say only one—and that's to you. Though synthetic vitamins and minerals have produced satisfactory results, the benefits from natural vitamins, on a variety of levels, surpass them. Chemical analysis of both might appear the same, but there's more to natural vitamins because there's more to those substances in nature. (See section 29.)

Synthetic vitamin C is just that, ascorbic acid and nothing more. Natural C from rose hips contains bioflavonoids, the entire C complex, which make the C much more effective.

Natural vitamin E, which includes all the tocopherols—alpha, beta, gamma, and delta—not just alpha, is more potent and better absorbed than its synthetic form of dl-alpha-tocopherol.

According to Dr. Theron G. Randolph, noted allergist: *"A synthetically derived substance may cause a reaction in a chemically susceptible person when the same material of natural origin is tolerated, despite the two substances having identical chemical structures."*

On the other hand, people who are allergic to pollen could experience an undesirable reaction to a natural vitamin C that has possible pollen impurities.

Nonetheless, as many who have tried both can attest, there are fewer gastrointestinal upsets with natural supplements, and far fewer toxic reactions when taken in a higher than recommended dosage.

The difference between inorganic and organic is not the same as the difference between synthetic and natural, though that is the common misconception. All vitamins are organic. They are substances containing carbon.

23. Chelation, and What It Means

First, pronounce it correctly: *Key-lation.* This is the process by which mineral substances are changed into their digestible form. Most mineral supplements are often not chelated and must first be acted upon in the digestive process to form chelates before they are of use to the body. The natural chelating process is not performed efficiently in many people, and because of this a good deal of the mineral supplements taken are of little use.

When you realize that the body does not use whatever it takes in, that most of us do not digest our foods efficiently, that only 2–10 percent of inorganic iron taken into the body is actually absorbed, and, even with this small percentage, 50 percent is then eliminated, you can recognize the importance of taking minerals that have been chelated. *Amino acid–bound chelated mineral supplements provide three to ten times greater assimilation than the nonchelated ones!*

24. Time Release

Time (or sustained) release is a process by which vitamins are enrobed in micropellets (tiny time pills) and then combined into a special base for their release in a pattern that assures three- to six-hour absorption. Most vitamins are water soluble and cannot be stored in the body. Without time release, they are quickly absorbed into the bloodstream, and, no matter how large the dose, are excreted in the urine within two to three hours.

Time-release supplements can offer optimum effectiveness, minimal excretory loss, and stable blood levels during the day and through the night. (Check label for release pattern because many time-release vitamins do so in two hours or less, making them no better than regular tablets, which are generally less expensive.)

25. Fillers and Binders—What Else Am I Getting?

There's more to a vitamin supplement than meets the eye—and sometimes more than meets the label. Fillers, binders, lubricants, and the like do not have to be listed and often aren't. But if you'd like to know what you're swallowing, the following list should help.

Diluents or fillers These are inert materials added to the tablets to increase their bulk, in order to make them a practical size for compression. Dicalcium phosphate, which is an excellent source of calcium and phosphorus, is used in better brands. It is derived from purified mineral rocks. It is a white powder. Sorbitol and cellulose (plant fiber) are used occasionally.

Binders These substances give cohesive qualities to the powdered materials; otherwise, the binders or granulators are the materials that hold the ingredients of the tablet together. Cellulose and ethyl cellulose are used most often. Cellulose is the main constituent of plant fiber. Occasionally, lecithin and sorbitol are used. Another binder that can be used, but that you should be aware of—and look out for—is *acacia* (gum arabic), a vegetable gum that has been declared GRAS (generally recognized as safe) by the FDA (Food and Drug Administration) but which can cause mild to severe asthma attacks and rashes in asthmatics, pregnant women, and anyone prone to allergies.

Lubricants Slick substances, added to a tablet to keep it from sticking to the machines that punch it out. Calcium stearate and silica are commonly used. Calcium stearate is derived from natural vegetable oils. Silica is a natural white powder. Magnesium stearate can also be used.

Disintegrators Substances such as gum arabic, algin, and alginate are added to the tablet to facilitate its breakup or disintegration after ingestion.

Colors They make the tablet more aesthetic or elegant in appearance. Colors derived from natural sources, like chlorophyll, are best.

Flavors and sweeteners Used only in chewable tablets, the sweeteners are usually fructose (fruit sugar), malto-dextrins, sorbitol, or maltose. Sucrose (sugar) is rarely used in better brands.

Coating materials These substances are used to protect the tablet from moisture. They also mask unpleasant flavor or odor and make the tablet easier to swallow. Zein is one of the substances. It is natural, derived from corn protein, and a clear film-coating agent. Brazil wax, which is a natural product derived from palm trees, is also frequently used.

Drying agents These substances prevent water-absorbing (hydroscopic) materials from picking up moisture during processing. Silica gel is the most common drying agent.

26. Storage and Staying Power

Vitamin and mineral supplements should be stored in a cool, dark place away from direct sunlight in a well-closed—preferably opaque—container. They do not have to be stored in the refrigerator unless you live in a desert climate. To guard against excessive moisture, place a few kernels of rice at the bottom of your vitamin bottle. The rice works as a natural absorbent.

If vitamins are kept cool and away from light, and remain well sealed, they should last for two to three years. To ensure freshness, though, your best bet is to buy brands that have an expiration date on the label. Once a bottle is opened you can expect a six-month shelf life.

Our bodies tend to excrete in urine substances we take in on a four-hour basis, and this is particularly true of water-soluble vitamins such as B and C. On an empty stomach, B and C vitamins can leave the body as quickly as two hours after ingestion.

The oil-soluble vitamins, A, D, E, and K, remain in the body for approximately twenty-four hours, though excess amounts can be stored in the liver for much longer. Dry A and E do not stay in the body as long.

27. When and How to Take Supplements

The human body operates on a twenty-four-hour cycle. Your cells do not go to sleep when you do, nor can they exist without continuous oxygen and nutrients. Therefore, for best results, space your supplements as evenly as possible during the day.

The prime time for taking supplements is with or after meals. Vitamins are organic substances and should be taken with other foods and minerals for best absorption. Because the water-soluble vitamins, especially B complex and C, are excreted fairly rapidly in the urine, a regimen of taking supplements with breakfast, with lunch, and with dinner will provide you the highest body levels. If taking them with or after each meal is not convenient, then half the amount should be taken after breakfast and the other half after dinner.

If you must take your vitamins all at once, then do so with the largest meal of the day.

And remember, minerals are essential for proper vitamin absorption, so be sure to take your minerals and vitamins together.

28. What's Right for You

Supplement needs vary depending on your sex, age, health, lifestyle, daily stresses, and dietary restrictions. Job changes, illness, and physical and emotional traumas all take a nutritional toll. With more supplements available today than ever before, and in more delivery systems than ever before, there's no reason why you can't reap maximum health benefits by selecting the nutrients you need in a form that works for you.

If you're unsure whether you'd be better off with a powder, a liquid, a gelcap, or a tablet, regular vitamin E or dry, or taking supplements three times a day, my advice to you is to experiment. If the supplement you're taking doesn't agree with you, try it in another form. Vitamin C powder mixed in a beverage might be much easier to take than several large pills when you're coming down with a cold. If your face breaks out with vitamin E, try the dry (water dispersible) form. Review section 20 to see the variety of supplement delivery systems available. Also:

- Make sure you know all you should about your supplement. (Check sections 30 through 74.)
- If you're taking any prescription or over-the-counter (OTC) medications, familiarize yourself with drugs that deplete nutrients as well as nutrients that may interfere with medications. (See sections 381 through 387.)
- Match your vitamin needs with those listed in chapter XI.

DID YOU KNOW?

- It is not possible to obtain all the nutrients we need in our daily food intake.
- Vitamins can last two to three years in a well-sealed container.
- Oil-soluble vitamins are available in water-soluble ("dry") form.

29. Any Questions About Chapter II?

When vitamins smell awful, does that mean they're spoiled, and could they be harmful?

Strong odors don't necessarily signify spoilage (putting six to twelve kernels of rice at the bottom of your vitamin container absorbs the smell), but it is possible. If you've been keeping your vitamins in sunlight and warmth (great for you but not for them), it's more than possible, it's probable. But even if your vitamins have spoiled, they won't harm you. The worst that can happen is that they lose their effectiveness.

What should I look for when buying a multivitamin-mineral complex supplement?

When it comes to selecting a multiple vitamin and mineral supplement, always look for one that contains at least 100–300 percent of the daily value for all essential vitamins and minerals.

Every so often I detect a sort of alcohol smell in a bottle of vitamins. Does this indicate some sort of deterioration, and are these vitamins still safe to take?

No, the vitamins are not deteriorating, and yes they are safe to take. Alcohol is often used as a drying agent to prevent any moisture contamination. Occasionally, if the product is packed too quickly, some of the alcohol smell remains. My advice is to put six to twelve kernels of rice at the bottom of the bottle. These will absorb the moisture and the smell.

Are the dyes used in vitamin coatings natural or artificial, and how can I tell?

Regrettably, a lot of synthetic vitamins use coal-tar dyes

in their coatings—and keep it a secret. (Look for FD&C dye number listings.) These dyes are not necessarily harmful, but they can cause allergic reactions. My advice is to play it safe and buy natural vitamins that have no artificial adulterants—and *say so on the labeling!*

Sometimes I find that a few of my B vitamin pills are cracked. Are these safe to take?

Yes they are, as are your Cs and any others. Poor tablet coating causes the cracks, but the vitamins themselves are still effective and safe. Look for another brand that has a better coating such as zein or a modified vegetable coating with alpha-lipoic acid as a universal antioxidant to prevent rancidity.

If binders like acacia gum and alginic acid have been declared GRAS (generally recognized as safe) by the FDA, why aren't they?

Just because an additive has been declared GRAS doesn't mean that it can't harm you. Here's why: When the food additive law requiring scientific testing of all chemicals for safe usage in foods went into effect in 1958, the FDA established the GRAS list to eliminate expensive testing of what were unquestionably assumed to be safe chemicals (sugar, starch, salt, baking soda, etc.). As a result of the FDA's action, all additives in use before that year were deemed GRAS; regrettably, many were later found to be otherwise.

Is there a way for me to tell if the supplement I'm taking is a good one?

Look for "CL Approved," "USP Verified," "Certificate of Analysis Available," or "GMP" (Good Manufacturing Practices) on supplements before you buy. I recommend buying certified organic supplements that are devoid of pesticides, insecticides, herbicides, and heavy toxic metals such as lead and arsenic. You can see the brands voluntarily being evaluated by the United States Pharmacopeia (the independent organization responsible for assuring quality of prescription drugs) by going online to www.prevention.com/links.

How can I tell if I'm getting a natural or a synthetic vitamin?

You will always get natural vitamins from whole foods, but when it comes to supplements you have to read the small print on the label. The following is a quick guide:

If the source for vitamin A is acetate, palmitate, or not given, the supplement is synthetic. If the source is fish oils, it's natural, and if it's lemongrass it's half natural.

For all natural vitamins in the B-complex family, the source should be either yeast, rice, bran, liver, or soybeans. Any other sources indicate that the vitamin is synthetic or only partly natural.

It's easy to be confused, especially when it turns out that if the source for the vitamin niacin is niacin the supplement is synthetic. (If the source is niacinamide it is half natural.) And if the source for biotin is d-Biotin, it is also synthetic.

For natural vitamin C look for citrus, rose hips, and acerola berries as the source; ascorbic acid means it's synthetic.

For natural vitamin D the source should be fish oils; irradiated ergosterol/yeast or calciferol indicate the supplement is synthetic.

For natural vitamin E the sources are vegetable oil, wheat germ oil, or mixed tocopherols and d-alpha tocopheral.

NOTE: dl-alpha tocopherol *indicates a synthetic. In fact, the "dl" form of any supplement is synthetic.*

III

Everything You Always Wanted to Know About Vitamins but Had No One to Ask

30. Vitamin A

Facts:

Vitamin A is fat soluble. It requires fats as well as minerals to be properly absorbed by your digestive tract.

It can be stored in your body and need not be replenished every day.

It occurs in two forms—preformed vitamin A, called retinol (found only in foods of animal origin); and provitamin A, known as carotene (provided by foods of both plant and animal origin).

Vitamin A is measured in USP (United States Pharmacopeia) units, IU (international units), and RE (retinol equivalents). (See section 240.)

The recommended daily dosage for adult males to prevent deficiency is 1,000 RE (or 5,000 IU). For females it's

800 RE (4,000 IU). During pregnancy the RDIs/RDAs do not recommend an increase, but for nursing mothers an additional 500 RE is suggested for the first six months and an additional 400 RE for the second six months.

There is no formal RDI/RDA for beta-carotene, because it is not (yet) officially recognized as an essential nutrient. But anywhere from 10,000 to 15,000 IUs of beta-carotene are needed to meet the RDI/RDA for vitamin A.

DRI (see section 241) is 900 mcg. (3,000 IU).

UL (see section 241) is 3,000 mcg. (10,000 IU).

NOTE: *Throughout this book, beta-carotene will be the preferred form of vitamin A. I find it preferable because it does not have the same toxicity potential of preformed vitamin A (retinol). Moreover, it has been shown to be a preventive for certain types of cancer, helpful in lowering levels of harmful cholesterol, effective in boosting the immune system by increasing the number of infection-fighting T lymphocytes (T cells), and a significant factor in reducing the risk of heart disease.*

WHAT IT CAN DO FOR YOU:

Counteract night blindness, weak eyesight, and aid in the treatment of many eye disorders. (It permits formation of visual purple in the eye.)

Build resistance against respiratory infections.

Aid in the proper function of the immune system.

Shorten the duration of diseases.

Keep the outer layers of your tissues and organs healthy.

Help in the removal of age spots.

Promote growth, strong bones, healthy skin, hair, teeth, and gums.

When applied externally can help treat acne, superficial wrinkles, impetigo, boils, carbuncles, and open ulcers.

Aid in the treatment of emphysema and hyperthyroidism.

DEFICIENCY DISEASE:

Xerophthalmia, night blindness. (For deficiency symptoms, see section 235.) Deficiency often occurs as a result of chronic fat malabsorption. It's most commonly found in children under five years, usually because of insufficient dietary intake.

BEST NATURAL SOURCES:

Fish liver oil, liver, carrots, dark green and yellow vegetables, eggs, milk and dairy products, margarine, and yellow fruits. (*NOTE*: The color intensity of a fruit or vegetable is not necessarily a reliable indicator of its beta-carotene content.)

SUPPLEMENTS:

Usually available in two forms, one derived from natural fish liver oil and the other water dispersible. Water-dispersible supplements are either acetate or palmitate and recommended for anyone intolerant to oil, particularly acne sufferers. The most common daily doses are 5,000 to 10,000 IU.

Vitamin A acid (retin A), which has often been used in the treatment of acne, and is now being marketed as a treatment for eradicating superficial wrinkles, is available only by prescription in the United States.

TOXICITY AND WARNING SIGNS OF EXCESS:

More than 50,000 IU daily, if taken for many months, can produce toxic effects in adults.

More than 18,500 IU daily can produce toxic effects in infants.

More than 34,000 IU beta-carotene daily can cause yellowing of the skin.

Symptoms of vitamin A excess include hair loss, nausea,

vomiting, diarrhea, scaly skin, blurred vision, rashes, bone pain, irregular menses, fatigue, headaches, and liver enlargement.

ENEMIES:

Polyunsaturated fatty acids with carotene work against vitamin A unless there are antioxidants present. (See sections 104–129 for antioxidants, and section 381 for drugs that deplete vitamins.)

PERSONAL ADVICE:

You need at least 10,000 IU of vitamin A if you take more than 400 IU of vitamin E daily.

If you are on the pill, your need for A is *decreased*.

If your weekly diet includes ample amounts of liver, carrots, spinach, sweet potatoes, or cantaloupe, it's unlikely you need an A supplement.

Vitamin A should *not* be taken with mineral oil.

Vitamin A works best with B complex, vitamin D, vitamin E, calcium, phosphorus, and zinc. (Zinc is what's needed by the liver to get vitamin A out of its storage deposits.)

A deficiency of vitamin A can lead to a loss of vitamin C.

Don't supplement your dog's or cat's diet with vitamin A unless a vet specifically advises it.

Oral forms of vitamin A prescribed for skin problems are potent drugs that can cause birth defects and should not be used by pregnant women.

INTERACTION WITH DRUGS:

Cholesterol-reducing medications (e.g., Questran)— decrease absorption of vitamin A; supplementation may be needed.

Retinoids—may cause hypervitaminosis A; use beta-carotene instead.

31. Vitamin B1 (Thiamin)

FACTS:

Water soluble. Like all the B-complex vitamins, any excess is excreted and not stored in the body. It must be replaced daily.

Measured in milligrams (mg.).

Being synergistic, B vitamins are more potent together than when used separately. B1, B2, and B6 should be equally balanced (e.g., 50 mg. of B1, 50 mg. of B2, and 50 mg. of B6) to work effectively.

The RDI/RDA for adults is 1.0 to 1.5 mg. (During pregnancy and lactation, 1.5 to 1.6 mg. is suggested.)

DRI (see section 241) is 1.2 mg.

Need increases during illness, stress, and surgery.

Known as the "morale vitamin" because of its beneficial effects on the nervous system and mental attitude.

Has a mild diuretic effect.

WHAT IT CAN DO FOR YOU:

Promote growth.

Aid digestion, especially of carbohydrates.

Improve your mental attitude.

Keep nervous system, muscles, and heart functioning normally.

Fight car sickness, as well as air- and seasickness.

Relieve dental postoperative pain.

Aid in treatment of herpes zoster.

DEFICIENCY DISEASE:

Beriberi. (For deficiency symptoms, see section 235.)

BEST NATURAL SOURCES:

Brewer's yeast, rice husks, unrefined cereal grains, whole wheat, soybeans, egg yolks, fish, oatmeal, peanuts, organic meats, lean pork, most vegetables, bran, milk.

SUPPLEMENTS:

Available in low- and high-potency dosages—usually 50 mg., 100 mg., and 500 mg. It is most effective in B-complex formulas, balanced with B2 and B6. It is even more effective when the formula contains antistress pantothenic acid, folic acid, and B12. The most common daily doses are 100 to 300 mg.

TOXICITY AND WARNING SIGNS OF EXCESS:

No known toxicity for this water-soluble vitamin. Any excess is excreted in the urine and not stored to any degree in tissues or organs.

Rare excess symptoms (when doses exceed 5–10 g. daily) include tremors, herpes outbreak, edema, nervousness, rapid heartbeat, and allergies.

ENEMIES:

Cooking heat easily destroys this B vitamin. Other enemies of B1 are caffeine, alcohol, food-processing methods, air, water, estrogen, antacids, and sulfa drugs. (See section 381 for drugs that deplete vitamins.)

PERSONAL ADVICE:

If you are a smoker, drinker, or heavy sugar consumer, you need more vitamin B1.

If you are pregnant, nursing, or on the pill, you have a greater need for this vitamin.

If you're in the habit of taking an after-dinner antacid,

you're losing the thiamin you might have gotten from the meal.

As with all stress conditions—disease, anxiety, trauma, postsurgery—your B-complex intake, which includes thiamin, should be increased.

INTERACTION WITH DRUGS:

Digoxin—may undermine the ability of heart cells to absorb and use thiamin.

Dilantin—may contribute to drug's side effects by lowering thiamin blood level.

Diuretics (water pills)—may reduce thiamin levels in the body.

32. Vitamin B2 (Riboflavin)

FACTS:

Water soluble. Easily absorbed. The amount excreted depends on bodily needs and may be accompanied by protein loss. Like the other B vitamins, it is not stored and must be replaced regularly through whole foods or supplements.

Also known as vitamin G.

Measured in milligrams (mg.).

Unlike thiamin, riboflavin is *not* destroyed by heat, oxidation, or acid. But it is easily destroyed by light.

For average adults, 1.2–1.7 mg. is the RDI/RDA. During pregnancy, 1.6 mg. is suggested. For nursing mothers, 1.8 mg. is recommended for the first six months and 1.7 mg. for the second six months.

DRI (see section 241) is 1.3 mg.

Increased need in stress situations.

America's most common vitamin deficiency is riboflavin.

WHAT IT CAN DO FOR YOU:

Aid in growth and reproduction.

Promote healthy skin, nails, and hair.

Help eliminate sore mouth, lips, and tongue.

Benefit vision, alleviate eye fatigue, and may help prevent cataracts.

Function with other substances to metabolize carbohydrates, fats, and proteins.

Help alleviate the pain of migraine headaches.

Work as an antioxidant, reducing cell damage from free radicals.

DEFICIENCY DISEASE:

Ariboflavinosis—mouth, lips, skin, genitalia lesions. (For deficiency symptoms, see section 235.)

BEST NATURAL SOURCES:

Milk, liver, kidney, cheese, leafy green vegetables, fish, eggs, yogurt, beans.

SUPPLEMENTS:

Available in both low and high potencies—most commonly in 100 mg. doses. Like most of the B-complex vitamins, it is most effective when in a well-balanced formula with the others.

The most common daily doses are 100–300 mg.

TOXICITY AND WARNING SIGNS OF EXCESS:

No known toxic effects.

Possible symptoms of minor excess include itching, numbness, and sensations of burning or prickling.

ENEMIES:

Light—especially ultraviolet light—and alkalies are destructive to riboflavin. (Opaque milk cartons now protect riboflavin that used to be destroyed in clear-glass milk bottles.) Other natural enemies are water (B2 dissolves in cooking liquids), sulfa drugs, estrogen, and alcohol.

PERSONAL ADVICE:

If you are taking the pill, pregnant, or lactating, you need more vitamin B2.

If you eat little red meat or dairy products, you should increase your intake.

There is a strong likelihood of your being deficient in this vitamin if you are on a prolonged restricted diet for ulcers or diabetes. (In all cases where you are under medical treatment for a specific illness, check with your doctor before altering your present food regimen or embarking on a new one.)

All stress conditions require additional B complex.

This vitamin works best with vitamin B6, vitamin C, and niacin.

Drinkers need more of this vitamin because alcohol interferes with proper absorption.

If you are taking high doses of vitamin B2 (more than 10 mg. daily), especially without antioxidant supplements, you may develop a sensitivity to sunlight. Be sure to wear sunglasses that protect your eyes from ultraviolet light.

Studies done at the New England Center for Headache in Stamford, Connecticut, have shown that patients who take 400 mg. of B2 daily have a 50 percent decrease in either the frequency, duration, or severity of migraines. But it takes three to four months of steady use to get results.

INTERACTION WITH DRUGS:

Tetracycline—absorption and effectiveness of this antibiotic are compromised if taken with riboflavin (or any B-complex supplement). Take B vitamin supplements at a different time from when you take tetracycline or other antibiotics.

Tricyclic antidepressants—can reduce levels of riboflavin in the body; conversely, riboflavin may increase the effectiveness of some antidepressants, including imipramine, desipramine, amitriptyline, and nortriptyline.

Phenothiazines—may lower riboflavin levels.

Doxorubicin—may be deactivated by riboflavin; conversely, doxorubicin may deplete levels of riboflavin in the body.

Antineoplastics—some may be rendered less effective by too much riboflavin.

Probenecid—may decrease absorption of riboflavin and increase its excretion in the urine.

Thiazide diuretics—may cause increased excretion of riboflavin in the urine.

33. Vitamin B3 (Niacin, Niacinamide, Nicotinic Acid, Nicotinamide)

FACTS:

Water soluble and a member of the B-complex family.

Usually measured in milligrams (mg.).

Using the amino acid tryptophan, the body can manufacture its own niacin.

A person whose body is deficient in B1, B2, and B6 will not be able to produce niacin from tryptophan.

Lack of niacin can bring about negative personality changes.

The RDI/RDA for niacin is 13–19 mg. for adults. For nursing mothers the recommendation is 20 mg.

DRI (see section 241) is 16 mg.

Essential for synthesis of sex hormones (estrogen, progesterone, testosterone), as well as cortisone, thyroxine, and insulin.

Necessary for healthy nervous system and brain functions.

One of the few vitamins that is relatively stable in foods and can withstand cooking and storage with little loss of potency.

What It Can Do for You:

Help reduce cholesterol and tryglycerides.

Aid in metabolizing fats and promoting a healthy digestive system, alleviate gastrointestinal disturbances.

Give you healthier-looking skin.

Help prevent and ease severity of migraine headaches.

Increase circulation and reduce high blood pressure.

Ease some attacks of diarrhea.

Reduce the unpleasant symptoms of vertigo in Ménière's disease.

Increase energy through proper utilization of food.

Help eliminate canker sores and, often, bad breath.

Deficiency Disease:

Pellagra, severe dermatitis. (For deficiency symptoms, see section 235.)

Best Natural Sources:

Fish, lean meat, whole wheat products, brewer's yeast, liver, wheat germ, fish, eggs, roasted peanuts, the white meat of poultry, avocados, dates, figs, prunes.

SUPPLEMENTS:

Available as niacin; inositol hexanicotinate (IHN), also called "no-flush" niacin; and niacinamide. (Niacin—nicotinic acid—might cause flushing; niacinamide and inositol hexanicotinate—which contain niacin and inositol—will not. If you prefer niacin, you can minimize the flushing by taking your pill on a full stomach or with an equivalent amount of inositol.)

Usually found in 50–1,000 mg. doses in tablet, capsule, and powder forms.

The better B-complex formulas and multivitamin preparations ordinarily contain 50–100 mg. (Check labels.)

TOXICITY AND WARNING SIGNS OF EXCESS:

Large amounts of niacin can interfere with the control of uric acid, bringing on attacks of gout in people who are prone to this disease (see section 349).

High levels of niacin can also interfere with the body's ability to dispose of sugar, causing possible deterioration of glucose control in borderline diabetes, precipitating the full-blown disease, and may promote liver abnormalities.

Except for possible side effects, such as flushing and itching resulting from doses above 100 mg., niacin is essentially nontoxic.

Do not give to animals, especially dogs. It can cause flushing and sweating and great discomfort for the animal.

ENEMIES:

Water, sulfa drugs, alcohol, sleeping pills, estrogen. (See section 381.)

PERSONAL ADVICE:

If you're taking antibiotics and suddenly find your niacin flushes becoming severe, don't be alarmed. It's quite common. (The flush usually disappears in about twenty minutes. Drinking a glass of water helps.) You'll probably be more comfortable, though, if you switch to a "no-flush" supplement with inositol hexanicotinate.

To avoid gastrointestinal upsets, do not take niacin on an empty stomach or with hot beverages.

If you have a cholesterol problem, increasing your niacin intake can help. (I recommend using it under the supervision of your physician if you are taking other medication—and, if so, never take them at the same time of day.)

Skin that is particularly sensitive to sunlight is often an early indicator of niacin deficiency.

CAUTION: *Niacin should not be taken by people with liver disease, stomach ulcers, or gout. Do not give niacin to your dog or cat; it causes flushing and greatly discomforts the animal.*

INTERACTION WITH DRUGS:

Tetracycline—absorption and effectiveness of this antibiotic are compromised if taken with niacin (or any B-complex supplement). Take B vitamin supplements at a different time from when you take tetracycline or other antibiotics.

Anticoagulants—effects of these medications may be potentiated, increasing the risk of bleeding.

Blood pressure medications; alpha-blockers—may dangerously strengthen the effect of medications to lower blood pressure.

Cholesterol-lowering drugs—effectiveness may be decreased if taken with niacin; take at different times of the day.

Diabetes medications—blood glucose levels may be increased.

34. VITAMIN B4 (Adenine)

FACTS:

Water soluble and a member of the B-complex family.
Acts as a coenzyme with other vitamins to produce energy.
Helps make up the code in DNA and RNA.
Performs important functions in cellular metabolism.

WHAT IT CAN DO FOR YOU:

Aid in regulating heart arrhythmias.
Help alleviate fatigue.
Strengthen the immune system.
Help prevent the formation of free radicals.
Help to balance blood sugar levels.

DEFICIENCY DISEASE:

Slowed growth rate, blood and skin disorders, hypoglycemia, weakened immune system, allergies, muscle weakness. (For deficiency symptoms, see section 235.)

BEST NATURAL SOURCES:

Brewer's yeast, whole grains (breads and cereals), raw unadulterated honey, bee pollen, royal jelly, propolis, most fresh fruit and vegetables. Also may be found in such herbs as blessed thistle, blue cohosh, capsicum (cayenne), cloves, ginger, kelp, sage, spearmint, and thyme. (See sections 161–227.)

SUPPLEMENTS:

Most commonly found in B-complex formulas.

TOXICITY AND WARNING SIGNS OF EXCESS:

No known toxic effects.

ENEMIES:

Alcoholic drinks, cola beverages, coffee (caffeinated and decaffeinated), tea, chocolate, refined sugar, sugar substitutes, and processed foods.

PERSONAL ADVICE:

If you are a nursing mother, adenine can be helpful in improving lactation. People who tire easily or suffer from a lack of energy may be helped by an increased intake of adenine.

35. Vitamin B5/Pantothenic Acid (Panthenol, Calcium Pantothenate)

FACTS:

Water soluble, another member of the B-complex family.

Helps in cell building, maintaining normal growth, and development of the central nervous system.

Vital for the proper functioning of the adrenal glands.

Essential for conversion of fat and sugar to energy.

Necessary for synthesis of antibodies, for utilization of PABA and choline.

The RDI/RDA (as set by the FDA) is 10 mg. for adults.

DRI (see section 241) is 5 mg.

Can be synthesized in the body by intestinal bacteria.

WHAT IT CAN DO FOR YOU:

Aid in wound healing.

Fight infection by building antibodies.

Treat postoperative shock.

Prevent fatigue.

Reduce adverse and toxic effects of many antibiotics.

Lower cholesterol and triglycerides.

DEFICIENCY DISEASE:

Hypoglycemia, duodenal ulcers, blood and skin disorders. (For deficiency symptoms, see section 235.)

BEST NATURAL SOURCES:

Meat, whole grains, wheat germ, bran, kidney, liver, heart, green vegetables, brewer's yeast, nuts, chicken, unrefined molasses.

SUPPLEMENTS:

Most commonly found in B-complex formulas in a variety of strengths from 10 to 100 mg.

The daily doses usually taken are 10–300 mg.

TOXICITY AND WARNING SIGNS OF EXCESS:

No known toxic effects.

ENEMIES:

Heat, food-processing techniques, canning, caffeine, sulfa drugs, sleeping pills, estrogen, alcohol. (See section 381.)

PERSONAL ADVICE:

If you frequently have tingling hands and feet, you might try increasing your pantothenic acid intake—in combination with other B vitamins.

People who need to cut their cholesterol may be given doses up to 1,000 mg. daily by their physicians.

Pantothenic acid can help provide a defense against a stress situation that you foresee or are involved in.

In some cases, 1,000 mg. daily has been found to be effective in reducing the pain of arthritis.

If you suffer from allergies, relief could be just a vitamin B5 and C away. Try taking 1,000 mg. of each—with food—morning and evening.

Interaction with Drugs:

Tetracycline—interferes with absorption of this antibiotic; take at different times.

Cholinesterase inhibitors (for Alzheimer's)—may increase the drugs' potency and lead to severe side effects.

36. Vitamin B6 (Pyridoxine)

Facts:

Water soluble. Excreted within eight hours after ingestion and, like the other B vitamins, needs to be replaced by whole foods or supplements.

B6 is actually a group of substances—pyridoxine, pyridoxal, and pyridoxamine—that are closely related and function together.

Measured in milligrams (mg.).

Requirement increased when high-protein diets are consumed.

Must be present for the production of antibodies and red blood cells.

There is some evidence of synthesis by intestinal bacteria, and that a vegetable diet supplemented with cellulose is responsible.

The recommended adult intake is 1.6–2.0 mg. daily, with 2.2 mg. doses suggested during pregnancy and 2.1 mg. for lactation.

DRI (see section 241) is 1.7 mg.

Required for the proper absorption of vitamin B12.

Necessary for the production of hydrochloric acid and magnesium.

Dairy products are relatively poor sources of B6.

What It Can Do for You:

In combination with folic acid, it can help break down the amino acid homocysteine, *significantly* lowering the risk of heart disease.

Strengthen the immune system.

Help prevent kidney stone formation.

Properly assimilate protein and fat.

Aid in the conversion of tryptophan, an essential amino acid, to niacin.

Help prevent various nervous and skin disorders.

Alleviate nausea (many morning-sickness preparations that doctors prescribe include vitamin B6).

Promote proper synthesis of antiaging nucleic acids.

Help reduce dry mouth and urination problems caused by tricyclic antidepressants.

Reduce night muscle spasms, leg cramps, hand numbness, certain forms of neuritis in the extremities.

Work as a natural diuretic.

Deficiency Disease:

Anemia, seborrheic dermatitis, glossitis. (For deficiency symptoms, see section 235.)

Best Natural Sources:

Brewer's yeast, wheat bran, wheat germ, liver, fish, soybeans, cantaloupe, cabbage, blackstrap molasses, unmilled rice, eggs, oats, peanuts, walnuts.

Supplements:

Readily available in a wide range of dosages—from 50 to 500 mg.—in individual supplements as well as in B-complex and multivitamin formulas.

To prevent deficiencies in other B vitamins, pyridoxine should be taken in equal amounts with B1 and B2.

Can be purchased in time-disintegrating formulas that provide for gradual release up to ten hours.

TOXICITY AND WARNING SIGNS OF EXCESS:

Daily doses of 2–10 grams can cause neurological disorders.

Possible symptoms of an oversupply of B6 are night restlessness, too-vivid dream recall, numb feet, and twitching.

Doses over 500 mg. are not recommended.

ENEMIES:

Long storage, canning, roasting or stewing of meat, freezing fruits and vegetables, water, food-processing techniques, alcohol, estrogen. (See section 381.)

PERSONAL ADVICE:

If you are on the pill, you are more than likely to need increased amounts of B6.

Heavy protein consumers need extra amounts of this vitamin.

To reduce your risk of heart attack, increase your B6 and folic acid.

Vitamin B6 might decrease a diabetic's requirement for insulin, and if the dosage is not adjusted, a low-blood-sugar reaction could result.

Arthritis sufferers being treated with Cuprimine (*penicillamine*) should be taking supplements of this vitamin.

This vitamin works best with vitamin B1, vitamin B2, pantothenic acid, vitamin C, and magnesium.

Supplements for this vitamin should *not* be taken by anyone under *levodopa* treatment for Parkinson's disease! (Ask your doctor about Sinemet, a drug that can bypass this particular adverse vitamin interaction.)

INTERACTION WITH DRUGS:

Antibiotics, tetracycline—all B vitamins can interfere with the absorption and effectiveness of tetracycline and should be taken at different times of the day.

Antidepressants—supplements of B6 may improve the effectiveness of many tricyclic antidepressants. On the other hand, MAO antidepressants may reduce blood levels of B6.

Chemotherapy drugs—may reduce some side effects without interfering with the medication's effectiveness. (Be sure to talk to your doctor before supplementing.)

Erythropoietin (EPO)—may decrease B6 levels in blood, requiring B6 supplementation.

Levodopa (L-dopa)—reduces the effectiveness of this medication for Parkinson's disease.

Phenytoin (Dilantin)—reduces the antiseizure effectiveness of this medication.

37. Vitamin B12 (Cobalamin, cyanocobalamin)

FACTS:

Water soluble and effective in very small doses.

Commonly known as the "red vitamin," also cyanocobalamin.

Cyanocobalamin is the commercially available form of vitamin B12 used in vitamin pills.

Measured in micrograms (mcg.).

The only vitamin that contains essential mineral elements.

Not well assimilated through the stomach. Needs to be combined with calcium during absorption to properly benefit the body.

Recommended adult dose is 2 mcg., with 2.2 mcg. suggested for pregnant women and 2.6 mcg. for nursing mothers.

DRI (see section 241) is 2.4 mcg.

A diet low in B1 and high in folic acid (such as a vegetarian diet) often hides a vitamin B12 deficiency.

A properly functioning thyroid gland helps B12 absorption. Symptoms of B12 deficiency may take more than five years to appear after body stores have been depleted.

In the human diet, vitamin B12 is supplied primarily by animal products, since plant foods (with minor exceptions) don't contain it.

Unique among water-soluble vitamins, it can be stored in the body; it can take up to three years to deplete your supply.

What It Can Do for You:

Form and regenerate red blood cells, thereby preventing anemia.

Help break down the amino acid homocysteine, lowering the risk of heart disease.

Promote growth and increase appetite in children.

Increase energy.

Help protect your brain from shrinking with age.

Help slow macular degeneration.

Aid in alleviating depression.

Help prevent and effectively treat canker sores.

Maintain a healthy nervous system.

Properly utilize fats, carbohydrates, and protein.

Relieve irritability.

Improve concentration, memory, and balance.

Help protect against smoking-induced cancer.

Small amounts (80 mcg.) help strengthen bones and aid in prevention of osteoporosis.

DEFICIENCY DISEASE:

Pernicious anemia, neurological disorders. (For deficiency symptoms, see section 235.)

BEST NATURAL SOURCES:

Liver, beef, pork, eggs, milk, cheese, fish.

SUPPLEMENTS:

Because B12 is not absorbed well through the stomach, I recommend the sublingual form of the vitamin, or the time-release form—accompanied by sorbitol—so that it can be assimilated in the small intestine.

Supplements are available in a variety of strengths from 50 mcg. to 10,000 mcg.

Doctors routinely give vitamin B12 injections. If there is a severe indication of deficiency or extreme fatigue, this method might be the supplementation that's called for.

Daily dosages most often used are 5–100 mcg.

TOXICITY AND WARNING SIGNS OF EXCESS:

There have been no cases reported of vitamin B12 toxicity, even on megadose regimens.

ENEMIES:

Acids and alkalies, water, sunlight, alcohol, estrogen, sleeping pills. (See section 381.)

PERSONAL ADVICE:

If you are vegan or a vegetarian who has excluded eggs and dairy products from your diet, then you need B12 supplementation.

If you keep regular "Happy Hours" and drink a lot, B12 is an important supplement for you.

Combined with folic acid, B12 can be a most effective revitalizer.

Surprisingly, heavy protein consumers may also need extra amounts of this vitamin, which works synergistically with almost all other B vitamins as well as vitamins A, E, and C.

The ability to absorb vitamin B12 from food declines with age. It's recommended that adults over the age of fifty obtain the RDA for this vitamin from supplements or fortified foods, which do not require stomach acid for absorption.

Women may find B12 helpful—as part of a B complex—during and just prior to menstruation.

INTERACTION WITH DRUGS:

Acid-lowering medications (Prilosec, Prevacid, Zantac)—can impair absorption of B12.

Antibiotics, tetracycline—all B vitamins may interfere with the absorption and effectiveness of tetracycline and should be taken at different times of the day.

Chloramphenicol—can significantly interfere with B12 absorption.

38. Vitamin B13 (Orotic Acid)

FACTS:

Not available in the United States.
Metabolizes folic acid and vitamin B12.
No RDI/RDA has been established.
Used as a feed supplement to add growth to calves.

WHAT IT CAN DO FOR YOU:

Possibly prevent certain liver problems and premature aging.
Aid in the treatment of multiple sclerosis.

DEFICIENCY DISEASE:

Deficiency symptoms and diseases related to this vitamin are still uncertain.

BEST NATURAL SOURCES:

Root vegetables, whey, the liquid portion of soured or curdled milk.

SUPPLEMENTS:

Available as calcium orotate in supplemental form outside the United States.

TOXICITY AND WARNING SIGNS OF EXCESS:

Too little is known about the vitamin at this time to establish guidelines.

ENEMIES:

Water and sunlight.

PERSONAL ADVICE:

Not enough research has been done on this vitamin for recommendations to be made.

39. B15 (Pangamic Acid, DMG, Dimethylglycine)

FACTS:

Water soluble.

Because its essential requirement for diet has not been proved, it is not a vitamin in the strict sense.

Measured in milligrams (mg.).

Works much like vitamin E in that it is an antioxidant.

Introduced by the Russians, who are thrilled with its

results, while the U.S. Food and Drug Administration has, at the time of this writing, taken it off the market.

Action is often improved by being taken with vitamins A and E.

WHAT IT CAN DO FOR YOU:

Extend cell life span.
Neutralize the craving for liquor.
Speed recovery from fatigue.
Lower blood cholesterol levels.
Protect against pollutants.
Relieve symptoms of angina and asthma.
Protect the liver against cirrhosis.
Ward off hangovers.
Stimulate immunity responses.
Aid in protein synthesis.

DEFICIENCY DISEASE:

Again, research has been limited, but indications point to glandular and nerve disorders, heart disease, and diminished oxygenation of living tissue.

BEST NATURAL SOURCES:

Brewer's yeast, whole brown rice, whole grains, pumpkin seeds, sesame seeds.

SUPPLEMENTS:

Usually available in 50 mg. strengths.
Daily doses most often used are 50–150 mg.

TOXICITY AND WARNING SIGNS OF EXCESS:

There have been no reported cases of toxicity. Some people say they have experienced nausea on beginning a B15 regimen, but this usually disappears after a few days and can be alleviated by taking the B15 supplements after the day's largest meal.

ENEMIES:

Water and sunlight.

PERSONAL ADVICE:

Despite the controversy, I have found B15 effective and believe most diets would benefit from supplementation.

If you are an athlete or just want to feel like one, I suggest one 50 mg. tablet in the morning with breakfast and one in the evening with dinner.

Do not take pangamic acid if you are pregnant, breast-feeding, or have kidney problems.

INTERACTION WITH DRUGS:

Thiazide diuretics—may cause there to be too much calcium in the body when taken with pangamic acid supplements that contain calcium.

Calcium channel blockers—effectiveness of these medications may be decreased if taken with calcium containing pangamic acid supplements.

Digoxin (Lanoxin)—pangamic acid with calcium may increase the drug's side effects.

40. B17 (Laetrile, Amygdalin, Nitrilosides)

For many years, this controversial compound of two sugar molecules (one benzaldehyde and one cyanide) was erroneously called "vitamin" B17, a thoroughly misleading term. Apricot kernels are the richest source of B17 and purported to have specific cancer-controlling and preventive properties. It is likely the cyanide that accounts for the controversy over this substance, particularly in regard to cancer therapy. It is still illegal in the United States.

Other foods that contain "vitamin" B17 are: bitter almonds, millet, wheatgrass, and lima beans.

I've cited B17 in this edition simply to clear up any residually held belief in its status as a vitamin.

41. Biotin (Coenzyme R or Vitamin H)

FACTS:

Water soluble, sulfur containing, and another member of the B-complex family.

Usually measured in micrograms (mcg.).

Synthesis of ascorbic acid requires biotin.

Essential for normal metabolism of fat and protein.

The RDI/RDA for adults is 100–300 mcg.

The adequate intake (AI) and DRI for adults is 30 mcg.

Can be synthesized by intestinal bacteria.

Raw eggs prevent absorption by the body.

Synergistic with B2, B6, niacin, A, and in maintaining healthy skin.

WHAT IT CAN DO FOR YOU:

Aid in keeping hair from turning gray.

Help in preventive treatment for baldness.

Ease muscle pains.

Alleviate eczema and dermatitis.

Help prevent and heal cracked, split, and brittle nails.

DEFICIENCY DISEASE:

Eczema of face and body, extreme exhaustion, impairment of fat metabolism, alopecia, depression. (For deficiency symptoms, see section 235.)

BEST NATURAL SOURCES:

Beef liver, egg yolk, soy flour, cauliflower, cheese, brewer's yeast, milk, peanut butter, salmon, spinach, and unpolished rice.

SUPPLEMENTS:

Biotin is usually included in most B-complex supplements and multivitamin tablets.

Daily doses most often used are 25–300 mcg. (300 mcg. supplies 100 percent of your RDA daily values [DV]).

TOXICITY AND WARNING SIGNS OF EXCESS:

There are no known cases of biotin toxicity.

ENEMIES:

Raw egg white (which contains avidin, a protein that prevents biotin absorption), water, sulfa drugs, estrogen, food-processing techniques, and alcohol. (See section 381.)

PERSONAL ADVICE:

If you drink high-protein shakes made with raw eggs, you probably need biotin supplementation.

Be sure you're getting at least 25 mcg. daily if you are on antibiotics or sulfa drugs.

Balding men might find that a biotin supplement will help them keep their hair longer.

Keep in mind that biotin works synergistically—and more effectively—with B2, B6, niacin, and A.

Biotin levels fall progressively throughout pregnancy. Although there's been no association with low birth weight, you might want to check with your doctor about a supplement that could help keep your spirits up.

Because biotin is expensive, supplement manufacturers often cut corners and include as little as 10 percent of your DV, so look for multivitamins that come closest to having 100 percent of your DV.

To help heal cracked, peeling, or brittle nails, try 300 mcg. daily for three months. If you notice an improvement, cut back on the daily dosage. On the other hand (no pun intended), if there's no improvement, stop taking the supplement and consult a dermatologist.

INTERACTION WITH DRUGS:

Antiseizure medications—can reduce blood levels of biotin.

Broad-spectrum antibiotics—can increase risk of deficiency.

Lipid-lowering drugs—their potency may be increased.

42. Choline

FACTS:

A member of the B-complex family and a lipotropic (fat emulsifier).

Works with inositol (another B-complex member) to utilize fats and cholesterol.

One of the few substances able to penetrate the so-called blood-brain barrier, which ordinarily protects the brain against variations in the daily diet, and go directly into the brain cells to produce a chemical that aids memory.

No RDI/RDA has yet been established, though it's estimated that the average adult diet contains between 500 and 900 mg. a day.

DRI (see section 241) is 550 mg.

Seems to emulsify cholesterol so that it doesn't settle on artery walls or in the gallbladder.

The utilization of choline in the body depends on vitamin B12, folic acid, and the amino acid L-carnitine.

WHAT IT CAN DO FOR YOU:

Help control cholesterol buildup.

Aid in the sending of nerve impulses, specifically those in the brain used in the formation of memory.

Assist in conquering the problem of memory loss in later years (doses of 1–5 g. a day).

Help eliminate poisons and drugs from your system by aiding the liver.

Produce a soothing effect.

Aid in the treatment of Alzheimer's disease.

DEFICIENCY DISEASE:

May result in cirrhosis and fatty degeneration of liver, hardening of the arteries, and possibly Alzheimer's disease. (For deficiency symptoms, see section 235.)

BEST NATURAL SOURCES:

Egg yolks, beef brain and heart, green leafy vegetables, yeast, liver, wheat germ, and, in small amounts, lecithin.

SUPPLEMENTS:

Choline may be sold under the name of phosphatidylcholine or phosphatidylinositol.

Six lecithin capsules, made from soybeans, contain 244 mg. each of inositol and choline.

The average B-complex supplement contains approximately 50 mg. of choline and inositol.

Daily doses most often used are 500–1,000 mg.

TOXICITY AND WARNING SIGNS OF EXCESS:

None known.

ENEMIES:

Water, sulfa drugs, estrogen, food processing, and alcohol. (See section 381.)

PERSONAL ADVICE:

Always take choline with your other B vitamins.

If you are often nervous or "twitchy," it might help to increase your choline.

If you are taking lecithin, you probably need a chelated calcium supplement to keep your phosphorus and calcium in balance, since choline seems to increase the body's phosphorus.

Try getting more choline into your diet as a way to improve memory.

Large doses of choline, taken over a long period of time, may produce a deficiency of vitamin B6.

If you're a heavy drinker, make sure you're giving your liver the choline it needs to do the extra work.

43. Folic Acid (Folacin, Folate)

FACTS:

Water soluble, another member of the B complex, also known as Bc or vitamin M.

Measured in micrograms (mcg.).

Essential to the formation of red blood cells.

Aid in protein metabolism.

The RDI/RDA for adults is 180 to 200 mcg., twice that amount for pregnant women, and for nursing mothers, 280 mcg. the first six months and 260 mcg. the second six months. (Babies are significantly protected from neural-tube defects, such as spina bifida, if women get the recommended double RDI/RDA at the time of conception and during early pregnancy.)

DRI (see section 241) is 400 mcg. from food, 200 mcg. synthetic.

Important for the production of nucleic acids (RNA and DNA).

Essential for division of body cells.

Needed for utilization of sugar and amino acids.

Can be destroyed by being stored, unprotected, at room temperature for extended time periods.

WHAT IT CAN DO FOR YOU:

Lower homocysteine levels and reduce risk of heart disease.

Help protect against birth defects.

Improve lactation.

Aid in protecting against intestinal parasites and food poisoning.

Promote healthier-looking skin.

Act as an analgesic for pain.

May delay hair graying when used in conjunction with pantothenic acid and PABA.

Increase appetite, if you are debilitated (run-down).

Act as a preventive for canker sores.

Help ward off anemia.

DEFICIENCY DISEASE:

Nutritional macrocytic anemia. (For deficiency symptoms, see section 235.)

BEST NATURAL SOURCES:

Deep green leafy vegetables, carrots, tortula yeast, liver,

egg yolk, cantaloupe, artichokes, apricots, pumpkins, avocados, beans, whole and dark rye flour.

Supplements:

Usually supplied in 400 mcg. and 800 mcg. strengths. Strength of 1 mg. (1,000 mcg.) is available only by prescription in the United States.

B-complex formulas sometimes supply 400 mcg., but often only 100 mcg. (Check labels.)

Daily doses most often used are 400 mcg. to 5 mg.

Look for supplements that contain both folate and B12.

Toxicity and Warning Signs of Excess:

No known toxic effects, though a few people experience allergic skin reactions.

Excess folic acid can mask anemia created by a B12 deficiency.

Enemies:

Water, sulfa drugs, sunlight, estrogen, food processing (especially boiling), heat. (See section 381.)

Personal Advice:

If you're a woman, be sure you're getting folic acid and vitamin B6. Just 400 mcg. of folic acid with 2–10 mg. of vitamin B6 can reduce your risk of heart attack by 42 percent!

If you're trying to become pregnant, 400 mcg. of folic acid daily can help increase fertility in women and aid in upping sperm counts in men. (See section 280.)

If you are a heavy drinker, it is advisable to increase your folic acid intake.

High vitamin C intake increases excretion of folic acid,

and anyone taking more than 2 g. of C should probably up his or her folic acid intake.

I've found that many people taking 1–5 mg. daily, for a short period of time, have reversed several types of skin discoloration. If this is a problem for you, it's worth checking out a nutritionally oriented doctor about the possibility.

If you are getting sick, or fighting an illness, make sure your stress supplement has ample folic acid. When folic acid is deficient, so are your antibodies.

INTERACTION WITH DRUGS:

Anticonvulsants/antiseizure medications—effectiveness may be decreased or increased when taken with folic acid; consult with your healthcare practitioner before taking supplements.

Anticancer drugs—absorption and bioavailability for many can be decreased, reducing effectiveness.

Aspirin—may deplete or interfere with folic acid absorption.

Oral contraceptives—can deplete folic acid or interfere with absorption; folic acid supplements may reduce likelihood and/or severity of side effects of medication.

Sulfonamides—if taken for more than two weeks can deplete or interfere with folic acid absorption.

44. Inositol

FACTS:

Water soluble, another member of the B-complex group, and a lipotropic.

Measured in milligrams (mg.).

Combines with choline to form lecithin.

Metabolizes fats and cholesterol.

Daily dietary allowances have not yet been established, but the average healthy adult gets approximately 1 g. a day.

Like choline, it has been found to be important in nourishing brain cells.

WHAT IT CAN DO FOR YOU:

Help lower cholesterol levels.

Promote healthy hair—aid in preventing loss.

Help in preventing eczema.

Aid in redistribution of body fat.

Produce a calming effect.

DEFICIENCY DISEASE:

Eczema. (For deficiency symptoms, see section 235.)

BEST NATURAL SOURCES:

Liver, brewer's yeast, dried lima beans, beef brain and heart, cantaloupe, grapefruit, raisins, wheat germ, unrefined molasses, peanuts, cabbage.

SUPPLEMENTS:

As with choline, 6 soy-based lecithin capsules contain approximately 244 mg. each of inositol and choline.

Available in lecithin powders that mix well with liquid. Most B-complex supplements contain approximately 100 mg. of choline and inositol.

Daily doses most often used are 250–500 mg.

TOXICITY AND WARNING SIGNS OF EXCESS:

No known toxic effects.

ENEMIES:

Water, sulfa drugs, estrogen, food processing, alcohol, and coffee. (See section 381.)

PERSONAL ADVICE:

Take inositol with choline and your other B vitamins.

If you are a heavy coffee drinker, you probably need supplemental inositol.

If you take lecithin, I advise a supplement of chelated calcium to keep your phosphorus and calcium in balance, as both inositol and choline seem to raise phosphorus levels.

A good way to maximize the effectiveness of your vitamin E is to take enough inositol and choline.

INTERACTION WITH DRUGS:

Carbamazepine (Carbatrol, Epitol, Equetro, Tegretol)— may lower inositol levels in the brain and reduce effectiveness of medications.

Lithium—may diminish the drug's effectiveness as well as lower inositol levels in the brain.

Valproic acid—may interfere with the drug's effectiveness while also lowering inositol levels in the brain.

45. PABA (Para-Aminobenzoic Acid)

FACTS:

Water soluble, one of the newer members of the B-complex family.

Usually measured in milligrams (mg.).

Can be synthesized in the body.

No RDI/RDA has yet been established.

Helps form folic acid and is important in the utilization of protein.

Helps in the assimilation—and therefore the effectiveness—of pantothenic acid.

What It Can Do for You:

Reduce the pain of burns.
Keep skin healthy and smooth.
Help in delaying wrinkles.
Help to restore natural color to your hair.

Deficiency Disease:

Eczema. (For deficiency symptoms, see section 235.)

Best Natural Sources:

Liver, brewer's yeast, kidney, whole grains, rice, bran, wheat germ, and molasses.

Supplements:

Good B-complex capsules as well as high-quality multivitamins often contain 30–100 mg.

Available in 30–1,000 mg. strengths in regular and time-release forms.

Doses most often used are 30–100 mg. three times a day.

Toxicity and Warning Signs of Excess:

No known toxic effects, but long-term programs of high dosages are not recommended.

Symptoms that might indicate an oversupply of PABA are usually nausea and vomiting.

ENEMIES:

Water, sulfa drugs, food-processing techniques, alcohol, estrogen. (See section 381.)

PERSONAL ADVICE:

Some people claim that the combination of folic acid and PABA has returned their graying hair to its natural color. It has worked on animals, so it is certainly worth a try for anyone looking for an alternative to hair dye. For this purpose, 1,000 mg. daily for six days a week is a viable regimen.

If you are taking penicillin, your PABA intake should be increased through natural foods or supplements.

Excessive amounts of PABA in certain individuals may have a negative effect on the liver, kidneys, and heart.

INTERACTION WITH DRUGS:

Antibiotics—effectiveness of sulfonamides (Gantanol, Azulfidine, Gantrisin, Bactrim, Septra) can be decreased. Can also decrease the effectiveness of dapsone in treating infections.

Cortisone—can increase effects and side effects of cortisone injections.

46. Vitamin C (Ascorbic Acid, Cevitamin Acid)

FACTS:

Water soluble and a potent antioxidant.

Most animals synthesize their own vitamin C, but humans, apes, and guinea pigs must rely upon dietary sources.

Plays a primary role in the formation of collagen, which is important for the growth and repair of body-tissue cells, gums, blood vessels, bones, and teeth.

Helps in the body's absorption of iron.

Measured in milligrams (mg.).

Used up more rapidly under stress conditions.

The RDI/RDA for adults is 60 mg. (higher doses recommended during pregnancy and lactation: 70–95 mg.).

Smokers and older persons have greater need of vitamin C. (Each cigarette destroys 25–100 mg.)

DRI (see section 241) is 90 mg.

Prevents the oxidation of bad (LDL) cholesterol.

WHAT IT CAN DO FOR YOU:

Heal wounds, burns, and bleeding gums.

Increase effectiveness of drugs used to treat urinary tract infections.

Accelerate healing after surgery.

Help in decreasing blood cholesterol.

Aid in preventing many types of viral and bacterial infections and generally potentiate the immune system.

Offer protection against many forms of cancer.

Help counteract the formation of nitrosamines (cancer-causing substances).

Act as a natural laxative.

Lower incidence of blood clots in veins.

Aid in treatment and prevention of the common cold.

Extend life by enabling protein cells to hold together.

Increase the absorption of inorganic iron.

Reduce effects of many allergy-producing substances.

Help lower systolic and diastolic blood pressure.

Reduce bone loss, particularly in older men.

Prevent scurvy.

DEFICIENCY DISEASE:

Scurvy. (For deficiency symptoms, see section 235.)

BEST NATURAL SOURCES:

Citrus fruits, berries, green and leafy vegetables, tomatoes, cantaloupe, cauliflower, potatoes, and peppers.

SUPPLEMENTS:

Vitamin C is one of the most widely taken supplements. It is available in just about every form a vitamin can take, including tablets, capsules, lozenges, time-release tablets, syrups, powders, and chewable wafers.

The form that is *pure* vitamin C is derived from corn dextrose (although no corn or dextrose remains).

The difference between "natural" or "organic" vitamin C and ordinary ascorbic acid is primarily in the individual's ability to digest it.

The best vitamin C supplement is one that contains the complete C complex of bioflavonoids, hesperidin, and rutin. (Sometimes these are labeled citrus salts.)

Tablets and capsules are usually supplied in strengths up to 1,000 mg., and in powder form sometimes 5,000 mg. per tsp.

Daily doses most often used are 500 mg. to 4 g.

Rose hips vitamin C contains bioflavonoids and other enzymes that help C assimilate. They are the richest natural source of vitamin C. (The C is actually manufactured under the bud of the rose—called a hip.)

Acerola C is made with acerola berries.

CAUTION: *Don't chew vitamin C tablets or let the vitamin C remain on your teeth. The ascorbic acid in the tablet can destroy your teeth.*

TOXICITY AND WARNING SIGNS OF EXCESS:

Excessive intake may cause oxalic acid and uric acid stone formation (though taking magnesium, vitamin B6, and a sufficient amount of water daily can rectify this). Occasionally, very high doses (more than 10 g. daily) can cause unpleasant side effects, such as diarrhea, excess urination, and skin rashes. If any of these occur, cut back on your dosage.

Vitamin C should not be used by cancer patients undergoing radiation or chemotherapy. It can change test results.

ENEMIES:

Water, cooking, heat, light, oxygen, smoking. (See section 381.)

PERSONAL ADVICE:

Because vitamin C is excreted in two to three hours, depending on the quantity of food in the stomach, and it is important to maintain a constant high level of C in the bloodstream at all times, I recommend taking it with breakfast and dinner.

Large doses of vitamin C can alter the results of laboratory tests, including Pap smears. If you're going to have any blood or urine testing, be sure to inform your doctor that you're taking vitamin C so that no errors will be made in diagnosis. (Vitamin C can mask the presence of blood in stool, compromising screening for colon cancer.)

Diabetics should be aware that testing the urine for sugar could be inaccurate if you're taking a lot of vitamin C. (But there are testing kits available that aren't affected by vitamin C. Ask your pharmacist or physician.)

People with type 2 diabetes—or anyone with high blood pressure—can lower both systolic and diastolic blood pressure significantly with just 500 mg. of vitamin C daily.

High doses are not recommended for people with genetic conditions that cause iron overload, like thalassemia and hemochromatosis.

If you take vitamin C in a powder, brush your teeth

afterward to avoid erosion of tooth enamel from the ascorbic acid.

If you're taking more than 750 mg. daily, I suggest a magnesium supplement. This is an effective deterrent against kidney stones.

Carbon monoxide destroys vitamin C, so city dwellers should definitely up their intake.

You need extra C if you are on the pill.

To maximize the effectiveness of vitamin C, remember that it works best in conjunction with bioflavonoids, calcium, and magnesium.

I recommend increasing C doses if you take aspirin, which triples the excretion rate of vitamin C.

If you take ginseng, it's better to take it two hours before or after taking vitamin C or foods that are high in the vitamin.

To reduce the severity of colds, take 1,000 mg. of vitamin C twice daily. It's been shown to decrease the histamine in the blood by 40 percent. (Histamine is the substance that causes those annoying watery eyes and runny noses.)

CAUTION: *Supplementing with vitamin C before starting chemotherapy may interfere with treatment.*

INTERACTION WITH DRUGS:

Antipsychotics—drug effectiveness may be reduced.

Aspirin and nonsteroidal anti-inflammatory drugs (NSAIDs)—may remain in the body longer and cause unwanted buildup while depleting needed vitamin C.

Acetaminophen—high doses of C can raise drug blood levels.

Aluminum-containing antacids—amount of aluminum absorbed by the body may be increased, worsening side effects.

Barbiturates—can decrease effectiveness of vitamin C.

Chemotherapy drugs—effectiveness of some may be impaired.

Diabetes medications (chlorpropamide)—effectiveness may be diminished when taken with vitamin C.

Nitrate medications for heart disease—effectiveness may be undermined by vitamin C.

Oral contraceptives and hormone replacement therapy (HRT)—vitamin C can raise estrogen levels, and oral estrogens can decrease effectiveness of vitamin C in the body.

Protease inhibitors—levels of indinavir, medication used to treat HIV and AIDS, may be reduced.

Sulfonamides—taken with high doses of C may cause kidney stones.

Tetracycline (and similar antibiotics)—can decrease effectiveness of vitamin C, which, nonetheless, may increase blood levels of the drug.

47. Vitamin D (Calciferol, Viosterol, Ergosterol, "Sunshine Vitamin")

FACTS:

Fat soluble. Acquired through sunlight or diet. (Ultraviolet sun rays act on the oils of the skin to produce the vitamin, which is then absorbed into the body.)

When taken orally, vitamin D is absorbed with fats through the intestinal walls.

Measured in international units (IU), or micrograms of cholecalciferol (mcg.).

The RDI/RDA for adults is 200–400 IU, or 5–10 mcg.

DRI (see section 241) is 15 mcg. or 600 IU.

The American Academy of Pediatrics recommends 400 IU of vitamin D per day for all breast-fed infants unless weaned and consuming more than 1,000 ml. per day of vitamin D–fortified formula or milk, and for all non-breast-fed infants getting less than 1,000 ml of vitamin D–fortified formula or milk.

Smog reduces the vitamin D–producing sunshine rays.

After a suntan is established, vitamin D production through the skin stops.

WHAT IT CAN DO FOR YOU:

Properly utilize calcium and phosphorus to keep bones and teeth strong and healthy.

Boost the immune system.

Help stave off seasonal affective disorder (SAD) by keeping the brain flush with mood-regulating serotonin.

Improve cognitive function in people over age sixty-five.

Help in the treatment of diabetes mellitus.

May substantially cut the risk of breast, colon, prostate, and ovarian cancers.

Higher blood levels may reduce risk of insulin resistance.

May help protect against Alzheimer's disease.

Taken with vitamins A and C, it can aid in preventing colds or flu.

Help in treatment of conjunctivitis.

Aid in assimilating vitamin A.

DEFICIENCY DISEASE:

Rickets, severe tooth decay, osteomalacia, senile osteoporosis. (For deficiency symptoms, see section 235.)

NOTE: *Vitamin D deficiency also increases the risk of autoimmune diseases such as type 1 diabetes, multiple sclerosis, rheumatoid arthritis, heart disease, stroke, dementia, and many cancers. Low vitamin D levels have also been linked to Parkinson's disease, although it's not known if increased* *levels can improve Parkinson's symptoms. And vitamin D deficiency may also have a negative effect on organ tissues, including bone marrow, breast, colon, intestine, kidney, lung, prostate, retina, skin, stomach, and the uterus.*

BEST NATURAL SOURCES:

Fish liver oils, sardines, herring, salmon, tuna, milk and dairy products.

SUPPLEMENTS:

Usually supplied in 400 IU capsules, the vitamin itself is derived from fish liver oil.

Daily doses most often taken are 400–1,000 IU.

TOXICITY AND WARNING SIGNS OF EXCESS:

A daily intake of 20,000 IU over an extended period of time can produce toxic effects in adults.

Dosages of more than 1,800 IU daily may cause hypervitaminosis D in children.

Signs of excess are unusual thirst, sore eyes, itching skin, vomiting, diarrhea, urinary urgency; abnormal calcium deposits in blood vessel walls, liver, lungs, kidney, and stomach.

ENEMIES:

Mineral oil, smog. (See section 381.)

PERSONAL ADVICE:

Vitamin D synthesis in the skin declines with age. If you're over sixty, it's likely that you need to take supplemental vitamin D—an additional 800 to 1,000 IU daily.

Everyone concerned about their overall health should monitor their blood levels of vitamin D. (Talk to your doctor about getting a "serum 25-hydroxyvitamin D" test.)

Anyone with Crohn's disease, cystic fibrosis, or celiac disease is at risk of being deficient in vitamin D and should have their blood levels tested.

Low levels of vitamin D can cause a dip in a hormone that regulates appetite, impairing the brain's signal that you're full, leading to unwanted weight gain.

Night workers, and others whose lifestyle keeps them from sunlight, should increase the D in their diet.

Children or adolescents who don't drink at least 500 ml. of D-fortified milk daily should increase their intake of other vitamin D–rich foods—or take a daily multivitamin supplement containing at least 200 IU of vitamin D.

Pregnant women who have low levels of vitamin D are more likely to give birth by cesarean section.

Sunscreen blocks UVB rays the body needs to make vitamin D. Letting children stay in the sun for ten minutes before applying SPF lotion will give them vitamin D and still keep skin safe. (You'd need thirty cups of fortified orange juice or 3¾ pounds of fresh salmon to get the vitamin D value of ten minutes of exposure to sunlight.)

Dark-skinned people living in northern climates usually need an increase in vitamin D.

If you are overweight, you may be at risk of deficiency because excess fat can absorb vitamin D, making it unavailable to the body.

To get vitamin D from sunlight, be sure to protect yourself by going out for a limited exposure (about one quarter the time it takes for your skin to start reddening) without sunscreen.

Weight-loss products such as orlistat (Alli) and olestra contain a substance intended to prevent the absorption of fat, which may also prevent the body's absorption of fat-soluble vitamins (namely D, A, E, and K).

Do not supplement your dog's or cat's diet with vitamin D unless your vet specifically advises it.

Vitamin D works best with vitamin A, vitamin C, choline, calcium, and phosphorus.

INTERACTION WITH DRUGS:

Antacids—may decrease levels and availability of vitamin D.

Anticonvulsants—may induce liver enzymes that inactivate vitamin D and cause a deficiency.

Calcium channel blockers—may decrease vitamin D production in the body.

Cholestyramine—interferes with the absorption of vitamin D.

Digoxin—effects of drug may be increased and lead to an irregular heartbeat.

Estrogen—can increase vitamin D levels in the blood.

Thiazide diuretics—can increase vitamin D activity to inappropriate calcium levels in the blood; may cause hypercalcemia.

48. Vitamin E (Tocopherols/Tocotrienols)

FACTS:

Fat soluble and stored in the liver, fatty tissues, heart, muscles, testes, uterus, blood, and adrenal and pituitary glands.

Formerly measured by weight, but now generally designated according to its biological activity in international units (IU). With this vitamin, 1 IU is the same as 1 mg.

DRI (see section 241) is 15 mg.

Composed of a family of natural compounds called tocopherols and tocotrienols. The four tocopherols are alpha, beta, gamma, and delta. The four tocotrienols are also designated as alpha, beta, gamma, and delta.

Of the eight compounds, alpha-tocopherol is the most biologically active, but gamma-tocopherol is more potent in increasing the antioxidant enzyme superoxide dismutase (SOD) (see section 129) and in protecting against diseases associated with chronic inflammation, including cancer, Alzheimer's disease, heart disease, and aging.

For nutritional supplements, the claimed IU content is from alpha-tocopherol. The other tocopherols and tocotrienols are assumed to have zero IU value.

IU amounts on a product do not tell you if it contains only alpha-tocopherol or other tocopherols and tocotrienols.

An active antioxidant, vitamin E prevents oxidation of fat compounds as well as that of vitamin A, selenium, two sulfur amino acids, and some vitamin C.

Enhances activity of vitamin A.

The RDI/RDA for adults is 8–10 IU.

Of daily doses, 60–70 percent is excreted in feces. Unlike other fat-soluble vitamins, E is stored in the body for a relatively short time, much like B and C. It is not stored in the liver.

Important as a vasodilator and an anticoagulant.

Products with 25 mcg. of selenium for each 200 units of E increase E's potency.

WHAT IT CAN DO FOR YOU:

Keep you looking younger by slowing cellular aging due to oxidation.

Prevent oxidation of "bad" cholesterol.

Supply oxygen to the body to give you more endurance.

Protect your lungs against air pollution by working with vitamin A.

Help prevent various forms of cancer.

Increase the power of disease-fighting T cells.

Help to inhibit breast cancer cell growth.

Prevent and dissolve blood clots.

Alleviate fatigue.

Reduce risk of cataracts.

Prevent thick scar formation externally (when applied topically—it can be absorbed through the skin) and internally.

Accelerate healing of burns.

Working as a diuretic, it can lower blood pressure.

Aid in prevention of miscarriages.

Help alleviate leg cramps and charley horses.

Lower risk of ischemic heart disease and stroke.

Decrease risk and progression of Alzheimer's disease.

DEFICIENCY DISEASE:

Destruction of red blood cells, muscle degeneration, some anemias and reproductive disorders. (For deficiency symptoms, see section 235.)

BEST NATURAL SOURCES:

Wheat germ, soybeans, vegetable oils, nuts (walnuts, pecans, and peanuts are particularly rich in gamma-tocopherol), brussels sprouts, leafy greens, spinach, enriched flour, whole wheat, whole-grain cereals, and eggs.

SUPPLEMENTS:

Available in oil-base capsules as well as water-dispersible dry tablets.

Natural alpha-tocopherol supplements are twice as biologically potent as synthetic ones.

Usually supplied in strengths from 100 to 1,500 IU. The dry form is recommended for anyone who cannot tolerate oil or whose skin condition is aggravated by oil. It's also best for people over forty.

Daily doses most often used are 200–1,200 IU.

TOXICITY AND WARNING SIGNS OF EXCESS:

Essentially nontoxic.

ENEMIES:

Heat, oxygen, freezing temperatures, food processing, iron, chlorine, mineral oil. (See section 381.)

PERSONAL ADVICE:

If you're on a diet high in polyunsaturated oils, you might need additional vitamin E.

If you are having surgery, I suggest that you discontinue vitamin E supplements for two weeks before and after your operation to ensure proper blood clotting, unless advised otherwise by your doctor.

Natural vitamin E supplements are absorbed twice as well as synthetic ones. (Natural supplements are labeled d-alpha-tocopherol; synthetics are dl.)

It is especially important to take tocotrienols with some form of oil or fat-containing food.

Taking large doses of alpha-tocopherol depletes plasma levels of gamma-tocopherol, which has the ability to protect against nitrogen-based free radicals. (Nitrogen free radicals are inolved in diseases such as cancer, Alzheimer's disease, and heart disease.)

Taking gamma-tocopherol increases the levels of *both* alpha-tocopherol and gamma-tocopherol.

Gamma-tocotrienol has been found to be the most effective in inhibiting cancer cell growth.

Inorganic iron (ferrous sulfate) destroys vitamin E, so the two should not be taken together. If you're using a supplement containing any ferrous sulfate, E should be taken at least eight hours before or after.

Ferrous gluconate, peptonate, citrate, or fumerate (organic iron complexes) do not destroy E.

Weight-loss products such as orlistat (Alli) and olestra contain a substance intended to prevent the absorption of fat that may also prevent the body's absorption of fat-soluble vitamins (namely E, A, D, and K).

If you have chlorinated drinking water, you need more vitamin E.

Pregnant or lactating women, as well as those on the pill or taking hormones, need increased vitamin E.

I advise women going through menopause to increase their E intake. (If you are under forty years of age, 400 IU is fine; over forty, I suggest 800 IU daily. Dry form preferred.)

INTERACTION WITH DRUGS:

Anticoagulants (including aspirin and nonsteroidal anti-inflammatories (NSAIDs)—high doses of vitamin E can increase the potency of anticoagulants and interfere with the absorption of vitamin K, which promotes blood clotting.

Antidepressants (tricyclics)—absorption can be obstructed.

Antipsychotics (phenothiazines)—absorption can be obstructed.

AZT—vitamin E may protect against toxicity and side effects of the medication.

Beta-blockers—absorption of propranolol may be impaired.

Cholesterol-lowering medications—may decrease the absorption of vitamin E.

49. Vitamin F (Unsaturated Fatty Acids— Linoleic, Linolenic, and Arachidonic)

FACTS:

Fat soluble, made up of unsaturated fatty acids obtained from foods.

Measured in milligrams (mg.).

No RDI/RDA has been established, but the National Research Council has suggested that at least 1 percent of total calories should include essential unsaturated fatty acids.

Unsaturated fat helps burn saturated fat, with intake balanced two to one.

Twelve teaspoons of sunflower seeds or eighteen pecan halves can furnish a day's complete supply.

If there is sufficient linoleic acid, the other two fatty acids can be synthesized.

Heavy carbohydrate consumption increases need.

WHAT IT CAN DO FOR YOU:

Aid in preventing cholesterol deposits in the arteries.

Promote healthy skin and hair.

Give some degree of protection against the harmful effects of X-rays.

Aid in growth and well-being by influencing glandular activity and making calcium available to cells.

Combat heart disease.

Aid in weight reduction by burning saturated fats.

DEFICIENCY DISEASE:

Eczema, acne. (For deficiency symptoms, see section 235.)

BEST NATURAL SOURCES:

Vegetable oils (wheat germ, flaxseed, sunflower, safflower,

soybean, and peanut), peanuts, sunflower seeds, walnuts, pecans, almonds, avocados.

SUPPLEMENTS:

Comes in capsules of 100–150 mg. strengths.

TOXICITY AND WARNING SIGNS OF EXCESS:

No known toxic effects, but an excess can lead to unwanted pounds.

ENEMIES:

Saturated fats, heat, oxygen. (See section 381.)

PERSONAL ADVICE:

For best absorption of vitamin F, take vitamin E with it at mealtimes.

If you are a heavy carbohydrate consumer, you need more vitamin F.

Anyone worried about cholesterol buildup should be getting the proper intake of F.

Though most nuts are fine sources of unsaturated fatty acids, Brazil nuts and cashews are *not*!

Watch out for fad diets high in saturated fats.

INTERACTION WITH DRUGS:

Anticoagulants (warfarin, Coumadin)—can reduce the required dosages of these medications.

50. Vitamin K (Menadione)

FACTS:

Fat soluble.
Usually measured in micrograms (mcg.).

There is a trio of K vitamins. K1 (phylloquinone), found in green leafy vegetables, and K2 (menaquinone) can be formed by natural, probiotic bacteria in the intestines. K3 (dihydrophylloquinone) is a synthetic.

Vitamins K1 and K2 are essential for different aspects of good health.

Natural vitamin K2 is the most effective as a supplement.

Vitamin K3 is a free radical producer that doesn't act like real vitamin K in the body and by itself is not a good source of the vitamin.

The RDI/RDA for adults is 65–80 mcg.

Essential in the formation of prothrombin, a blood-clotting chemical.

What It Can Do for You:

Help in preventing internal bleeding and hemorrhages.

Aid in reducing excessive menstrual flow.

Promote proper blood clotting.

Help protect against diabetes by reducing risk of insulin resistance.

Improve bone mineral content and increase bone mass.

Help prevent bone loss after menopause.

Aid in preventing cardiovascular disease.

Deficiency Disease:

Celiac disease, sprue, colitis. (For deficiency symptoms, see section 235.)

Best Natural Sources:

Leafy green vegetables, yogurt, alfalfa, egg yolk, safflower oil, soybean oil, fish liver oils, kelp, natto.

SUPPLEMENTS:

Available in 100 mcg. tablets (though the abundance of natural vitamin K generally makes supplementation unnecessary).

It is not included ordinarily in multivitamins.

TOXICITY AND WARNING SIGNS OF EXCESS:

Although vitamin K, unlike other fat-soluble nutrients, does not build up in the body, more than 500 mcg. of synthetic vitamin K is not recommended.

ENEMIES:

X-rays and radiation, frozen foods, aspirin, air pollution, mineral oil. (See section 381.)

PERSONAL ADVICE:

People with gallstones, liver disease, or gastrointestinal disease are prone to vitamin K deficiency.

High doses of vitamin E can interfere with vitamin K absorption.

Excessive diarrhea can be a symptom of vitamin K deficiency, but before self-supplementing, see a doctor. Green leafy vegetables are your best defense against a vitamin K deficiency.

If you have nosebleeds often, try increasing your K through natural food sources. Alfalfa tablets might help.

Even natural foods containing vitamin K can reverse the effects of blood thinners.

Cholesterol-lowering drugs may cause a vitamin K deficiency. If you are on a chronic broad-spectrum antibiotic regimen, you're at high risk for a vitamin K deficiency. Increase the K-rich foods in your diet—and I suggest you check with a nutritionally oriented doctor about a supplement (see section 462).

INTERACTION WITH DRUGS:

Antibiotics (particularly cephalosporins)—reduce the absorption of vitamin K in the body.

Anticoagulants—can reverse the blood-thinning effects of these medications.

Anticonvulsants (phenytoin)—interfere with the body's ability to use vitamin K.

Bile acid sequestrants—may reduce absorption of vitamin K.

Orlistat (Xenical, Alli) and olestra—substances added to products to prevent the absorption of fat are now required to add vitamin K (and other fat-soluble vitamins), enabling those products to reverse the blood-thinning effects of anticoagulants.

51. Vitamin P (C Complex, Citrus Bioflavonoids, Rutin, Hesperidin)

FACTS:

Water soluble and composed of citrin, rutin, and hesperidin, as well as flavones and flavonals.

Usually measured in milligrams (mg.).

Necessary for the proper function and absorption of vitamin C.

Flavonoids are the substances that provide the yellow and orange colors in citrus foods. (See section 108.)

Also called the capillary permeability factor. (P stands for permeability.) The prime function of bioflavonoids is to increase capillary strength and regulate absorption.

Aids vitamin C in keeping connective tissues healthy.

No daily allowance has been established, but most nutritionists agree that for every 500 mg. of vitamin C you should have at least 100 mg. of bioflavonoids.

Works synergistically with vitamin C.

WHAT IT CAN DO FOR YOU:

Prevent vitamin C from being destroyed by oxidation.

Strengthen the walls of capillaries, thereby preventing bruising.

Help build resistance to infection.

Aid in preventing and healing bleeding gums.

Increase the effectiveness of vitamin C.

Help in the treatment of edema and dizziness due to disease of the inner ear.

DEFICIENCY DISEASE:

Capillary fragility. (For deficiency symptoms, see section 235.)

BEST NATURAL SOURCES:

The white skin and segment part of citrus fruit— lemons, oranges, grapefruit. Also in apricots, buckwheat, blackberries, cherries, and rose hips.

SUPPLEMENTS:

Available usually in a C complex or by itself. Most often there are 500 mg. of bioflavonoids to 50 mg. of rutin and hesperidin. (If the ratio of rutin and hesperidin is not equal, it should be twice as much rutin.)

All C supplements work better with bioflavonoids.

Most common doses of rutin and hesperidin are 100 mg. three times a day.

TOXICITY AND WARNING SIGNS OF EXCESS:

No known toxicity.

ENEMIES:

Water, cooking, heat, light, oxygen, smoking. (See section 381.)

PERSONAL ADVICE:

Menopausal women can usually find some effective relief from hot flashes with an increase in bioflavonoids taken in conjunction with vitamin D.

If your gums bleed frequently when you brush your teeth, make sure you're getting enough rutin and hesperidin.

Anyone with a tendency to bruise easily will benefit from a C supplement with bioflavonoids, rutin, and hesperidin.

52. Vitamin T

There is very little known about this vitamin, except that it helps in blood coagulation and the forming of platelets. Because of these attributes it is important in warding off certain forms of anemia and hemophilia. No RDI/RDA has been established, and there are no supplements for the public on the market. It is found in sesame seeds and egg yolks, and there is no known toxicity.

53. Vitamin U

Even less is known about vitamin U than vitamin T. It is reputed to play an important role in healing ulcers, but medical opinions vary on this. It is found in raw cabbage and no known toxicity exists.

DID YOU KNOW?

- Vitamin B6, folic acid, and vitamin B12 may save your life.
- Aspirin can triple the rate of excretion of vitamin C.
- After age fifty, vitamin D needs *increase*.
- Production of vitamin D through the skin stops once you have a suntan.

54. Any Questions About Chapter III?

Can you tell me what the difference is between vitamin D3 and vitamin D2?

Vitamin D3 (cholecalciferol) is produced by the skin when exposed to ultraviolet B (UVB) rays. Created whenever skin is exposed to sunlight, it is considered the best form of vitamin D. Vitamin D2 (ergocalciferol) comes from plants exposed to UV light. The liver and kidneys synthesize both forms to make them active in the body, but the average diet does not provide the required amount of vitamin D, making supplements your most viable alternative.

My mother is seventy years old and healthy in most ways except she seems to catch every cold or "bug" that comes around. Is she missing a particular vitamin?

It's quite likely. Immune function declines as we age, and recent studies have shown that older people with low blood-serum levels of vitamin E are often more vulnerable to developing infections. In fact, a study in the *American Journal of Clinical Nutrition* found that short-term supplementation with high doses of vitamin E significantly enhanced immune responsiveness in healthy individuals over sixty. I'd suggest that your mom do her immune system a favor and supplement her diet with a high-potency multivitamin with amino acid–chelated minerals—and at least 400–500 IU of vitamin E dry form, plus tocotrienol complex, daily.

Are there any new vitamins or combinations of nutrients that have been found to help people with Alzheimer's disease?

The most recent and potentially hopeful combo, according to the *Journal of Alzheimer's Disease,* is vitamin D2 and curcumin. (See sections 47 and 134.)

I've read that diets high in broccoli, brussels sprouts, and carrots can help reduce the risk of cancer, but I just hate these vegetables. What vitamins can I take instead?

You can get concentrated forms of cruciferous (cabbage, broccoli, brussels sprouts, cauliflower) and carotene-rich (spinach and carrots) vegetables in tablet form. I'd advise taking these supplements daily. Since they are made from vegetables that are picked ripe, carefully washed, and quickly dehydrated without cooking—as well as being fortified with vitamins A, C, and E, beta-carotene, and selenium—they'll provide you with optimal nutritional value.

Can you tell me how choline is helpful in the treatment of Alzheimer's disease?

Alzheimer's disease, which is a slow loss of mental faculties, seems to be caused by a depletion in central nervous system reserves of the neurotransmitter acetylcholine.

It has been found that patients with Alzheimer's disease are not only deficient in acetylcholine, but also the enzyme that catalyzes its production—choline acetyltransferase. Ingestion of more choline can apparently prevent existing acetylcholine from being broken down.

Phosphatidylcholine, a more potent form of this, is now recommended.

What sort of vitamin is beta-carotene? And why is there no RDA for it?

I'll answer the second part first. The reason there is no RDI/RDA for it is because it is not in itself a vitamin. Only after it's inside your body does it transform into vitamin A. Beta-carotene comes, primarily, from yellow and orange plant sources (carrots, pumpkins, sweet potatoes, cantaloupe) and has been found to be significantly helpful in the prevention of heart disease and many cancers. Levels decrease with old age, but beta-carotene can also be unnecessarily depleted by dieting, smoking, and heavy drinking. (See section 107.)

In my research, I have found that these are the top calorie sources in the US diet:

- grain-based desserts
- yeast breads
- chicken dishes
- soda/energy/sport drinks
- pizza
- alcoholic beverages
- pasta dishes
- tortillas, burritos, and tacos
- beef dishes
- dairy desserts

IV

YOUR MINERAL ESSENTIALS

55. Calcium

FACTS:

There is more calcium in the body than any other mineral.

Calcium and phosphorus work together for healthy bones and teeth.

Calcium and magnesium work together for cardiovascular health.

Almost all of the body's calcium (two to three pounds) is found in the bones and teeth.

Twenty percent of an adult's bone calcium is reabsorbed and replaced every year. (New bone cells form as old ones break down.)

Calcium must exist in a two-to-one relationship with phosphorus (two parts calcium to one part phosphorus).

In order for calcium to be absorbed, the body must have sufficient vitamin D.

The RDI/RDA for adults has been elevated from

800 mg. to 1,200 mg. And the National Institutes of Health now recommends 1,200–1,500 mg. for pregnant and nursing mothers, and 1,500 mg. for women over fifty and men over sixty-five years of age.

DRI (see section 241) is 1,300 mg.

Calcium and iron are the two minerals in which the American woman's diet is most deficient.

What It Can Do for You:

Maintain strong bones and healthy teeth.

Decrease risk of bone loss and fractures.

Help lower risk of colon cancer.

Keep your heart beating regularly.

Alleviate insomnia.

Help metabolize your body's iron.

Aid your nervous system, especially in impulse transmission.

Help in weight management.

Deficiency Disease:

Rickets, osteomalacia, osteoporosis—commonly known as brittle bones. (See section 235 for symptoms.)

Best Natural Sources:

Milk and milk products, all cheeses, soybeans, tofu, sardines, salmon, peanuts, walnuts, sunflower seeds, dried beans, kale, broccoli, collard greens.

Supplements:

Most often available in 250–500 mg. tablets.

The best form is coral calcium tablets. (Calcium citrate provides the most usable calcium per tablet.)

Chewable calcium citrate supplements are available in flavors.

Calcium citrate is also available as effervescent tablets that dissolve in water and become a pleasant-tasting drink.

Bonemeal, formerly one of the most popular supplements, is no longer recommended—especially for children—because of its possible high lead content. (You can check with the manufacturer for an analysis.)

Calcium gluconate (a vegetarian source) and calcium lactate (a milk sugar derivative) are definitely lead-free and easy to absorb. (Gluconate is more potent than lactate.)

The letters USP (United States Pharmacopeia) on the label indicate that the calcium in the product has met quality standards for dissolving within thirty minutes.

When combined with magnesium, the ratio should be twice as much calcium as magnesium.

Although most multivitamin supplements contain calcium, none contain the RDA (1,000–1,200 mg. daily), so an extra calcium supplement is advised to make up the difference

TOXICITY AND WARNING SIGNS OF EXCESS:

Excessive daily intake of more than 2,500 mg. might lead to hypercalcemia. Overly high intakes may also cause constipation and increase the risk of kidney stones and urinary tract infections.

ENEMIES:

Large quantities of fat, oxalic acid (found in chocolate, spinach, Swiss chard, parsley, beet greens, and rhubarb), and phytic acid (found in grains) are capable of preventing proper calcium absorption. (See section 381.)

PERSONAL ADVICE:

If you have chronic back pain, chelated calcium supplements might help.

Menstrual-cramp sufferers can often find relief by increasing their calcium intake.

If you enjoy chewing on chicken or turkey drumsticks, you're in luck. The tips of poultry leg bones are high in calcium.

If you're taking daily doses of 1,500 mg. calcium, and are prone to urinary tract infections, I'd advise taking your supplements with cranberry juice. This juice coats the bacteria and helps stop it from sticking to the urinary tract.

Teenagers who suffer from "growing pains" will usually find that they disappear with an increase in calcium consumption.

Long-term high dairy calcium intakes may increase the rate at which dietary fat is burned.

Hypoglycemics could use more calcium. (I recommend calcium citrate for best absorption, in doses of 1,000–1,500 mg. daily.)

If you consume lots of soft drinks, be aware that, because they're high in phosphorus, you may be depleting your body of calcium and increasing your chances of osteoporosis.

Calcium works best with vitamins A, C, and D; iron, magnesium, and phosphorus. (Too much phosphorus, as I've mentioned above, can deplete calcium.)

Calcium supplements are absorbed best when taken with meals. If you take your supplements on an empty stomach, or are over sixty years of age, calcium citrate is your best calcium choice.

Taking poorly assimilated supplements can create more problems than it will solve, such as stiffening your joints and hardening your arteries.

The body does not effectively absorb more than 500 mg. of supplemental calcium at one time, so divide doses. In fact, daily absorption may be enhanced even by taking smaller doses throughout the day. You need extra calcium if you've been bedridden for a week or more. (The body loses bone density during extended bed rest.)

Taking calcium and magnesium at bedtime can help you get a good night's rest.

INTERACTION WITH DRUGS:

Antacids that contain aluminum—aluminum absorbed in the blood may be increased; dangerous for anyone with kidney disease.

Antibiotics—calcium supplements can interfere with the body's ability to absorb them. Take supplements two to four hours before or after taking antibiotics.

Anticonvulsants—can lower calcium levels in the body; supplementation with vitamin D may be recommended. Take medication and supplements at least two hours apart for effective absorption of both.

Antihypertensives—can interfere with blood levels of beta-blockers; concomitantly, beta-blockers can interfere with blood levels of calcium. Same may be true of calcium channel blockers.

Cholesterol-lowering medications—can interfere with calcium absorption and increase calcium loss in the urine. Supplementation with calcium and vitamin D may be recommended.

Corticosteroids—calcium supplements may be needed.

Diuretics—thiazide diuretics can raise blood levels of calcium and loop diuretics can decrease them; potassium-sparing diuretics may decrease the amount of calcium excreted in urine, thereby increasing calcium levels in the blood.

Gentamicin—calcium supplements may increase potential for toxic effects on the kidneys.

Oral contraceptives, estrogens—can increase calcium blood levels.

56. Chlorine

FACTS:

Regulates the blood's alkaline-acid balance.

Works with sodium and potassium in a compound form.

Aids in the cleaning of body wastes by helping the liver to function.

No dietary allowance has been established, but if your daily salt intake is average, you are getting enough.

WHAT IT CAN DO FOR YOU:

Aid in digestion.

Help keep you limber.

DEFICIENCY DISEASE:

Loss of hair and teeth.

BEST NATURAL SOURCES:

Table salt, kelp, olives.

SUPPLEMENTS:

Most good multimineral preparations include it.

TOXICITY AND WARNING SIGNS OF EXCESS:

More than 15 g. can cause unpleasant side effects.

PERSONAL ADVICE:

If you have chlorine in your drinking water, you aren't

getting all the vitamin E you think. (Chlorinated water destroys vitamin E.)

Anyone who drinks chlorinated water should be well advised to eat yogurt—a good natural way to replace the intestinal bacteria the chlorine destroys.

57. Chromium

FACTS:

Works with insulin in the metabolism of sugar.

Helps bring protein to where it's needed.

No official dietary allowance has been established, but 50–200 mcg. is the tentatively recommended adult intake.

As you get older, you retain less chromium in your body.

WHAT IT CAN DO FOR YOU:

Aid growth.

Help prevent and lower high blood pressure.

Work as a deterrent of diabetes.

Help prevent sugar cravings and sudden drops in energy.

DEFICIENCY DISEASE:

A suspected factor in arteriosclerosis and diabetes.

BEST NATURAL SOURCES:

Calves' livers, wheat germ, brewer's yeast, chicken, corn oil, clams.

SUPPLEMENTS:

May be found in better multimineral preparations. (Chromium dinicotinate glycinate is the preferred form.)

TOXICITY AND WARNING SIGNS OF EXCESS:

No known toxicity.

PERSONAL ADVICE:

If you are low in chromium (90 percent of adults are not getting enough in their diet), you might try a zinc supplement. For some reason, chelated zinc seems to substitute well for deficient chromium.

The best assurance of an adequate chromium intake is a varied diet that provides a sufficient intake of other essential nutrients.

INTERACTION WITH DRUGS:

Insulin—may decrease blood sugar, causing it to drop too low.

Levothyroxin (Synthroid)—can decrease amount absorbed and make drug less effective.

Nonsteroidal anti-inflammatory drugs (NSAIDs)—may increase risk of adverse effects if taken at the same time.

58. Cobalt

FACTS:

A mineral that is part of vitamin B12.

Usually measured in micrograms (mcg.).

Essential for red blood cells.

Must be obtained from food sources.

No daily allowance has been set for this mineral, and only very small amounts are necessary in the diet (usually no more than 8 mcg.).

WHAT IT CAN DO FOR YOU:

Stave off anemia.

DEFICIENCY DISEASE:

Anemia.

BEST NATURAL SOURCES:

Meat, kidney, liver, milk, oysters, clams.

SUPPLEMENTS:

Rarely found in supplement form.

TOXICITY AND WARNING SIGNS OF EXCESS:

No known toxicity.

ENEMIES:

Whatever is antagonistic to B12.

PERSONAL ADVICE:

If you're a strict vegetarian, you are much more likely to be deficient in this mineral than someone who includes meat and shellfish in his or her diet.

59. Copper

FACTS:

Required to convert the body's iron into hemoglobin.

Can reach the bloodstream fifteen minutes after ingestion.

Makes the amino acid tyrosine usable, allowing it to work as the pigmenting factor for hair and skin.

Present in cigarettes, birth control pills, and automobile pollution.

Essential for the utilization of vitamin C.

No RDI/RDA has been established by the National Research Council, but 1.5–3.0 mg. for adults is currently recommended.

WHAT IT CAN DO FOR YOU:

Keep your energy up by aiding in effective iron absorption.

DEFICIENCY DISEASE:

Anemia, edema, skeletal defects, and possibly rheumatoid arthritis.

NATURAL FOOD SOURCES:

Dried beans, peas, whole wheat, prunes, organ meats, shrimp, and most seafood.

SUPPLEMENTS:

Usually available in multivitamin and mineral supplements in 2 mg. doses.

TOXICITY AND WARNING SIGNS OF EXCESS:

Rare.

ENEMIES:

Not easily destroyed.

PERSONAL ADVICE:

As essential as copper is—and most Americans are not getting enough in their diet—I rarely suggest special supplementation. An excess seems to lower zinc levels and produce insomnia, hair loss, irregular menses, and depression. On the other hand, high levels of supplemental zinc, taken over an extended period of time, may result in a copper deficiency.

If you eat enough whole-grain products and fresh green leafy vegetables, or organ meats, you don't have to worry about your copper intake.

Cooking or storing acidic foods in copper pots can add to your daily intake.

INTERACTION WITH DRUGS:

Nonsteroidal anti-inflammatory drugs (NSAIDs)— increases anti-inflammatory effects.

Penicillamine—reduces copper levels in the body.

Allopurinol—may reduce copper levels in the body.

Cimetidine (Tagamet)—may elevate copper levels, leading to damage of the liver and other organs.

60. Fluorine

FACTS:

Part of the synthetic compound sodium fluoride (the type added to drinking water) and calcium fluoride (a natural substance).

Decreases chances of dental caries, though too much can discolor teeth.

No RDI/RDA has been established, but most people get about 1 mg. daily from fluoridated drinking water. (1.5–4.0 mg. is suggested by the National Academy of Sciences–National Research Council.)

WHAT IT CAN DO FOR YOU:

Reduce tooth decay.

Strengthen bones.

DEFICIENCY DISEASE:

Tooth decay.

BEST NATURAL SOURCES:

Fluoridated drinking water, seafood, and tea.

SUPPLEMENTS:

Not ordinarily found in multimineral supplements.

Available in prescription multivitamins for children in areas without fluoridated water.

TOXICITY AND WARNING SIGNS OF EXCESS:

Levels of 20–80 mg. per day.

ENEMIES:

Aluminum cookware.

PERSONAL ADVICE:

Don't take additional fluoride unless it is prescribed by a physician or dentist.

The fluoride content of food is increased significantly if it's cooked in fluoridated water or a Teflon-treated utensil.

61. Iodine (Iodide)

FACTS:

Two-thirds of the body's iodine is in the thyroid gland.

Since the thyroid gland controls metabolism, and iodine influences the thyroid, an undersupply of this mineral can result in slow mental reaction, weight gain, and lack of energy.

The RDI/RDA, as established by the National Research Council, is 150 mcg. for adults (1 mcg. per kilogram of body weight) and 175–200 mcg. for pregnant and lactating women respectively.

DRI (see section 241) is 150 mcg.

WHAT IT CAN DO FOR YOU:

Help you with dieting by burning excess fat.
Promote proper growth.
Give you more energy.
Improve mental alacrity.
Promote healthy hair, nails, skin, and teeth.

DEFICIENCY DISEASE:

Goiter, hypothyroidism.

BEST NATURAL SOURCES:

Kelp, vegetables grown in iodine-rich soil, onions, and all seafood.

SUPPLEMENTS:

Available in multimineral and high-potency vitamin supplements in doses of 0.15 mg.
Natural kelp is a good source of supplemental iodine.

TOXICITY AND WARNING SIGNS OF EXCESS:

No known toxicity from natural iodine, though intakes above 2 mg. are not recommended and iodine as a drug can be harmful if prescribed incorrectly.

ENEMIES:

Food processing, nutrient-poor soil.

PERSONAL ADVICE:

Aside from kelp, and the iodine included in multimineral and vitamin preparations, I don't recommend additional supplements unless you're advised by a doctor to take them.

If you use salt and live in the Midwest, where iodine-poor soil is common, make sure the salt is iodized.

If you are inclined to eat excessive amounts of raw cabbage, you might *not* be getting the iodine you need, because there are elements in the cabbage that prevent proper utilization of the iodine. This being the case, you might consider a kelp supplement.

Keep in mind that most iodine supplements contain potassium. See interactions below.

INTERACTION WITH DRUGS:

Antithyroid medications—iodine might decrease the thyroid too much.

Amiodarone—contains iodine and with supplements may cause side effects that affect the thyroid.

Lithium—can increase iodine's effect on the thyroid and *decrease* thyroid function.

ACE inhibitors—combined with iodine, these medications for high blood pressure might decrease how quickly the body gets rid of potassium, causing too much to be retained in the body.

Diuretics—combination may cause too much potassium to be in the body.

62. Iron

FACTS:

Essential and required for life, necessary for the production of hemoglobin (red blood corpuscles), myoglobin (red pigment in muscles), and certain enzymes.

Only about 8 percent of your total iron intake is absorbed and actually enters your bloodstream.

An average 150-pound adult has about 4 g. of iron in his or her body. Hemoglobin, which accounts for most of the iron, is recycled and reutilized as blood cells are replaced every 120 days. Iron bound to protein (ferritin) is stored in the body, as is tissue iron (present in myoglobin) in very small amounts.

The RDI/RDA, according to the National Research Council, is 10–15 mg. for adults, and 30 mg. for pregnant women. Nursing mothers' RDI/RDA is the same as for nonpregnant women (15 mg.).

DRI (see section 241) for adults is 8–18 mg., 27 mg. for pregnant women, and 10 mg. for nursing mothers.

Copper, cobalt, manganese, and vitamin C are necessary to assimilate iron.

Iron is necessary for proper metabolization of B vitamins.

Excessive amounts of zinc and vitamin E interfere with iron absorption.

Too much iron in the blood can promote formation of free radicals and increase the risk of heart disease—especially for men.

WHAT IT CAN DO FOR YOU:

Aid growth.
Promote resistance to disease.
Prevent fatigue.
Cure and prevent iron-deficiency anemia.
Bring back good skin tone.

DEFICIENCY DISEASE:

Iron-deficiency anemia. (For deficiency symptoms, see section 235.)

BEST NATURAL SOURCES:

Pork, beef, liver, red meat, clams, dried peaches, farina, egg yolks, oysters, nuts, beans, asparagus, molasses, oatmeal.

SUPPLEMENTS:

The most assimilable form of iron is amino acid chelate, which means organic iron that has been processed for fastest assimilation. This form is nonconstipating and easy on sensitive systems.

Ferrous sulfate, inorganic iron, appears in many vitamin and mineral supplements and can destroy vitamin E (they should be taken at least eight hours apart). Check labels; many drugstore formulas contain ferrous sulfate.

Supplements with organic iron—ferrous gluconate, ferrous fumarate, ferrous citrate, or ferrous peptonate—do not neutralize vitamin E. They are available in a wide variety of doses, usually up to 320 mg.

TOXICITY AND WARNING SIGNS OF EXCESS:

Rare in healthy individuals. Adult doses, though, can be a hazard for children. A dose of 3 g. can be lethal for a two-year-old child. Individuals with idiopathic hemochromatosis are genetically at risk from iron overload. Keep children's chewable vitamins with iron safely out of their reach. Teach them that these are not candies.

ENEMIES:

Phosphoproteins in eggs and phytates in unleavened whole wheat reduce iron availability to body.

PERSONAL ADVICE:

If you are a woman who experiences very heavy menstrual bleeding, a strict vegetarian, or are an extreme low-calorie dieter, you might need an iron supplement. Check the label on your multivitamin or mineral preparation and see what you are already getting so you can guide yourself accordingly. (You might want to have your blood iron status tested by your doctor to be sure you're not getting too much.)

If you're on the anti-inflammatory drug Indocin, or take aspirin on a daily basis, you might need more iron. (Check with your physician.)

Keep your iron supplements safely out of the reach of children.

Coffee drinkers, as well as tea drinkers, be aware that if you consume large quantities of either beverage, you are most likely inhibiting your iron absorption.

If you are pregnant, check with your doctor before taking iron or iron-fortified vitamin supplements. (Iron poisoning has been found in children whose mothers have taken too many pills during pregnancy.)

Do not take iron supplements if you have an infection. Bacteria require iron for growth and extra iron would encourage their increase.

If you're a premenopausal woman, look for a multivitamin supplement that provides at least 18 mg. of iron.

As a rule, men and postmenopausal women should look for supplements without iron.

INTERACTION WITH DRUGS:

Antithyroid—can potentiate medication and decrease thyroid function too much.

Amiodarone (Cordarone)—can result in too much iodine in the blood.

Lithium—taking this medication with iron may decrease thyroid function too much.

63. Magnesium

FACTS:

Necessary for calcium and vitamin C metabolism, as well as that of phosphorus, sodium, and potassium.

Measured in milligrams (mg.).

Essential for effective nerve and muscle functioning.

Important for converting blood sugar into energy.

Known as the antistress mineral.

Alcoholics are usually deficient.

Adults need 250–500 mg. daily. For pregnant and lactating women, the recommendation, according to the National Research Council, is 300–355 mg.

DRI (see section 241) is 310–420 mg. for adults, 350–460 mg. for pregnant women, and 310–360 mg. for nursing mothers.

The human body contains approximately 21 g. of magnesium.

What It Can Do for You:

Help burn fat and produce energy.

Aid in fighting depression.

Promote a healthier cardiovascular system and help prevent heart attacks.

Keep cholesterol levels under control.

Help prevent muscle spasms.

Aid in relieving severity of angina pain.

Help prevent premature labor.

Keep teeth healthier.

Help prevent calcium deposits, kidney and gallstones.

Bring relief from indigestion.

Combined with calcium can work as a natural tranquilizer.

Alleviate premenstrual syndrome (PMS).

Deficiency Disease:

For deficiency symptoms, see section 235.

BEST NATURAL SOURCES:

Unmilled grains, figs, almonds, nuts, seeds, dark green vegetables, bananas.

SUPPLEMENTS:

Magnesium and calcium in perfect balance (half as much magnesium as calcium) is the preferred form.

Available in multivitamin and mineral preparations.

Can be purchased as magnesium oxide: 250 mg. strength equals 150 mg. per tablet.

Commonly available in 133.3 mg. strengths and taken four times a day.

Supplements of magnesium should not be taken after meals, since the mineral does neutralize stomach acidity.

TOXICITY AND WARNING SIGNS OF EXCESS:

Large amounts, over an extended period of time, can be toxic if your calcium and phosphorus intakes are high or if you have impaired kidney function.

ENEMIES:

Diuretics, alcohol. (See section 381.)

PERSONAL ADVICE:

If you are a drinker, I suggest you increase your intake of magnesium.

If your daily workouts are exhausting, you probably need more magnesium.

Women who are on the pill or taking estrogen in any form would be well advised to eat more magnesium-rich foods. (Keep in mind that meat, fish, and dairy products are relatively poor sources.)

If you are a heavy consumer of nuts, seeds, and green vegetables, you probably get ample magnesium—as does anyone who lives in an area with hard water.

If you are an insulin-resistant diabetic, eating a magnesium-rich diet can help lower your blood pressure. (Talk to your physician before taking a supplement.)

Magnesium works best with vitamin A, calcium, and phosphorus.

Magnesium by itself can cause diarrhea, so be sure to take it in combination with calcium, in a multivitamin, or in the form of magnesium glycinate, gluconate, or citrate.

Keep in mind that because magnesium turns on the enzymes that use vitamins B1, B2, and B6, a deficiency of the mineral can cause symptoms associated with an insufficiency of B vitamins—often convulsions.

CAUTION: *If you're on the medicine digitalis to treat heart disease, the medication can be toxic if you are deficient in magnesium or potassium. Be aware that many drugs can deplete magnesium (see section 381), especially aminoglycosides, cisplatin, corticosteroids, cyclosporine, diuretics, foscarnet, gentamicin, and pentamidine.*

INTERACTION WITH DRUGS:

Antibiotics—may diminish absorption and effectiveness; take one hour before or after medication to avoid interference.

Blood pressure medications, calcium channel blockers—negative side effects of these medications may be increased.

Diabetic medications—absorption of these may be increased, requiring a reduction in dosage.

Digoxin—low levels of magnesium can increase adverse effects of the drug. Additionally, digoxin can increase the loss of magnesium, requiring supplementation.

Diuretics—may deplete magnesium and require supplementation.

Levothyroxin (Synthroid)—antacids and laxatives containing magnesium may reduce the effectiveness of this medication.

Penicillamine—may reduce medication's side effects.

Tiludronate and alendronate—may interfere with absorption of these osteoporosis drugs; take one hour before or after medication.

64. Manganese

FACTS:

Helps activate enzymes necessary for the body's proper use of biotin, B1, and vitamin C.

Needed for normal bone structure.

Measured in milligrams (mg.).

Important in the formation of thyroxin, the principal hormone of the thyroid gland.

Necessary for the proper digestion and utilization of food.

No official daily allowance has been established, but 2–5 mg. is the National Research Council's recommended average adult requirement.

DRI (see section 241) is 9–11 mg. for adults.

Important for reproduction and normal central nervous system function.

WHAT IT CAN DO FOR YOU:

Help eliminate fatigue.

Aid in muscle reflexes.

Help prevent osteoporosis.

Improve memory.

Reduce nervous irritability.

DEFICIENCY DISEASE:

Ataxia.

BEST NATURAL SOURCES:

Whole-grain cereals, nuts, green leafy vegetables, peas, beets.

SUPPLEMENTS:

Most often found in multivitamin and mineral combinations in dosages of 1–9 mg.

TOXICITY AND WARNING SIGNS OF EXCESS:

Rare, except from industrial sources.

ENEMIES:

Large intakes of calcium and phosphorus will inhibit absorption, as can the fiber and phytic acid contained in bran and beans. (See section 381.)

PERSONAL ADVICE:

If you suffer from recurrent dizziness, you might try adding more manganese to your diet.

I advise absentminded people, or anyone with memory problems, to make sure they are getting enough of this mineral.

Heavy dairy milk drinkers and meat eaters need increased manganese.

INTERACTION WITH DRUGS:

Antibiotics—may interfere with absorption. Take one hour before or after medication.

Tetracycline antibiotics—decreases the amount absorbed,

reducing effectiveness. Take two hours before or after medication.

65. Molybdenum

FACTS:

Aids in carbohydrate and fat metabolism.

A vital part of the enzyme responsible for iron utilization.

No RDA/RDI has been set, but the estimated daily intake of 75–250 mcg. has generally been accepted as the adequate human requirement.

DRI (see section 241) is 45 mcg.

WHAT IT CAN DO FOR YOU:

Help in preventing anemia.

Promote general well-being.

DEFICIENCY DISEASE:

None known.

BEST NATURAL SOURCES:

Dark green leafy vegetables, whole grains, legumes.

SUPPLEMENTS:

Not ordinarily available.

TOXICITY AND WARNING SIGNS OF EXCESS:

Rare, but 5–10 mg. a day can be considered toxic.

PERSONAL ADVICE:

As important as molybdenum is, there seems no need for supplementation unless all the food you consume comes from nutrient-deficient soil.

66. Phosphorus

FACTS:

Present in every cell in the body.

Vitamin D and calcium are essential to proper phosphorus functioning.

Calcium and phosphorus should be balanced two to one to work correctly (twice as much calcium as phosphorus).

Involved in virtually all physiological chemical reactions.

Necessary for normal bone and tooth structure.

Niacin cannot be assimilated without phosphorus.

Important for heart regularity.

Essential for normal kidney functioning.

Needed for the transference of nerve impulses.

The RDI/RDA is 800–1,200 mg. for adults, the higher levels for pregnant and lactating women.

DRI (see section 241) for adults is 700–1,250 mg.

WHAT IT CAN DO FOR YOU:

Aid in growth and body repair.

Provide energy and vigor by helping in the metabolization of fats and starches.

Lessen the pain of arthritis.

Promote healthy gums and teeth.

DEFICIENCY DISEASE:

Rickets, pyorrhea.

BEST NATURAL SOURCES:

Fish, poultry, meat, whole grains, eggs, nuts, seeds.

SUPPLEMENTS:

Bonemeal is a fine natural source of phosphorus. (Make

sure vitamin D has been added to help assimilation, *and that the bonemeal is lead-free*!)

TOXICITY AND WARNING SIGNS OF EXCESS:

No known toxicity.

ENEMIES:

Too much iron, aluminum, and magnesium can render phosphorus ineffective. (See section 381.)

PERSONAL ADVICE:

When you get too much phosphorus, you throw your mineral balance off and decrease your calcium. Our diets are usually high in phosphorus—since it does occur in almost every natural food—and therefore calcium deficiencies are frequent. Be aware of this and adjust your diet accordingly.

Alcohol may pull phosphorus from the bones and deplete it from the body.

If you're over forty, you should cut down on your weekly meat consumption and eat more leafy vegetables. The reason for this is that after forty, our kidneys don't help excrete excess phosphorus, and calcium is again depleted. Be on the lookout for foods preserved with phosphates and consider them as part of your phosphorus intake.

CAUTION: *Using phosphorus supplements with potassium supplements can result in high blood levels of potassium (hyperkalemia), resulting in serious heart rhythm abnormalities.*

INTERACTION WITH DRUGS:

Antacids—can prevent phosphorus absorption.

Anticonvulsants—may lower phosphorus levels and increase levels of an enzyme that helps remove phosphate from body.

Bile acid sequestrants—can decrease absorption of phosphates from the diet and supplements. Take phosphorus at least one hour before or four hours after taking these drugs.

Corticosteroids—may increase urinary phosphorus levels.

Diuretics—can increase elimination of phosphorus from the body in the urine, causing a deficiency.

Insulin—high doses may decrease blood levels of phosphorus.

67. Potassium

FACTS:

Works with sodium to regulate the body's water balance and normalize heart rhythms. (Potassium works inside the cells, sodium works only outside them.)

Nerve and muscle functions suffer when the sodium-potassium balance is off.

Hypoglycemia (low blood sugar) causes potassium loss, as does a long fast or severe diarrhea.

No dietary allowance has been set, but 1,600–2,000 mg. is considered a sufficient daily intake for healthy adults.

DRI (see section 241) is 4.7 grams for adults.

Both mental and physical stress can lead to a potassium deficiency.

WHAT IT CAN DO FOR YOU:

Aid in clear thinking by sending oxygen to brain.

Reduce risk of stroke and cardiovascular disease.

Help dispose of body wastes.

Assist in lowering blood pressure.

Aid in allergy treatment.

DEFICIENCY DISEASE:

Edema, hypoglycemia. (For deficiency symptoms, see section 235.)

BEST NATURAL SOURCES:

Citrus fruits, cantaloupe, tomatoes, watercress, all green leafy vegetables, mint leaves, sunflower seeds, bananas, sweet potatoes, white beans, lima beans, cooked halibut, plain nonfat yogurt, winter squash.

SUPPLEMENTS:

Available in most high-potency multivitamin and multimineral preparations.

Inorganic potassium salts are the sulfate (alum), the chloride, the oxide, and the carbonate. Organic potassium refers to the gluconate, the citrate, the fumerate.

Can be bought separately as potassium, citrate, gluconate, or chloride in dosages up to nearly 600 mg. (99 mg. elemental potassium). Glycinated potassium citrate is the preferred form.

TOXICITY AND WARNING SIGNS OF EXCESS:

An intake of 18 g. can cause toxicity.

ENEMIES:

Alcohol, coffee, sugar, diuretics. (See section 381.)

PERSONAL ADVICE:

If you drink large amounts of coffee, you might find that the fatigue you're fighting is due to the potassium loss you're suffering from.

Increasing your potassium consumption, while lowering

your dietary sodium intake, can help reduce the incidence of cardiovascular disease.

If you like bananas, you can get the entire recommended 4.7 grams of potassium a day by eating ten of them.

Heavy drinkers and anyone with a hungry sweet tooth should be aware that their potassium levels are probably low.

If you have low blood sugar, you are likely to be losing potassium while retaining water. And if you take a diuretic, you'll lose even more potassium! Watch your diet, increase your green vegetables, and take enough magnesium to regain your mineral balance.

On a low-carbohydrate diet, weight might not be the only thing you're losing. Chances are your potassium level is down. Watch out for weakness and poor reflexes.

You can get plenty of potassium without supplements by eating a wide variety of high-potassium foods. (See Best Natural Sources above.)

Excess potassium is normally excreted by the kidneys. However, people with impaired kidney function should not eat foods high in potassium or take potassium supplements.

INTERACTION WITH DRUGS:

Nonsteroidal anti-inflammatory drugs (NAIDs)—may cause potassium levels to rise.

Ace inhibitors—can cause potassium levels to rise. If taken with NSAIDS may result in hyperkalemia and serious heart rhythm abnormalities.

Heparin, cyclosporin, Bactrim, Septra, and beta-blockers—can increase potassium levels.

Diuretics, corticosteroids, antacids, insulin, fluconazole, theophylline, and laxatives—can cause potassium levels to decrease.

Digoxin—low potassium levels can increase the likelihood of toxic effects from medication.

68. Selenium

FACTS:

Vitamin E and selenium are synergistic. This means that each increases the potency of the other.

Both vitamin E and selenium are antioxidants, preventing or at least slowing down aging and hardening of tissues through oxidation.

Selenium is critical for the production of glutathione peroxidase, the body's primary antioxidant that is found in every cell.

Males appear to have a greater need for selenium. Almost half their body's supply concentrates in the testicles and portions of the seminal ducts adjacent to the prostate gland. Also, selenium is lost in the semen.

The RDI/RDA for this mineral is 50 mcg. for women, 70 mcg. for men, 65 mcg. for pregnant women, and 75 mcg. for nursing mothers.

DRI (see section 241) is 55 mcg. for adults.

WHAT IT CAN DO FOR YOU:

Help protect against various types of cancer.
Aid in reducing risk of stroke.
May help prevent heart disease.
Help keep youthful elasticity in tissues.
Alleviate hot flashes and menopausal distress.
Help in treatment and prevention of dandruff.
Raise sperm count and increase fertility in men.

DEFICIENCY DISEASE:

Premature stamina loss; Keshan disease.

BEST NATURAL SOURCES:

Seafood, kidney, liver, wheat germ, bran, tuna fish, onions, tomatoes, broccoli, garlic, brown rice.

SUPPLEMENTS:

Available in small microgram doses: 25, 50, 100, and 200 mcg.

Also available combined with vitamin E and other antioxidants.

Selenomethionine is the preferred form.

TOXICITY AND WARNING SIGNS OF EXCESS:

High doses can produce toxic effects, including gastro-intestinal disorders, garlicky breath odor, brittle nails, a metallic taste in the mouth, and yellowish skin. I suggest you do not exceed 300 mcg. daily. (Studies so far have shown toxicity at levels of 2,400 mcg. daily, but I suggest you err on the side of caution until safe levels have been firmly established.)

ENEMIES:

Food-processing techniques. (See section 381.)

PERSONAL ADVICE:

If normally selenium-rich foods are grown in selenium-depleted soil, you're not getting enough of this mineral from food.

If you're trying to become pregnant, you and your partner can increase your chances of conception by eating selenium-rich foods and taking 50–100 mcg. supplemental selenium daily.

In addition to eating selenium-rich foods, I suggest taking selenium supplements—between 100 and 200 mcg. daily as a preventive against disease. The FDA has finally granted health-claim status to selenium as being protective against some cancers—namely, bladder, prostate, and thyroid. This is a step in the right direction, but the recommended dietary requirements are still astonishingly low.

Although selenium may help reduce side effects of chemotherapy drugs, consult your oncologist before taking it—or any supplement.

INTERACTION WITH DRUGS:

Anticoagulants—may increase risk of bleeding.

Barbiturates—can make sedative effects of these medications last longer.

Cholesterol-lowering medications—may reduce their effectiveness.

69. Sodium

FACTS:

Sodium and potassium were discovered together and both found to be essential for normal growth.

High intakes of sodium (salt) will result in a depletion of potassium.

Diets high in sodium usually account for many instances of high blood pressure.

There is no official allowance, but the National Research Council's estimated sodium chloride requirement for healthy adults is 500 mg. daily.

The Centers for Disease Control and Prevention (CDC) recently announced that most adults should limit their sodium intake to 1,500 mg. daily.

Sodium aids in keeping calcium and other minerals in the blood soluble.

WHAT IT CAN DO FOR YOU:

Aid in preventing heat prostration or sunstroke.
Help your nerves and muscles function properly.

DEFICIENCY DISEASE:

Impaired carbohydrate digestion, possibly neuralgia.

BEST NATURAL SOURCES:

Salt, shellfish, carrots, beets, artichokes, dried beef, brains, kidney, bacon.

SUPPLEMENTS:

Rarely needed, but if so, kelp is a safe and nutritive supplement.

TOXICITY AND WARNING SIGNS OF EXCESS:

More than 14 g. of sodium chloride daily can produce toxic effects.

PERSONAL ADVICE:

If you think you don't eat much salt, see sections 427 and 428 and think again.

If you have high blood pressure, cut down on your sodium intake by reading the labels on the foods you buy. Look for SALT, SODIUM, or the chemical symbol *Na*.

Adding sodium to your diet is as easy as a shake of salt, but subtracting it can be difficult. Avoid luncheon meats, frankfurters, salt-cured meats such as ham, bacon, corned beef, as well as condiments—ketchup, chili sauce, soy sauce, mustard. Don't use baking powder or baking soda in cooking.

INTERACTION WITH DRUGS:

Antihypertensives—can alter and/or undermine effects of these medications.

70. Sulfur

FACTS:

Essential for healthy hair, skin, and nails.

Helps maintain oxygen balance necessary for proper brain function.

Works with B-complex vitamins for basic body metabolism, and is part of tissue-building amino acids.

Aids the liver in bile secretion.

No RDI/RDA has been set, but a diet sufficient in protein will generally be sufficient in sulfur.

WHAT IT CAN DO FOR YOU:

Tone up skin and make hair more lustrous.

Help fight bacterial infections.

DEFICIENCY DISEASE:

None known.

BEST NATURAL SOURCES:

Lean beef, dried beans, fish, eggs, cabbage, kale, garlic, brussels sprouts.

SUPPLEMENTS:

MSM (methylsulfonylmethane), an organic sulfur, in 1,000 mg. tablets with a vitamin C complex is available as a supplement.

MSM is used in lotion form for skin problems.

TOXICITY AND WARNING SIGNS OF EXCESS:

No known toxicity from organic sulfur, but ill effects may occur from large amounts of inorganic sulfur.

PERSONAL ADVICE:

Organic sulfur, MSM, is nonallergenic. Do not confuse it with the synthetic *sulfa* drugs, which can trigger allergic reactions in many people.

Taken with glucosamine, another sulfur compound, MSM can significantly reduce the pain and stiffness of arthritis.

For allergies, parasitic infections, and faster recovery after working out, MSM with a vitamin C complex is terrific. (For allergies, I suggest taking 1,000–3,000 mg. two to three times daily with food during flare-ups or when there is a high pollen count.)

Sulfur creams and ointments have been remarkably successful in treating a variety of skin problems. Check the ingredients in the preparation you are now using. There are many fine natural preparations available at health-food centers.

DMSO (dimethyl sulfoxide) may interact with other medications, so talk to your doctor before using it.

71. Vanadium

FACTS:

Inhibits the formation of cholesterol in blood vessels.
Necessary for the formation of teeth and bones.
No dietary allowance set.
Mimics the action of the hormone insulin.

WHAT IT CAN DO FOR YOU:

Aid in preventing heart attacks.
Help control insulin-resistant and type 2 diabetes.
Improve nutrient transport into cells and increase energy.

DEFICIENCY DISEASE:

None known.

BEST NATURAL SOURCES:

Fish, olives, whole grains.

SUPPLEMENTS:

Vanadium amino acid chelate is the preferred form.

Also available in the form of vanadyl sulfate, the biologically active form of vanadium.

Usual daily dose is 50 mcg. of elemental vanadium daily.

Diabetics should check with their doctor for specific dosage.

TOXICITY AND WARNING SIGNS OF EXCESS:

Can easily be toxic if taken in synthetic form.

PERSONAL ADVICE:

This is not one of the minerals that need to be supplemented. A good fish dinner will supply you with the vanadium you need.

There is a biologically active form of vanadium, vanadyl sulfate. It's a trace mineral that mimics the action of the hormone insulin and has been used by alternative physicians in the treatment of diabetes.

CAUTION: *If you have diabetes, do not self-medicate. Vanadyl can lower blood sugar levels too quickly, causing problems. See section 462 for a listing of alternative practitioners.*

Vanadyl sulfate is available as a supplement, and bodybuilders claim that it helps build muscle, increasing strength and definition. The recommended dosage for bodybuilding is 10 mg. a half hour before working out.

INTERACTION WITH DRUGS:

Anticoagulants—may increase drug potency and risk of bleeding.

Diabetes drugs—may lower blood sugar levels to hypoglycemic levels.

72. Zinc

FACTS:

Zinc acts as a traffic director, overseeing the efficient flow of body processes, the maintenance of enzyme systems and cells.

Essential for protein synthesis and collagen formation.

Governs the contractibility of muscles.

Helps in the formation of insulin.

A constituent of many vital enzymes, including the antioxidant superoxide dismutase (SOD).

Important for blood stability (keeps the proper concentration of vitamin E in the blood) and in maintaining the body's acid-alkaline balance.

Exerts a normalizing effect on the prostate and is important in the development of all reproductive organs.

Some studies indicate its importance in brain function and the treatment of schizophrenia.

Strong evidence of its requirement for the synthesis of DNA.

The RDI/RDA, as set by the National Research Council, is 12–15 mg. for adults (slightly higher allowances for nursing mothers).

DRI (see section 241) is 8–11 mg. for adults.

Excessive sweating can cause a loss of as much as 3 mg. of zinc per day.

Most zinc in foods is lost in processing, or never exists in substantial amounts because of nutrient-poor soil.

WHAT IT CAN DO FOR YOU:

Accelerate healing time for internal and external wounds.

Get rid of white spots on the fingernails.

Help restore loss of taste.

Aid in the treatment of infertility.

Help avoid prostate problems.

Promote growth and mental alertness.

Help decrease cholesterol deposits.

Aid in the treatment of mental disorders.

Help reduce length and severity of colds.

DEFICIENCY DISEASE:

Possibly prostatic hypertrophy (noncancerous enlargement of the prostate gland), arteriosclerosis, hypogonadism.

BEST NATURAL SOURCES:

Meat, liver, seafood (especially oysters), wheat germ, brewer's yeast, pumpkin seeds, eggs, nonfat dry milk, ground mustard.

SUPPLEMENTS:

Available in all good multivitamin and multimineral preparations.

Can be bought as zinc sulfate, zinc gluconate, or zinc picolinate in doses ranging from 15 to 50 mg. of elemental zinc. Zinc sulfate and zinc gluconate seem to be equally effective, but zinc gluconate appears to be more easily tolerated.

Glycinated zinc citrate is the best form of supplemental zinc.

Zinc is also available in combination with vitamin C, magnesium, and the B-complex vitamins.

Zinc lozenges, for colds, must dissolve in your mouth—otherwise they are ineffective.

TOXICITY AND WARNING SIGNS OF EXCESS:

Excessive intake can cause gastrointestinal irritation, impaired immune function, and copper deficiency. Doses of 1,000 mg. or more can produce toxic effects.

ENEMIES:

Phytates, compounds found in grains and legumes, bind with zinc so that it cannot be absorbed. (See section 381.)

PERSONAL ADVICE:

You need higher intakes of zinc if you are taking large amounts of vitamin B6. This is also true if you are an alcoholic or a diabetic.

Men with prostate problems—and without them—would be well advised to keep their zinc levels up.

I have seen success in cases of erectile dysfunction and impotence with a supplement program of B6 and zinc.

Elderly people concerned about senility might find a zinc and manganese supplement beneficial.

If you are bothered by irregular menses, you might try a zinc supplement before resorting to hormone treatment to establish regularity.

Your zinc levels may be lowered by diarrhea and consumption of large amounts of fiber.

Remember, if you are adding zinc to your diet, you will increase your need for vitamin A. (Zinc works best with vitamin A, calcium, and phosphorus.)

If you're taking both iron and zinc supplements, take them at different times as they can interfere with each other's activity.

CAUTION: *Although zinc is an immune system booster, doses of more than 150 mg. daily may inhibit immune response.*

INTERACTION WITH DRUGS:

Amiloride (Midamor)—can increase zinc levels in blood. (Do not take zinc if you take amiloride unless directed to do so by your physician.)

Blood pressure medications/Ace inhibitors—may decrease zinc levels in your blood.

Antibiotics—may decrease the body's absorption of two types of antibiotics, quinolones and tetracyclines (ask your pharmacist what type you're taking). However, zinc does not interact with doxycyline.

Cisplatin—this chemotherapy drug may cause more zinc to be excreted in urine, but do not take a zinc supplement (or any other supplement) without consulting your oncologist.

Immunosuppresants—zinc strengthens the immune system and should not be taken with any medication intended to suppress the immune system.

Nonsteroidal anti-inflammatory drugs (NSAIDs)—may reduce effectiveness of these medications.

Penicillamine—decreases zinc levels in the blood.

Thiazide diuretics—lowers the amount of zinc in the blood.

73. Water

FACTS:

The simple truth is that this is our most important nutrient. One-half to four-fifths of the body's weight is water.

A human being can live for weeks without food, but only a few days without water.

Water is the basic solvent for all the products of digestion.

Regulates body temperature.

Essential for removing wastes.

There is no specific dietary allowance since water loss varies with climate, situations, and individuals, but under ordinary circumstances six to eight 8-ounce glasses daily is considered healthy. I recommend 8–10 glasses of filtered water daily. (See advice below.) Nursing mothers have increased water requirements because of the amount that's secreted in their milk.

Older people are less able to feel thirsty when they need fluids.

Dark yellow urine may indicate a need for more fluids.

WHAT IT CAN DO FOR YOU:

Maintain all your bodily functions.

Aid in dieting by depressing appetite before meals.

Help prevent constipation.

Aid in preventing kidney stones.

DEFICIENCY DISEASE:

Dehydration.

BEST NATURAL SOURCES:

Drinking water and juices; eating fruits and vegetables.

SUPPLEMENTS:

Most drinkable liquids can substitute for our daily water requirements.

TOXICITY AND WARNING SIGNS OF EXCESS:

No known toxicity, but an intake of one and a half gallons (that's 16–24 glasses) in about an hour could be dangerous to an adult. It could kill an infant.

PERSONAL ADVICE:

I advise 8–10 glasses of filtered water daily, to be drunk a half hour before meals, especially for anyone who's dieting. If you're running a fever, be sure to drink lots of water to prevent dehydration and to flush the system of wastes.

Drink more water whenever you notice your urine color is darker than usual.

The more water you drink with a drug that can cause stomach distress—aspirin, ibuprofen, antibiotics—the less your chance of stomach upset.

Coffee and alcohol tend to promote dehydration and should not be counted as fluid intake.

Milk is a food and should not be considered a substitute for water.

Don't drink water from your hot water tap. Hot water dissolves more lead than cold water. And in the morning, always let the water run a few minutes to get the lead out of overnight accumulations.

If you live in an area where there is hard water, you're probably getting more calcium and magnesium than you think.

The least expensive water filtration route is a pitcher with a filter attached. All you do is pour the water through.

Obviously a more sophisticated system that eliminates heavy metals and other carcinogens is preferable but filtering your drinking water with a filtered pitcher is affordable and better than not filtering your water at all.

HOW TO DETERMINE YOUR DAILY WATER NEEDS

To determine approximately how many ounces of water your body needs per day, divide your body weight by 2. For example:

185 lb. male ÷ 2 = 92 ounces or 11 (8 oz.) glasses daily
145 lb. female ÷ 2 = 72 ounces or 9 (8 oz.) glasses daily
(Some water will be obtained from food or other beverages.)

Special Water Cautions:

Don't freeze your plastic water bottles with water in them, as this may release dioxins—highly toxic carcinogens—in the plastic.

If you live in an old home containing lead pipes, have your water analyzed by the local county health department. Water with the wrong pH can dissolve lead from pipes, subjecting children to possible lead poisoning. (Even homes with copper plumbing can have lead-soldered joints that might affect tap water.)

If there are chlorinated solvents or pesticides in your water, they can be absorbed through the skin and are volatile. *Taking a fifteen-minute shower can be as toxic as drinking 8 glasses of contaminated water!*

Most home water-filtering systems have drawbacks, and many can be hazardous to your health. For instance:

- Activated carbon filters can become fouled with harmful contaminants if they are not changed on a regular basis.
- Reverse-osmosis systems, which remove chemicals, but not necessarily inorganic contaminants, must be tested periodically because the filter can be loaded with bacteria without evidencing a reduced flow rate.
- Distillers, which are generally more effective in removing inorganic than organic contaminants, must be descaled regularly. If not, the product water can be *worse* instead of better! If you use a home filtering system, remember that it must be properly maintained and checked periodically. Stick to well-known or national brands.

DID YOU KNOW?

- Water softeners can unhealthily increase your daily salt intake.
- Milk is a food and should not be considered a substitute for water.
- Men who drink more than 4 glasses of water daily can lower their risk of colon cancer by 32 percent.
- Anyone bedridden for a week or more needs extra calcium because the body loses bone density during extended bed rest.

---

74. Any Questions About Chapter IV?

Is there really a difference between plain water and electrolyte water—and which is better for you?

There is a difference; it just depends on what you need. A study published in *Wilderness & Environmental Medicine* found that if you want or need faster, better hydration, you should drink eletrolyte-fortified water. People exposed to severe environmental conditions require 75 percent more plain water to stay as hydrated as those who drink the electrolyte-fortified H_2O.

I'm a forty-year-old woman and drink 3 glasses of milk every day. Do I still need more calcium?

If that's your sole source of calcium, you do! Three 8-ounce glasses of whole milk give you only 776 mg. of calcium—not enough and certainly not worth the 360 mg. of sodium, 33 mg. of cholesterol, 15 g. of saturated fat, and 577 calories that you also get. Skim milk, low-fat milk, or buttermilk will lower the amount of calories and fat, but still won't provide you with sufficient calcium. (See section 55 for other natural sources.)

I've read that chlorinated drinking water can cause cancer. Is this true? If so, why do they chlorinate water?

Unfortunately, chlorination has indeed been linked to a group of cancer-causing chemicals (trihalomethanes) in our water. But according to the Environmental Protection Agency, the risk to the public is far outweighed by the benefits—primarily the prevention of widespread outbreaks of typhoid and other waterborne diseases. Home water-filtering systems can remove chlorine from tap water after bacteria have been killed, but see section 73 for water cautions to be aware of.

I'm worried about all the pollution in our rivers and streams. How do I know that my tap water is safe to drink?

The best thing to do if you want to find out if there

are contaminants in your water is to contact your local water superintendent and ask for the results of water-sampling tests and sanitary surveys. Ask to see the Public Health Service standards, too, so that you'll be able to compare the former with the latter. You can also have your water tested for contaminants at most local hospital laboratories.

Meanwhile, until you are sure that your water is safe, I recommend taking the following emergency measures:

- Let your water run for three to four minutes before using it. This helps flush out any lead, cadmium, or cobalt that may lodge in your pipes.
- Boil your water (uncovered) for at least twenty minutes before using it. Boiling can kill bacteria and remove some organic chemicals.
- If you're worried about trihalomethanes (which are carcinogens found in chlorinated water), whip your water in a blender for fifteen minutes with the top off. Aeration removes chlorine and chlorinated organics.
- Buy a water filter.

I get very confused in the supermarket. Is mineral water better for me than springwater?

Better? Not really. Some bottled mineral waters may actually have fewer dissolved minerals than many city water supplies. In fact, the term "mineral water" is frequently used to describe all bottled water, with the exception of bulk water, club soda, and seltzer. Springwater must, under truth-in-labeling laws, come from a spring. But that spring has minerals in it, too. What you want to watch out for are mineral waters without the word *natural* on the label. This means that minerals may have been removed or added—and if you're going to buy a nutrient cocktail, you're better off making it yourself!

I know I need calcium, but I'm allergic to dairy products. Can you recommend alternative dietary sources?

Lots! Orange juice (6 oz.) fortified with calcium will give you approximately 200 mg. A 3-ounce can of sardines or salmon (with bones) will give you another 200–300 mg. Tofu, made with calcium sulfate, will also supply calcium (150 mg. per 4-oz. serving) as will almonds, Brazil nuts, and hazelnuts (approximately 200–300 mg. per cup). You might also want to try nori and other seaweeds. They're an acquired taste, but they are high in calcium.

I've been told that calcium will help me lose weight. If this is true, how much should I be eating or taking in supplements?

Sorry to tell you, but it's not true. Calcium will not help you lose weight, but it will help you achieve greater weight loss and fat loss on a reduced-calorie diet. If that sounds contradictory, I'll explain. Studies have shown that as dietary calcium increases, calcium levels within fat cells decrease. Because of this, lower calcium levels within cells impact the metabolism of fat in favor of weight loss. Fat synthesis decreases and fat breakdown increases, resulting in less fat storage and a reduction in body weight. Obese adults following a reduced-calorie diet higher in calcium lost more weight and fat than those on a reduced-calorie, lower-calcium diet. And, interestingly, the impact of calcium on weight loss seems to be even greater when it comes from low-fat dairy products as opposed to calcium supplements. (See section 55 for best natural sources.)

V

PROTEIN—AND THOSE AMAZING AMINO ACIDS

75. The Protein–Amino Acid Connection

Protein is a life necessity in the diet of man and all animals. Actually, though, it is not protein itself that is required, but the amino acids, which are the building blocks of protein.

Amino acids, which combined with nitrogen form thousands of different proteins, are not only the units from which proteins are formed, but are also the end products of protein digestion.

There are twenty-three commonly known amino acids. Eight of these are called *essential amino acids.* These essential amino acids *cannot,* like the others, be manufactured by the human body and *must* be obtained from food or supplements. A ninth amino acid, histidine, is considered essential only for infants and children.

Unlike other nutrients, the human body cannot store

amino acids for later use; therefore, they must be consumed every day in foods or supplements.

In order for the body to effectively use and synthesize protein, all the essential amino acids must be present and in the proper proportions. Even the temporary absence of a single essential amino acid can adversely affect protein synthesis. In fact, whatever essential amino acid is low or missing will proportionately reduce the effectiveness of all the others.

THE AMINO ACIDS

(Essential amino acids are marked with asterisks.)

Alanine	*Leucine
Arginine	*Lysine
Asparagine	*Methionine
Aspartic acid	Ornithine
Cysteine	*Phenylalanine
Cystine	Proline
Glutamic acid	Serine
Glutamine	Taurine
Glycine	*Threonine
*Histidine (for infants and children)	*Tryptophan
	Tyrosine
*Isoleucine	*Valine

76. How Much Protein Do You Need, Really?

Everyone's protein requirements differ, depending on a variety of factors including health, age, and size. Actually, the larger and younger you are, the more you need. To estimate your own personal daily recommended allowance, see the chart below.

Age	1–3	4–6	7–10	11–14	15–18	19 and over
Pound Key	0.82	0.68	0.55	0.45	0.40	0.36

- Find the pound key under your age group.
- Multiply that number by your weight.
- The result will be your daily protein requirement in grams.

Example: You weigh 100 pounds and are 33 years old. Your pound key is 0.36.
0.36 x 100 = 36 g.—your daily protein requirement.

An average minimum protein requirement is around 45 g. a day. That's 15 g. or about half an ounce per meal. And you don't need to eat a lot of meat to get it. A 4-ounce serving of chicken breast has about 30–35 g., a cup of yogurt will give you 12 g., and a cup of 2 percent milk with two shredded-wheat biscuits will give you a breakfast boost of 14 g.

77. Types of Protein—What's the Difference?

All proteins are not the same, though they're manufactured from the same twenty-three amino acids. They have different functions and work in different areas of the body.

There are basically two types of protein—complete protein and incomplete protein.

Complete protein provides the proper balance of eight necessary amino acids that build tissue, and is found in foods of animal origin such as meats, poultry, seafood, eggs, milk, and cheese.

Incomplete protein lacks certain essential amino acids

and is not used efficiently when eaten alone. However, when it is combined with small amounts of animal-source protein, it becomes complete. It is found in seeds, nuts, peas, grains, and beans.

Mixing complete and incomplete proteins can give you better nutrition than either one alone. A good rice-and-beans dish with some cheese can be just as nourishing, less expensive, and lower in fat than a steak.

78. Protein Myths

A lot of people seem to think that protein is nonfattening. This misconception has frustrated many a determined dieter who forgoes bread but eats healthy portions of steak and wonders where the weight is coming from. The fact is

- 1 g. protein = 4 calories
- 1 g. carbohydrate = 4 calories
- 1 g. fat = 9 calories

In other words, protein and carbohydrates have the same gram-for-gram calorie count.

It is also thought that protein can burn up fat. This is another erroneous assumption that leaves dieters staring uncomprehendingly at their scales. It just is not true that the more protein you eat the thinner you'll get. And, believe it or not, one homemade beef taco or a slice of cheese pizza will give you more protein than two eggs or four slices of bacon or even a whole cup of milk. (Of course, if the taco or pizza is made with all sorts of additives, you're better off taking a cut in protein and sticking with the eggs.)

79. Protein Supplements

For anyone who isn't able to get his or her daily protein requirement from whole food, protein supplements are helpful. The best formulas are derived from soybeans, egg white, whey, and nonfat milk, which contain all the essential amino acids. They come in liquid and powdered forms, are available without carbohydrates or fats, and generally supply about 26 g. of protein an ounce (2 tbsp.). That would be about the same amount of protein you get from a 3-ounce T-bone.

Supplements can easily be added to beverages and foods. Texturized vegetable protein (TVP) can be added to ground beef to extend and enhance hamburgers, which will be more economical and better for you because of the cut in saturated fat.

80. Amino Acid Supplements

Free-form amino acids are now available in balanced formulas or as individual supplements, because so many have been found to offer specific health-enhancing properties—from improving the immune system to reducing dependence on drugs. (See individual listings, sections 81 through 89.)

It's wise when taking amino acid supplements to also take the major vitamins that are involved in their metabolization, for instance, vitamins B6, B12, and niacin. And if you're going to take an amino acid formula, make sure it's well-balanced. *Read the label!* For protein synthesis to occur, there must be a balance between "essential" and "nonessential" amino acids, and the essentials in proper proportion to one another. (Lysine should be in a 2:1 ratio to methionine, 3:1 to tryptophan, and so on. When in doubt, ask your pharmacist or consult a reliable nutrition-ist. See section 462.) What you want is a formula that's modeled after naturally occurring proteins so that you can get the proper therapeutic value.

CAUTION: *It's dangerous to use any supplement in place of food on a regular basis or take a supplement in megadoses without the advice of a physician. Always keep supplements out of the reach of children.*

81. Let's Talk Tryptophan—and 5-HTP

Tryptophan is an essential amino acid that's used by the brain—along with vitamin B6, niacin (or niacinamide), and magnesium—to produce serotonin, a neurotransmit-ter that carries messages between the brain and one of the body's biochemical mechanisms of sleep.

WHAT IT CAN DO FOR YOU:

Help induce natural sleep.
Reduce pain sensitivity.
Act as a nondrug antidepressant.
Alleviate migraines.
Aid in reducing anxiety and tension.
Help relieve some symptoms of alcohol-related body-chemistry disorders and aid in the control of alcoholism.

BEST NATURAL SOURCES:

Cottage cheese, milk, meat, fish, turkey, bananas, dried dates, peanuts, all protein-rich foods.

SUPPLEMENT GUIDE:

L-tryptophan is no longer available as an over-the-counter supplement, and can be obtained only by prescription. (It was recalled by the U.S. FDA in 1988 after a tainted batch from Japan caused several deaths. The problem was not with the tryptophan itself but with seriously flawed manufacturing procedures.)

But let's talk 5-HTP (5-hydroxytryptophan), a supplement very similar to tryptophan that is also being hailed as a natural alternative to Prozac. It is a selective serotonin reuptake inhibitor (SSRI) that, like Prozac, enhances the activity of serotonin. But unlike prescription antidepressants and sleep aids, 5-HTP does not cause unpleasant side effects, such as dry mouth and loss of libido. *And* not only has 5-HTP been found to alleviate depression and function as a sleep aid, it's been shown to help suppress appetite as well. (For dieters, that can be a mood elevator right there.)

As a supplement, I recommend one or two 50 mg. capsules daily on an empty stomach.

PERSONAL ADVICE:

For best results with 5-HTP (or L-tryptophan), be sure that you are also taking a complete balanced B-complex formula (50–100 mg. of B1, B2, and B6) with your morning and evening meals.

82. The Phenomenal Phenylalanine

Phenylalanine is an essential amino acid that is a neurotransmitter, a chemical that transmits its signals between the nerve cells and the brain. In the body it's turned into norepinephrine and dopamine, excitatory transmitters, which promote alertness and vitality. (Do not confuse with DL-phenylalanine; see section 83.) It is also half the artificial sweetener aspartame (phenylalanine and aspartic acid) and in virtually all diet soft drinks with the exception of Dr Pepper, as well as most dietetic foods and medicines.

What It Can Do for You:

Reduce hunger.
Increase sexual interest.
Improve memory and mental alertness.
Alleviate depression.

Best Natural Sources:

All protein-rich foods, bread stuffing, soy products, cottage cheese, dry skim milk, almonds, peanuts, lima beans, pumpkin seeds, and sesame seeds.

Supplement Guide:

Available in 250–500 mg. tablets. For appetite control, tablets should be taken one hour before meals with juice or water (no protein).

For general alertness and vitality, tablets should be taken between meals, but again with water or juice (no protein).

CAUTION: *Phenylalanine is contraindicated during pregnancy and for people with PKU (phenylketonuria) or skin cancer.*

Personal Advice:

Before resorting to prescription or recreational drugs, I'd advise giving this natural "upper" a chance. (Keep in mind, though, that it cannot be metabolized if you are deficient in vitamin C.)

Phenylalanine is nonaddictive, *but it can raise blood pressure*! If you are hypertensive or have a heart condition, I'd advise checking with your doctor before using phenylalanine. (In most cases, persons with high blood pressure are able to take phenylalanine *after* meals, but clear it with your doctor first.)

83. DL-Phenylalanine (DLPA)

This form of the essential amino acid phenylalanine is a mixture of equal parts D (synthetic) and L (natural) phenylalanine. By producing and activating morphinelike hormones called *endorphins,* it intensifies and prolongs the body's own natural painkilling response to injury, accident, and disease.

Certain enzyme systems in the body continually destroy endorphins, but DL-phenylalanine effectively inhibits these enzymes, allowing the painkilling endorphins to do their job.

People who suffer from chronic pain have lower levels of endorphin activity in their blood and cerebrospinal fluid. Since DLPA can restore normal endorphin levels, it can thereby assist the body in reducing pain naturally—without the use of drugs.

Moreover, because DLPA is capable of selective pain-blocking, it can effectively alleviate chronic long-term discomfort while leaving the body's natural defense mechanisms for short-term acute pain (burns, cuts, etc.) unhindered.

The effect of DLPA often equals or exceeds that of morphine and other opiate derivatives, but DLPA differs from prescription and over-the-counter medicines in that:

- It is nonaddictive.
- Pain relief becomes *more* effective over time (without development of tolerance).
- It has strong antidepressant action.

- It can provide continuous pain relief for up to a month without additional medication.
- It's nontoxic.
- It can be combined with any other medication or therapy to increase benefits without adverse interactions.

What It Can Do for You:

Act as a natural painkiller for conditions such as whiplash, osteoarthritis, rheumatoid arthritis, lower back pain, migraines, leg and muscle cramps, postoperative pain, and neuralgia.

Supplement Guide:

DL-phenylalanine is generally available in 375 mg. tablets. Correct dosages vary according to the individual's own experience of pain.

Six tablets per day (2 tablets taken approximately fifteen minutes before each meal) is the best way to begin a DLPA regimen. Pain relief should occur within the first four days, though it may, in some cases, take as long as three to four weeks. (If no substantial relief is noticed in the first three weeks, double the initial dosage for an additional two to three weeks. If treatment is still not effective, discontinue the regimen. It's been found that 5–15 percent of users do not respond to DLPA's analgesic properties.)

CAUTION: *DLPA is contraindicated during pregnancy and for people with phenylketonuria. Because it elevates blood pressure, people with heart conditions or hypertension should check with a doctor before starting any DLPA regimen. Usually, though, it's allowed if taken after meals.*

PERSONAL ADVICE:

On a DLPA regimen, pain usually diminishes within the first week. Dosages can then be reduced gradually until a minimum requirement is determined. Whatever yours turns out to be, doses should be regularly spaced throughout the day.

Some people require only one week of DLPA supplements a month; others need it on a continuous basis. (I found it interesting to discover that many people who do not respond to such conventional prescription painkillers as Empirin and Valium *do* respond to DLPA.)

84. Looking at Lysine

This essential amino acid is vital in the makeup of critical body proteins. It's needed for growth, tissue repair, and the production of antibodies, hormones, and enzymes.

WHAT IT CAN DO FOR YOU:

Help reduce the incidence of and/or prevent herpes simplex infection (fever blisters and cold sores).

Promote better concentration.

Properly utilize fatty acids needed for energy production.

Aid in the absorption of calcium.

Help in the prevention and treatment of osteoporosis.

Aid in alleviating some fertility problems.

BEST NATURAL SOURCES:

Fish, milk, lima beans, meat, cheese, yeast, eggs, soy products, all protein-rich foods.

SUPPLEMENT GUIDE:

L-lysine is generally available in 500 mg. capsules or

tablets. The usual dose is 1–2 daily, half an hour before mealtimes.

PERSONAL ADVICE:

If you're often tired, unable to concentrate, prone to bloodshot eyes, nausea, dizziness, hair loss, and anemia, you could have a lysine deficiency.

Older persons, particularly men, require more lysine than younger persons.

Lysine is lacking in certain cereal proteins such as gliadin (from wheat) and zein (from corn). Supplementation of wheat-based foods with lysine improves their protein quality. (See complete and incomplete proteins in section 77.)

Lysine supplements should not be taken by children under ten years of age unless recommended by a physician. (Undiagnosed allergies in young children may cause unwanted side effects.)

If you have herpes, lysine supplements in doses of 3–6 g. daily—plus lysine-rich foods—are strongly recommended. For cold sores or fever blisters, 500–1,000 mg. daily, between meals, is a good preventive.

85. All About Arginine, "A Natural Viagra"

This amino acid is necessary for the normal function of the pituitary gland. Along with ornithine, phenylalanine, and other neurochemicals, arginine is required for the synthesis and release of the pituitary gland's growth hormone. (See section 87.) It is frequently recommended by natural healers as a supplement for men who have problems maintaining an erection long enough to engage in sex. It increases the blood flow to the penis, which results in harder erections. Regrettably, it does not work for everyone and the effect is short-lived, but for maximum effectiveness in improving sexual performance it should be taken about forty-five minutes before having sex. Arginine can also increase sperm count (seminal fluids contain as much as 80 percent of this protein building block) and may help in treating male infertility. Additionally, arginine can improve immune function by stimulating the thymus gland, where disease-fighting T cells (T lymphocytes) are stored until they are called into action. In fact, studies show that arginine can increase the number of T cells, and may even trigger the production of natural killer cells that can aid in the body's defense against cancer.

What It Can Do for You:

Stimulate release of human growth hormone. (See section 87.)

Increase sperm count and enhance sexual performance in men.

Aid in immune response and healing of wounds.

Help metabolize stored body fat and tone up muscle tissue.

Promote physical and mental alertness.

Help in lowering LDL, the "bad" cholesterol.

Best Natural Sources:

Nuts, popcorn, carob, gelatin desserts, chocolate, brown rice, oatmeal, raisins, sunflower seeds, sesame seeds, whole wheat bread, meat, and all protein-rich foods.

Supplement Guide:

L-arginine is available in tablets or powder and should be taken on an empty stomach, with juice or water (no protein). Time release is the preferred form (1,500 mg. twice daily). As an immune booster and to promote physical and mental alertness, take a 2 g. (2,000 mg.) dose immediately before retiring. For muscle-toning, take 2 g. (2,000 mg.) one hour prior to engaging in vigorous physical exercise. For sex-enhancing benefits, take 3–6 g. (3,000–6,000 mg.) of L-arginine forty-five minutes before having sex.

CAUTION: *Do not give to growing children (could cause giantism) or persons with schizophrenic conditions. Arginine supplements—and arginine-rich foods—are contraindicated for anyone who has herpes or who is taking ACE inhibitors. Arginine may temporarily increase the size of blood vessels and affect treatment dosages of hypertensive medications, as well as alter the effects and treatment dosages of nitrate medications such as* nitroglycerin, isosorbide mononitrate, isosorbide dinitrate, *and* amyl nitrate. *(Check with a nutrtionally oriented professional before using supplements.) Dosages exceeding 20–30 g. daily are not recommended (could cause enlarged joints and deformities of bones).*

PERSONAL ADVICE:

Arginine is necessary for adults because after the age of thirty there is almost a complete cessation of its secretion from the pituitary gland.

If you notice a thickening or coarsening of your skin, you're taking too much arginine. Several weeks of extremely high doses can cause this side effect, but it is reversible. Just cut back on your intake.

Any physical trauma increases your need for dietary arginine.

Arginine and lysine are absorbed into cells by the same process. Taking too much of either arginine or lysine can decrease the level of the other in the body, necessitating supplementation with the affected nutrient.

L-arginine taken in conjunction with L-ornithine can help stimulate weight loss. (See section 88.)

86. Taurine

Synthesized in the body, this nonessential amino acid is the building block of all the other amino acids. Taurine is abundant in the tissues of the heart, the skeletal muscles, and the central nervous system. It is needed for the digestion of fats, the absorption of fat-soluble vitamins, and the control of serum cholesterol levels. It also has a protective effect on the brain.

WHAT IT CAN DO FOR YOU:

Strengthen heart function.
Help bolster vision and prevent macular degeneration.
Aid in treatment of anxiety and epilepsy.

BEST NATURAL SOURCES:

Eggs, fish, meat, milk.

SUPPLEMENT GUIDE:

Taurine is available in 500 mg. capsules. Take up to three 500 mg. capsules daily, with juice or water (no protein), half an hour before mealtimes.

PERSONAL ADVICE:

Taurine is not in vegetable proteins. But it can be effectively synthesized in the body as long as there are sufficient quantities of vitamin B6.

Excessive alcohol consumption causes the body to lose its ability to utilize taurine properly.

Diabetes increases requirements for taurine.

Taurine taken in conjunction with cystine may decrease the need for insulin.

87. Growth Hormone (GH) Releasers

Growth hormone (GH) releasers are nutrients that stimulate the production of growth hormone in the body. The human growth hormone is stored in the pituitary gland and the body releases it in response to sleep, exercise, and restricted food intake.

WHAT IT CAN DO FOR YOU:

Help burn fat and convert it into energy and muscle.
Improve resistance to disease.
Accelerate wound healing.
Aid in tissue repair.
Strengthen connective tissue for healthier tendons and ligaments.
Enhance protein synthesis for muscle growth.
Reduce urea levels in blood and urine.

Important GH releasers are the amino acids ornithine, arginine, tryptophan, glutamine, glycine, and tyrosine, which work synergistically (more effectively together than separately) with vitamin B6, niacinamide, zinc, calcium, magnesium, potassium, and vitamin C to trigger the nighttime release of growth hormone. Peak secretion of GH is reached about ninety minutes after we fall asleep.

Natural growth hormone levels decrease as we grow older. Somewhere around age fifty, GH production virtually stops. But by supplementing your diet with the amino acids and vitamins that stimulate release of growth hormone, production can be brought back up to the levels of a young adult.

88. The Ornithine-Arginine Connection

Ornithine and arginine, two of the amino acids involved in the release of human growth hormone, are a dynamic duo and among the most popular amino acid supplements today, mainly because they can help you slim down and shape up while you sleep (which is when GH is secreted). While some hormones encourage the body to store fat, growth hormone acts as a mobilizer of fat, helping you to not only look trimmer but have more energy as well.

Ornithine stimulates insulin secretion and helps insulin work as an anabolic (muscle-building) hormone, which has increased its use among bodybuilders. Taking extra ornithine will help increase the levels of arginine in your body. (Actually, arginine is constructed from ornithine; ornithine is released from arginine in a continuing cyclic process.)

Because ornithine and arginine are so closely related, the characteristics and cautions for one apply to the other. (See section 85, "All About Arginine.") As a supplement, ornithine works best when taken at the same time and in the same manner as arginine (on an empty stomach, with juice or water—no protein).

89. Other Amazing Amino Acids

GLUTAMINE and GLUTAMIC ACID

Glutamic acid serves primarily as a brain fuel. It has the ability to pick up excess ammonia—which can inhibit high-performance brain function—and convert it into the buffer glutamine. Since glutamine produces marked elevation of glutamic acid, a shortage of the former in the diet can result in a shortage of the latter in the brain.

Glutamine is also a component of glutathione, the body's primary antioxidant, which is present in virtually every cell. So if you are deficient in glutamine, you're likely to be deficient in glutathione. And glutamine can also help boost the level of human growth hormone.

Aside from improving intelligence (even the IQs of intellectually disabled children), glutamine has been shown to help in the control of alcoholism. It has also been found to shorten healing time for ulcers and alleviate fatigue, depression, and erectile dysfunction. Additionally, it has helped promote healing in burn victims and may prevent muscle wasting in the chronically ill. Most recently it's been used successfully in the treatment of schizophrenia, senility, and on cancer patients undergoing bone marrow transplants, shortening their hospital stay and reducing their risk of infection. It has also been shown to enhance muscle size in healthy people who work out.

L-glutamine (the natural form of glutamine) is available as a supplement in 500 mg. capsules. My recommended dosage is up to three 500 mg. capsules or tablets either half an hour before or two hours after eating. (I'd suggest starting with 500–1,000 mg. for the first few weeks and building up to 1,500 mg. over the course of a month.)

CAUTION: *Though glutamine and glutamic acid are not the same as monosodium glutamate (MSG), persons with a sensitivity to the latter could experience an allergic reaction and are advised to consult a physician before using these supplements.*

ASPARTIC ACID

Aspartic acid aids in the expulsion of harmful ammonia from the body. (When ammonia enters the circulatory system, it acts as a highly toxic substance.) By disposing of ammonia, aspartic acid helps protect the central nervous system. Recent research indicates that it may be an important factor in increased resistance to fatigue. When salts of aspartic acid were given to athletes, they showed decidedly improved stamina and endurance.

L-aspartic acid (the natural form of aspartic acid) is available as a supplement in 250 mg. and 500 mg. tablets. The usual dosage is 500 mg. one to three times daily with juice or water (no protein).

CYSTINE and CYSTEINE

Cystine is the *stable form* of the sulfur-containing amino acid cysteine (an important antiaging nutrient). The body readily converts one into the other as needed, and the two forms can be considered as a single amino acid in metabolism. When cystine is metabolized, it yields sulfuric acid, which reacts with other substances to help detoxify the system.

Sulfur-containing amino acids, particularly cystine and methionine, have been shown to be effective protectors against copper toxicity. (An excessive accumulation of copper in humans is a sign of Wilson's disease.) Cystine/cysteine can also help "tie up" and protect the body from other harmful metals as well as destructive free radicals that are formed by smoking and drinking. A cysteine supplement (L-cysteine) taken daily with vitamin C (three times as much vitamin C as cysteine) is the regimen that's been suggested for smokers and alcohol drinkers. (Supplements need not be taken on an empty stomach.) Recent research also indicates that therapeutic doses of cysteine can offer an important degree of protection against X-ray and nuclear radiation.

CAUTION: *Large doses of cysteine/cystine along with vitamins C and B1 are not recommended for anyone with diabetes mellitus, and should be undertaken only on the advice of* *a physician. (The combination of these nutrients could negate insulin effectiveness.)*

CARNITINE

A potentially life-extending amino acid biosynthesized from lysine (see section 84) and methionine (see entry below), carnitine's primary job is to provide heart and skeletal cells with energy. It can help in the treatment of heart disease, reduce angina attacks, aid in the control of hypoglycemia, and may help slow the progression of Alzheimer's disease as well as benefit patients with diabetes, liver, or kidney disease.

It plays an important role in converting stored body fat into energy and is being used by athletes, enabling longer periods of intense workouts. Additionally, it may prove useful in the treatment of male infertility, since the carnitine content of seminal fluid is directly related to sperm count and motility, and early studies have shown increases of both.

Pregnant women are prone to diminished carnitine levels (as early as twelve weeks), often because of inadequate iron, and may need low-dose supplementation to prevent gestational diabetes. (Be sure to check with your physician before taking any supplements.)

Meat, fish, poultry and dairy products are the major natural sources of L-carnitine. There is no recommended daily allowance for this amino acid, but the average American consumes between 100 and 300 mg. of it daily. As a supplement, I suggest two 500 mg. capsules a day. In rare cases, people taking over 1 g. of carnitine daily may develop a fishy odor (caused by the breakdown of carnitine by intestinal bacteria). This usually disappears when the dose is cut back.

CAUTION: *There are two kinds of carnitine: L-carnitine and D-carnitine. Stick to products containing only L-carnitine, as some studies suggest that D-carnitine may be toxic. If you have an existing heart condition, do not take this or any other supplement without first consulting your physician. Taking antibiotics for long-term prevention of infections may deplete carnitine levels.*

METHIONINE

An essential amino acid that helps in the breakdown of fats, methionine is a powerful antioxidant. Like cystine, it is another sulfur-containing amino acid, and helps protect the body from toxic substances as well as destructive free radicals. Methionine helps in some cases of schizophrenia by lowering the blood level of histamine, which can cause the brain to relay wrong messages. When combined with choline and folic acid, it has been shown to offer protection against certain tumors. It is also beneficial for women who take oral contraceptives because it promotes the excretion of estrogen.

An insufficiency of methionine can break down the body's ability to process urine and result in edema (swelling due to retention of fluids in tissues) and susceptibility to infection. A methionine deficiency has also been linked to cholesterol deposits, atherosclerosis, and hair loss in laboratory animals.

Because methionine is not synthesized in the body, it must be obtained from food or supplements. Good food sources of this amino acid are beans, fish, eggs, garlic, soybeans, meat, onions, seeds, and yogurt.

GLYCINE

Sometimes referred to as the simplest of the amino acids, glycine has been shown to yield quite a few remarkable benefits. It has been found helpful in the treatment of low pituitary gland function, and, because it supplies the body with additional creatine (essential for muscle function), it has also been found effective in the treatment of progressive muscular dystrophy. Interestingly, having too much of this amino acid can cause fatigue, but the proper amount produces more energy.

Glycine is necessary for central nervous system function and has been used in the treatment of manic depression and hyperactivity; it can also help in preventing epileptic seizures.

Many nutritionally oriented doctors now use glycine in the treatment of hypoglycemia. (Glycine stimulates the release of glucagon, which mobilizes glycogen, which is then released into the blood as glucose.)

Additionally, it is effective as a treatment for gastric hyperacidity (and is included in many gastric antacid drugs). It has also been used to treat certain types of acidemia (low pH of the blood), especially one caused by a leucine imbalance, which results in an offensive body and breath odor (a condition formerly treated only by a dietary restriction of leucine).

TYROSINE

Though this is a nonessential amino acid, it's a high-ranking neurotransmitter, and important because of its role in stimulating and modifying brain activity. For instance, in order for phenylalanine to be effective as a mood elevator or an appetite depressant (see section 82), it must first convert into tyrosine. If this conversion does not take place, because of either some enzyme insufficiency or a great need elsewhere in the body for phenylalanine, insufficient quantities of norepinephrine will be produced by the brain and depression will result.

Tyrosine promotes healthy functioning of the adrenal, pituitary, and thyroid glands. It also stimulates the release of growth hormone and it produces norepinephrine, which suppresses appetite.

Clinical studies have shown that tyrosine supplementation has helped control medication-resistant depression and anxiety, and has enabled patients taking amphetamines (as mood elevators or diet drugs) to reduce their dosages to minimal levels in a matter of weeks.

Tyrosine has also helped cocaine addicts to kick their habit by helping to avert the depression, fatigue, and extreme irritability that accompany withdrawal. A regimen of tyrosine, dissolved in orange juice, taken along with vitamin C, tyrosine hydroxylase (the enzyme that lets the body use tyrosine), and vitamins B1, B2, and niacin seems to work.

Supplements of L-tyrosine should be taken with high-carbohydrate meals, or at bedtime, so as not to compete for absorption with other amino acids. Good natural sources are dairy products, bananas, avocados, lima beans, almonds, pumpkin seeds, and sesame seeds.

DID YOU KNOW?

- Amino acids can't be stored in the body and must be consumed daily in foods or supplements.
- Eating half an onion a day can lower your risk of stomach cancer.
- Arginine supplements can help strengthen erections and increase sperm count.
- Carnitine may help slow the progression of Alzheimer's.

90. Any Questions About Chapter V?

I'd really like to stay a vegetarian, but I worry about getting enough bodybuilding benefits from my food. Is there anything that compares favorably with complete meat protein?

I'm happy to tell you that there is! And it's delicious, too! I'm talking about quinoa (pronounced *keen-wa*). This "superfood" looks, cooks, and tastes like a grain, but it isn't a grain at all. It's actually the dried fruit of an herb and has been a staple in the diet of native South Americans for centuries. (The Incas thought so highly of it they named it the "mother grain.") And what's truly unusual—and wonderful—about it is that it's rich in all eight essential amino acids that compose a "complete protein" and are normally found only in red meat, eggs, and dairy products. What makes it even better than those other foods is that it's much lower in calories and fat and is abundant in fiber. One serving of quinoa (about 1 cup) has only 129 calories, 2 g. of fat, and 4.6 g. of fiber. It's also an excellent source of potassium and iron, and a good source of zinc and B vitamins. Mild in flavor, it cooks in about ten to fifteen minutes.

Mixed with a dash of olive oil, some herbs, and steamed veggies, quinoa is a treat. If you want to spice it up, you can add sesame seeds or sunflower seeds, or tamari. You can also stir-fry the veggies and seeds in sesame oil, then toss in the quinoa. It's easy to be creative with quinoa because it tastes so good and is so good for you!

I'm prone to convulsions, and my doctor put me on Dilantin (phenytoin) a year ago. Recently, a friend told me about taurine, which she said was a nonessential amino acid that was natural and could help me the same way. What I want to know is, if it's nonessential, why would I need it? And why would it work?

Let me begin by clearing up a major point of misunderstanding: Where amino acids are concerned, nonessential does *not* mean unnecessary. All the amino acids are necessary; it's just that the ones deemed essential can't be synthesized by the body in sufficient quantities to promote effective protein synthesis. If these essential ones are not supplied in the diet, *all* amino acids are reduced in the same proportion as the one that's low or missing. As for substituting taurine for an anticonvulsant medication, that's a decision only your doctor can make. I can say, though, that taurine has been shown to be quite successful as an anticonvulsant when taken in combination with glutamic and aspartic acids, but I would not recommend undertaking it without consulting a health professional. (For listings of nutritionally oriented doctors in your area, see section 462.)

I've read that exercise stimulates the release of growth hormone. I do at least twenty minutes of dance exercises every day, so does this mean that I probably don't need a GH supplement?

On the contrary, you probably do. Only certain exercises, such as weight lifting, where there is what's known as muscular "peak output" (even briefly sustained), promote a significant release of GH. Other exercises, even prolonged ones, produce negligible amounts (if any) of growth hormone—unless they are performed with peak muscular effort. In fact, because amino acids are lost through the skin when you sweat, exercise *increases* your need for amino acids that will stimulate growth hormone.

Is there such a thing as an antiaging amino acid?

As a matter of fact, L-glutathione (GSH) has been called a triple-threat antiaging amino acid. It's actually a tripeptide, synthesized from three amino acids—L-cysteine, L-glutamic acid, and glycine—and it has been shown to act as an antioxidant and deactivate free radicals that speed up the aging process. It is also an antitumor agent, a respiratory accelerator in the brain, and has been used to help in the treatment of allergies, cataracts, diabetes, hypoglycemia, and arthritis, as well as in helping to prevent the harmful side effects of high-dose radiation in chemotherapy and X-rays. Additionally, it helps to protect against the harmful effects of cigarette smoke and alcohol.

Glutathione is present in fruits and vegetables; however, cooking can reduce its potency. I recommend taking a 50 mg. capsule once or twice daily. (Taking this supplement on a daily basis helps avoid the ups and downs of glutathione levels that can leave you vulnerable to oxidative damage.)

Is there anything that can be done to significantly improve an individual's immune system to help prevent diseases such as cancer and AIDS?

Fortunately, lots! (See section 459 for an extensive list.) But when it comes to amino acids, growth hormone releasers are your best defense.

What happens is that as we get older, our immune system—that ever-ready army of white blood cells (called T cells because they're under the command of the thymus gland), which are told where and when to attack and what antibodies their cofighters (called B cells because they're made in the bone marrow) should produce—begins to break down due to the decreasing power and size of the thymus gland. This causes not only an ineffectual defense system, but often dangerous confusion where the T cells mistake friends for enemies and attack you, resulting in autoimmune disorders. (It's been suggested that diseases such as multiple sclerosis, myasthenia gravis, and arthritis may be due to this.)

What's been discovered, though, is that this is most likely due to a reduced rate of growth hormone, which is produced by the pituitary gland and necessary to the function of the thymus gland and therefore the immune system. But supplements of antioxidants, vitamin C, alpha- and beta-carotene, lutein, lycopene, selenium, grape-seed extract, green tea extract, alpha-lipoic acid, soy isoflavonoids (genistein and daidzein), zinc, and enzymes such as papain have been found to work wonders in reversing this degenerative syndrome.

I'm a professional bodybuilder and would like to know if there are any legal, natural supplement alternatives to steroids.

There certainly are. Branched chain amino acids (BCAAs)—which are composed of leucine, valine, and isoleucine—are natural anabolic muscle-building supplements. They regulate how protein is used by the body and play a unique role in protein metabolism in muscles. While all other amino acids are broken down in the liver, BCAAs are oxidized in peripheral muscle.

BCAAs are, in effect, a principal source of calories for human muscle. Intense physical exercise produces a rapid excretion of nitrogen, which causes a decrease in muscle protein synthesis. BCAAs limit this decrease.

During strenuous exercise, such as weight training, the stress on a muscle causes it to break down (catabolism). BCAAs not only act to prevent this, but actually reverse the process. They are, therefore, *anabolic* because they build up muscle.

BCAA facts that can help your workout:

- BCAAs can reduce appetite while preserving basic protein storage in the body.

- One-half of your body weight is muscle, and 15–20 percent of muscle is branched chain amino acids.
- In one hour, 50 percent of ingested BCAA is available to your muscles, 100 percent in two hours.
- BCAAs produce glycogen, which helps balance insulin secretion.
- BCAAs directly affect muscle and body weight changes, promoting lean muscle distribution.

Supplements should only be taken a half hour before workouts.

I'm a bit confused about N-acetylcysteine (NAC) and what it does. Is it a worthwhile amino acid supplement?

It sure is! NAC is an amino acid and a precursor to glutathione, the body's most abundant antioxidant. Studies have shown that NAC can help protect against such respiratory ailments as bronchitis, bronchial asthma, emphysema, chronic sinusitis—and may even help protect against lung damage caused by cancer-causing chemicals in cigarette smoke. NAC has also been used successfully to treat people with serious inner-ear infections. And bodybuilders have found that it helps them recover faster from their workouts. As a supplement, 1–3 capsules or tablets (500 mg.) can be taken with meals.

CAUTION: *Do not use NAC if you have peptic ulcers, or use drugs known to cause gastric lesions.*

VI

Fat and Fat Manipulators

91. Lipotropics—What Are They?

Methionine, choline, inositol, and betaine are all lipotropics, which means their prime function is to prevent abnormal or excessive accumulation of fat in the liver.

Lipotropics also increase the liver's production of lecithin, which keeps cholesterol more soluble, detoxifies the liver, and increases resistance to disease by helping the thymus gland carry out its functions.

92. Who Needs Them and Why

We all need lipotropics, some of us more than others. Anyone on a high-protein diet falls into the latter category.

Methionine and choline are *necessary* to detoxify the amines that are by-products of protein metabolism.

Because nearly all of us consume too much fat (the average consumption in the United States is now 36–42 percent of total calories), and a substantial part of that is saturated fat, lipotropics are indispensable. By helping the liver produce lecithin, they're helping to keep cholesterol from forming dangerous deposits in blood vessels, lessening chances of heart attack, arteriosclerosis, and gallstone formation as well.

We also need lipotropics to stay healthy, since they aid the thymus in stimulating the production of antibodies, the growth and action of phagocytes (which surround and gobble up invading viruses and microbes), and in destroying foreign or abnormal tissue.

93. The Cholesterol Story

Like everything else, there's a good side and a bad side to fats. The general misconception that all of them are bad for you, prevalent as it may be, simply is not true. And the most maligned of all is cholesterol.

Practically everyone knows that cholesterol can be responsible for arteriosclerosis, heart attacks, and a variety of illnesses, but very few are aware of the ways that it is *essential* to health.

At least two-thirds of your body cholesterol is produced by the liver or in the intestine. It is found there as well as in the brain, the adrenals, and nerve fiber sheaths. And when it's good, it's very, very good:

- Cholesterol in the skin is converted to essential vitamin D when touched by the sun's ultraviolet rays.
- Cholesterol aids in the metabolism of carbohydrates. (The more carbohydrates ingested, the more cholesterol produced.)
- Cholesterol is a prime supplier of life-essential adrenal steroid hormones, such as cortisone.
- Cholesterol is a component of every membrane and necessary for the production of male and female sex hormones.

Differences in the behavior of cholesterol depend upon the protein to which it is bound. Lipoproteins are the factors in our blood that transport cholesterol.

Low-density lipoproteins (LDL) carry about 65 percent of blood cholesterol and are the bad guys who deposit it in the arteries where, joined by other substances, it becomes artery-blocking plaque. (*NOTE*: Eating 1 oz. a day of pistachio nuts can help significantly lower your LDL.)

Very-low-density lipoproteins (VLDL) carry only about 15 percent of blood cholesterol but are the substances the liver needs and uses to produce LDL. The more of them, the more LDL the liver sends out and the greater your chance of heart disease.

High-density lipoproteins (HDL) carry about 20 percent of blood cholesterol and, composed principally of lecithin, are the good guys whose detergent action breaks up plaque and can transport cholesterol through the blood without clogging arteries. (A recent study found that people with big hips and trim waists have higher HDL cholesterol levels than do those with potbellies, which might explain why females, on the average, live eight years longer than males.)

In short: The higher your HDL, the lower your chances of developing heart disease.

It is also worth mentioning that though egg consumption in the United States is one-half of what it was in 1945, there has *not* been a comparable decline in heart disease. And though the American Heart Association deems eggs hazardous, a diet without them can be equally hazardous. Not only do eggs have the most perfect protein components of any food, but they contain lecithin, which aids in fat assimilation. And, most important, they *raise* HDL levels!

94. Leveling About Cholesterol Levels

When people talk about their cholesterol levels, they're referring to the total amount of cholesterol in their blood (serum cholesterol). The amounts are measured in milligrams per deciliter; the accepted levels—for *everyone*—should not exceed 200 mg./dl.

The ratio of HDL (good cholesterol) to LDL (bad cholesterol) is as important as the ratio of HDL to your total cholesterol level. The more HDL you have, therefore, the more protection you have against clogged arteries.

Blood cholesterol tests will usually also measure your levels of *triglycerides.* These fats differ from cholesterol, but there is a connection between them: Although you can have high triglyceride levels without high cholesterol (and vice versa), lowering triglyceride levels does seem to help bring down cholesterol.

Keeping your daily fat intake to no more than 30 percent (and preferably 20 percent) of total calories consumed is vital to leveling off elevated cholesterol levels. And no more than 10 percent of that fat should be saturated.

95. Saturated Fat vs. Unsaturated Fat

Saturated fat comes from animal sources (with a few exceptions, notably coconut and palm oils, and hydrogenated or partially hydrogenated vegetable oils), and *all* animal fats contain cholesterol. Saturated fats are solid at room temperature.

Unsaturated fat (be it mono- or polyunsaturated) comes from vegetable sources—and *no* vegetables or fruits contain cholesterol. Unsaturated fats are liquid at room temperature.

NOTE: *Even if foods don't contain cholesterol, that doesn't mean they don't contain fat. Avocados, for instance, are free of cholesterol, but just one used for guacamole will give you more than 30 g. of fat!*

LABEL ALERT: *A product labeled "Low Fat" means that it has less than 3 g. of fat per serving. Keep in mind, though, when fat is removed from a food it needs to be replaced with something to keep its taste. That "something" is usually sugar or refined starch. Dieters take note: Just because a food is lower in fat does* not *mean it is lower in calories.*

96. The Really Bad Guys: Trans-Fatty Acids

When foodmakers realized that consumers were becoming aware that saturated fats were bad for them, they began replacing "sat fats" with trans-fatty acids—unsaturated oils to which hydrogen has been added, making them thick enough to use in baked goods and margerine. Trans fat also gave packaged foods a longer shelf life and was thought to make all food safer. But on the label it did not have to be listed as fat. All consumers saw on the ingredient list was a "hydrogenated" oil—and that didn't sound bad at all.

It was soon learned that even small quantities of trans-fatty acids could raise LDL (bad) cholesterol levels, lower HDL (good) cholesterol levels, and seriously increase the risk of diabetes. But because of old labeling laws, dozens of cookies, crackers, snacks, and fast foods loaded with trans-fatty acids could legally be called "fat-free"—with the average consumer none the wiser or healthier for it.

It took an obesity epidemic and a slew of possible lawsuits to get some action, but the Food and Drug Administration has finally ruled that trans-fat grams must now be listed right below the sat-fat line on Nutrition Facts labels.

Trans fats are sometimes where you least expect them, so reading labels is essential. Your combined daily intake of saturated and trans fats should not rise above 20 g., and if you're at risk for heart disease, you should keep it at 15 g. or less.

NOTE: *In response to health concerns, many companies have already developed varieties of margerines that do not contain trans-fats. Check the Nutrition Facts label and choose one with 0 trans fat and no more than 2 g. of saturated fats per tbsp. and with liquid vegetable oil as the first ingredient (e.g., Benecol, Promise, Smart Balance Light).*

LABEL ALERT: *If a label says 0 g. trans fat, the product can still contain trans fats, but there is less than 1 g. per serving.*

97. CLA (Conjugated Linoleic Acid): The Good Fat

A potent antioxidant and cancer fighter, CLA is found in foods such as whole milk, butter, beef, and lamb obtained from grass-grazing animals. Grazing animals have from three to five times more CLA than animals fattened on grain. Simply switching from grain-fed to grass-fed products can greatly increase your intake of CLA, and below are some reasons why you should.

WHAT IT CAN DO FOR YOU:

- Potentially block all three stages of cancer (initiation, promotion, and metastasis).
- Slow the growth of a wide variety of tumors.

- Reduce the risk of cardiovascular disease.
- Help fight inflammation.
- Lower cholesterol and triglycerides.
- Help reduce appetite.
- Aid in reducing body fat (especially abdominal fat).
- Improve muscle tone.

Milk from grass-fed cows is healthier than milk from grain-fed cows because it contains more key nutrients, including omega-3 fatty acids, beta-carotene, and vitamin E (alpha-tocopherol), as well as conjugated linoleic acid—CLA.

NOTE: *Cooking or heating increases rather than decreases the CLA content in foods.*

CAUTION: *The use of synthetic CLA supplements by overweight people may tend to cause or aggravate insulin resistance, which can increase the risk of developing diabetes.*

98. Foods, Nutrients, and Supplements That Can Lower Your Cholesterol Naturally

The following is a list of natural foods, nutrients, and cholesterol-lowering supplements. (*Name-brand supplements appear in italics. Their inclusion is to provide information about what they are and should not be construed as any sort of product endorsement.*)

Before using any supplement to reduce high cholesterol, consult your doctor. Switching from prescription drugs to supplements or adding a supplement to a drug regimen on your own is potentially dangerous. And remember, no food, nutrient, or supplement is a magic bullet; a low-fat diet and regular exercise are still necessary to lower high cholesterol.

- Barley
- Vitamin C (1,000 mg. three times daily. If diarrhea occurs, cut back until it clears up.)
- Cayenne (Take a daily supplement or use liberally on your food.)
- *Cholestatin* (Contains phytosterols, compounds in food such as rice and soybeans, mainly sitosterol. Suggested dosage is 6–8 capsules daily, taken before meals.)
- Chromium picolinate (Most absorbable form of chromium; works particularly well with "no-flush" niacin. Take up to three 200 mcg. tablets daily.)
- Corn bran
- Cruciferous vegetables (broccoli, cauliflower)
- Eggplant
- Evening primrose oil (Contains gamma-linolenic acid [GLA]. I'd suggest 250 mg. one to three times daily.)
- *Evolve* (Contains tocotrienols extracted from rice bran. Recommended dosage is one to two 25 mg. capsules daily. *NOTE*: Vitamin E supplements may reduce this supplement's cholesterol-lowering effect.)
- Fenugreek seed (*CAUTION*: Do not use fenugreek during pregnancy.)
- Fiber (25–30 g. daily)
- Fish oils: EPA and DHA (omega-3 fatty acids; take up to six 1,000 mg. capsules daily. *CAUTION*: Can interfere with normal blood clotting. Do not use if you are taking blood thinners, such as coumadin or heparin, unless advised by your physician.)
- Garlic (As a supplement, take 1 capsule up to three times daily.)
- Ginger (As a supplement, take 1 capsule up to three times daily.)

- Green tea (As a supplement, take 1 capsule up to three times daily.)
- Guar gum (An extract from the seeds of the guar plant. Tablets must be chewed thoroughly or sucked gradually, and taken with lots of water. *CAUTION*: Should not be taken by anyone who has difficulty swallowing or who's had gastrointestinal surgery.)
- Gugulipid (An extract from the mukul myrrh tree, native to India, and used for centuries in ayurvedic medicine. Take one 25 mg. capsule with meals three times daily. *CAUTION*: May cause a rash or hives in susceptible individuals.)
- Lemongrass oil ·
- Lentils (pinto beans, lima beans, navy beans, kidney beans
- *LipoGuard* (Contains a combination of fish oil and garlic. The recommended dosage is 4–10 capsules daily. *CAUTION*: Should not be taken by anyone with a bleeding disorder, or on blood thinners, unless advised by a physician.)
- Monounsaturated oils (olive, peanut, canola)
- N-acetylcysteine (NAC) (500 mg. three times daily)
- Niacin (Use "no-flush" supplements with inositol hexanicotinate, IHN. Take up to three 500 mg. capsules daily. *CAUTION*: May bring on attacks of gout in people prone to the disease, and high doses may promote liver abnormalities.)
- Oat bran
- Onions
- Pectin (apples, grapefruit)
- *PhytoQuest* (Contains phytosterols, mainly sitosterol, which blocks cholesterol's absorption sites in the small intestine. Suggested dosage is 6–8 capsules daily, before meals.)

- Phytosterols: beta-sitosterol, stigmasterol, campesterol (naturally occurring compounds in plant foods such as rice and soybeans)
- Polyunsaturated oils (sunflower, corn, safflower)
- Prunes
- Psyllium husk (Three rounded tsp. supply 10 g. of cholesterol-lowering soluble fiber.)
- Raw carrots
- Red pepper
- Rice bran
- Soybeans and soy foods (See section 143.)
- Vitamin E
- Whole grains
- Yogurt

CAUTION: *If your cholesterol becomes too low (way below 150 mg./dl.), your risk of stroke increases.*

99. Do You Know What's Raising Your Cholesterol?

Many things that you might not be aware of can be raising your cholesterol levels or undermining your efforts to lower them. Here are a few you should think about:

- Smoking
- Caffeine
- Stress
- The pill
- Refined sugar
- Food additives
- Environmental pollutants

If you're watching your cholesterol, you probably know that turkey is a good dinner choice. Just remember that although 3 ounces of light-meat turkey has only about 67 mg. of cholesterol, the same amount of dark meat has 75 mg. And a cup of chopped turkey liver has about 830 mg.!

100. Omega-3 Fatty Acids: What They Are, Where They're Found, and What They Can Do for You

Not all omega-3 fatty acids are the same. EPA and DHA (eicosapentaenoic and docosahexaenoic acid) are a unique component of fish and fish oils. ALA (alpha-linolenic acid), found in plant sources like walnuts, flaxseed, soybean oil, and canola oil, as well as green leafy vegetables, works more slowly because it needs to be converted by the body into EPA and DHA in order for the body to make use of it.

Krill oil is a relatively new and exciting omega-3 supplement. Extracted from shrimplike crustaceans that feed mainly on phytoplankton (algae), krill oil is not only a powerful source of EPA and DHA, it also contains the potent antioxidant astaxanthin, one of the few that crosses the blood-brain barrier, expanding protection from free radicals to the brain and central nervous system. Additionally, krill oil is absorbed more quickly and efficiently by the body than ordinary fish oil and provides all the benefits without fishy burps. (*CAUTION*: People with seafood allergies should not use krill oil.)

All omega-3s have remarkable preventive and curative properties. They provide health benefits primarily by reducing inflammation, which contributes to numerous serious ailments. Already shown to significantly diminish the risk of coronary heart disease, omega-3s are now considered potential treatments for other serious conditions, ranging from Alzheimer's to epilepsy and rheumatoid arthritis. For example, they can:

- help reduce harmful cholesterol and trygliceride levels, lowering the risk of heart attack or stroke.
- stabilize cells and help prevent fatal heart rhythm disturbances.
- reduce blood levels of C-reactive protein (CRP), a marker for inflammation and a risk factor for cardiovascular disease.
- may have a more beneficial effect than statins on symptomatic heart-failure patients.
- help reduce brain levels of amyloid proteins associated with Alzheimer's disease.
- supplements of omega-3 fat docosahexaenoic acid (DHA) given to lactating mothers may save premature infants from developing mental delays.
- Swedish researchers found that boys who ate fish more than once a week wound up with an 11 percent increase in intelligence.
- reduce the "stickiness" of blood platelet cells and the amount of fibrin in the blood, reducing the risk of clot formation.
- help reduce risk of breast cancer and possibly aid in treatment of the disease.
- provide relief from the itching and scaling of psoriasis.
- reduce the body's rejection of tissue grafts.
- aid in the reduction and severity of migraine headaches.
- fight harmful effects of prostaglandins (which lower immunity and encourage tumor growth) and help prevent breast cancer.

- help in preventing arteriosclerosis.
- keep skin, hair, and nails healthy.
- aid in alleviating rheumatoid arthritis.

If you don't like fish or cannot eat it on a regular basis, fish oil supplements are an alternative. Ten capsules of concentrated marine lipids usally supply 1.8 g. of EPA. (A 4-oz. serving of salmon contains about 1 g.) *Alpha-linolenic acid* (ALA), found abundantly in flaxseeds, walnuts, and pumpkin seeds, is converted into EPA and DHA, the fatty acids more readily used by the body, albeit more slowly.

NOTE: *Unless a product specifies which fatty acids it contains, the ones you're getting are probably from ALA, meaning you need more than you would of DHA or EPA.*

Although the FDA has approved an omega-3 pill as a prescription medicine called Lovaza that can deliver DHA and EPA at levels of 4 g. or more, the simplest effective way to maximize your omega-3 intake is to take daily supplements that contain 500–1,100 mg. of EPA and DHA.

CAUTION: *Taking large doses of omega-3 supplements may cause excessive bruising and bleeding after minor trauma in some individuals. Anyone with a tendency to experience such bruising and bleeding is advised to avoid these supplements entirely. As with large doses of vitamin E, this could result in internal bleeding. If you are taking blood thinners, such as aspirin, Coumadin, or heparin; or any nonsteroidal anti-inflammatory drugs (NSAIDs), such as Motrin, Aleve, Advil, etc, do not use omega-3 supplements unless advised by your physician. I suggest you check with your healthcare provider before starting on an omega-3 regimen or any other supplement regimen.*

101. The Scoop on Omega-6

Omega-6 oils (found in olive, sunflower, and other seed oils) compete in the body with omega-3s. To get all the health benefits of the latter you need to reduce your intake of the former.

The recommended dietary ratio for these oils is about 4:1 (that's 4 omega-3s to 1 omega-6). Unfortunately, in the typical American diet the ratio is a hefty 10:1, undermining the effectiveness of omega-3s.

PERSONAL ADVICE:

When buying supplements, you want omega-3 only! Any that boast about also containing omega-6 are most likely a waste of money. Furthermore, omega-6 fatty acids may cause elevated triglyceride levels, diarrhea, and vitamin E deficiency.

CAUTION: *Omega-6 supplements may interact with blood-thinning medications and increase the risk of bleeding. They may also interact adversely with phenothiazines (medication used to treat schizophrenia and other mental or emotional conditions), leading to increased seizure risk.*

102. Warnings and Recommendations About Fish Sources of Omega-3s

Just because certain fish are high in omega-3s doesn't mean that those are the ones you should be eating a lot of. Large fish that feed on other fish accumulate the highest amount of mercury as well as toxic PCBs (polychlorinated biphenyls). (Mercury poisoning can cause memory loss, depression, nerve damage, birth defects, heart problems, and more.) For this reason the FDA and EPA, although still not in agreement over what "safe" levels of mercury in fish are, have put out a list of fish that should be avoided by children and pregnant women—and, in my opinion, anyone who's concerned about staying healthy.

Fish to Avoid

Shark, swordfish, king mackerel, tilefish (sometimes sold as snapper), tuna steaks (fresh), sea bass, marlin, halibut, walleye, largemouth bass, amberjack, and grouper.

Fish to Fill Up On

Sardines, salmon, shrimp, tilapia, catfish, clams, and oysters. (Shellfish are generally low in mercury. Scallops are a good choice, too, but Ben Raines, a reporter for the *Mobile* (Alabama) *Register*, who has received awards for investigating the issue of mercury in fish, cautions that some unscrupulous fishermen create look-alike versions using mercury-rich shark meat. Real scallops have a small "stalk" at one end.) In general, farm-raised fish have lower levels of mercury than their wild counterparts.

Other Fish for Thought

Flounder, mahimahi, red snapper, and trout are considered safe for men, and women finished with childbearing, as occasional, once-a-week meals. (Mahimahi and red snapper have medium levels of mercury, though, and should be limited to children and women in their reproductive years to just once a month.)

DID YOU KNOW?

- Moderate wine consumption can boost heart-healthy omega-3s.
- Labels saying "0 grams Trans Fat" can still contain them.
- Omega-3 fatty acids may make you feel happier.
- Your risk of stroke increases if your cholesterol becomes *too* low.

---

103. Any Questions About Chapter VI?

I'd like to know if there is any difference between being hyperlipidemic and hypercholesterolemic?

There is, but unfortunately not much when it comes to being a candidate for coronary heart disease. A person who is hyperlipidemic has elevated fats in general in the blood, and someone who is hypercholesterolemic just has elevated cholesterol levels. It's sort of a semantic moot point where health is concerned.

What are omega-9 fatty acids, and how do I know if I'm getting enough?

I'm fairly certain you are getting enough omega-9s, as they are the most abundant fatty acids in nature (found in animal fats and vegetable oils) and quite plentiful in our diets. They are not considered essential because we can make them from unsaturated fat in our bodies. The body will, if necessary, use omega-9 fatty acids as substitutes for omega-3s or omega-6s if these essential fatty acids are not present, but omega-9s are not the best replacement, and your health will eventually suffer from the substitution.

I'm confused. Some products say low-fat and some say low-cholesterol. Is there a difference?

A major difference! In fact, a product that's marked cholesterol-free can be loaded with fat. You have to understand that cholesterol and fat are not synonymous. Unlike fat, cholesterol is not used for energy; it's used primarily to transport fat to cells throughout the body.

What's the difference, as far as lowering cholesterol is concerned, between polyunsaturated and monounsaturated oils?

Polyunsaturated oils (sunflower, corn, safflower, soy) lower both the bad and the good (LDL and HDL) cholesterol. Monounsaturated oils (olive, peanut, canola), on the other hand, not only reduce the bad cholesterol, but raise the good (HDL) levels.

Are lipotropics available as supplements, and if so, what's the recommended dosage and are there any special instructions for taking them?

Lipotropics are available as supplements in tablet form. (Usually 3 tablets equal 1,000 mg.—or 1 g. of each lipotropic agent.) The dosage most often recommended is 1–2 tablets taken three times daily, *with* food.

Is it true that I can increase my omega-3 blood levels by drinking red wine? I don't particularly like fish.

Here's to your health! Studies have shown that women between the ages of twenty-six and sixty-five who drink a glass of red wine daily can indeed increase their omega-3 levels. But there is a caveat: If you have a family history of breast cancer, even one drink a day can increase your risk of getting it.

Is there an established daily value for essential fatty acid intake?

There's been a lot of confusion surrounding appropriate dosing of these "good fats," especially in supplement form. But the conclusions of a nutritional workshop held in Washington, DC, in 2008 that focused on establishing dietary reference intakes (DRI) for EPA and DHA found that between 200 and 500 mg. a day was achievable and sufficient to provide protection against coronary heart disease. It did acknowledge, though, that higher doses could well provide additional protection, recommending five to seven servings of fish weekly or 650–900 mg. of EPA+DHA daily in supplement form. For optimal health benefits, I'd suggest taking the higher route.

Do you consider lipotropic supplements more important for some people than for others?

Definitely, especially meat eaters. Lipotropics are the substances that can liquefy or homogenize fats. I feel that supplementation is particularly important for anyone on a high-protein diet, the reason being that lipotropics detoxify amines, which are by-products of protein metabolism. Also, anyone worried about gallstone formation would be wise to consider these supplements.

My daughter-in-law is taking a hemp oil supplement, which I know nothing about. I know marijuana comes from a hemp plant. Does this supplement have similar hallucinogenic effects?

Not at all! Hemp is a member of the *Cannabis sativa* family, but the products derived from it for supplements are not hallucinogenic.

Hemp oil is a rich source of the two essential fatty acids, omega-3 and omega-6 (particularly omega-3);

"good" fats. In fact, it has the highest level of EFAs of any vegetable source. It is also a rare source of gamma-linolenic acid (GLA) and many other key nutrients. Containing the optimal ratio of omega-3s to omega-6s, hemp oil's EFA profile is closer to fish oil than any other vegetable oil. It can be used in salad dressings and other foods, but not during cooking (omega-3s are destroyed by heating). The hemp oil capsules that your daughter-in-law is taking are one of the easiest ways to reap some essential health benefits.

I'm a vegetarian and I don't eat fish. Are there vegetable sources that have omega-3 fatty acids?

A small handful of walnuts or flaxseed mixed in yogurt, salad, or cereal will up your omega-3s, as will spinach (sauté and add to pasta for a treat) and winter squash. Vegetable oils such as soybean, canola, flaxseed, and hemp are other sources of omega-3s—but the conversion to EPA and DHA is much slower. You can also look for supplements derived from algae, the omega-3 source for fish.

What's the difference between omega-3 and omega-6 fatty acids in general and in a cholesterol-lowering regimen in particular?

In general, their differences are that omega-3 fatty acids reduce inflammation while omega-6s increase inflammation, and that omega-3s help prevent the formation of blood clots while omega-6s increase blood clotting. In relation to a cholesterol-lowering regimen, only omega-3 fatty acids will lower triglycerides as well as cholesterol.

If tuna is high in mercury, how much canned tuna is safe to eat?

The FDA's current standards say that two regular cans

of tuna (12 oz.) a week are safe for women of childbearing age and kids, but the Environmental Protection Agency recommends eating less. In fact, the EPA suggests that small children eat no more than one-third of a can per week.

I take fish oil gelcap supplements. They're easy to swallow, but they make my burps smell really fishy. Is there anything I can take to counteract this?

You can avoid those fishy burps by freezing your gel capsules and taking them at bedtime. Or you might think about switching to krill oil capsules, which are more quickly absorbed by the body and also contain the powerful antioxidant astaxanthin.

Could you please explain "prostaglandins" and their connection to fats, oils, aspirin, and heart attacks? I am very confused by being told that blocking them can help prevent heart attacks and reading that they're necessary to every cell in the body.

Your confusion is understandable, but I think I can clear it up. Prostaglandins are hormonelike substances that regulate every cell in the body in many of their complex interactions. But there are "good" and "bad" prostaglandins. Some prostaglandins, when made in excess in the body, play a role in promoting heart disease, inflammation, and pain. This is where the aspirin connection comes in. Aspirin blocks the production of prostaglandins. Unfortunately, it blocks the formation of both the "good" and the "bad." And by suppressing the good prostaglandins, aspirin also suppresses the immune system.

While bad prostaglandins can make blood more likely to clump together and cause a stroke or heart attack, good prostaglandins lower blood pressure, inhibit blood aggregation—and the production of cholesterol—and reduce inflammation reactions. In other words, "good" prostaglandins, most of which are made from omega-3 oils, can provide the same heart benefits that aspirin does without gastric and other unwanted side effects.

What's the skinny on fake fats?

Still pretty thin nutritionally. The synthetic fat called olestra (also known as Olean and sucrose polyester) is made with sucrose and fatty acids and was designed so that it couldn't be broken down by the body's enzymes and would, therefore, not be absorbed by the body. Great in theory, but this faux fat, which has been used primarily in snacks such as chips and cheese puffs, has some not-so-great side effects. Aside from the widely publicized "brown stain" effect (from many reports of people experiencing loose stools and fecal urgency), it depletes the body of fat-soluble vitamins A, D, E, and K—and carotenoids. Olestra is now fortified with these vitamins—but only to the US government's determinations of the bare minimum amount to prevent deficiency, not to maximize health. (Early studies of olestra found that six chips a day could reduce a person's beta-carotene level by 50 percent!) Admittedly, olestra does reduce the total grams of fat consumed, but it's a risky nutritional price to pay for reducing a serving of potato chips from 150 to 70 calories.

Alli is the only over-the-counter weight-loss product approved by the FDA. It promotes weight loss by decreasing the absorption of fat by the intestines, reducing the number of calories you absorb. (It also inhibits the absorption of fat-soluble vitamins, which can be a risky trade-off.) Alli is taken with fat-containing meals, up to three times a day. But here's the catch, you'd better not eat more than 15 g. of fat with each meal, or you could experience the same unwanted effects that can occur with Olestra, namely urgent bowel movements, diarrhea, and gas with oily spotting. If that's not enough to give you pause before starting a regimen with Alli, be aware that the FDA is currently investigating reports of liver damage from Alli.

CAUTION: *There are counterfeit Alli capsules being sold on the internet that contain a controlled substance, sibutramine, that can cause a potentially lethal interaction with other medications you may be taking. The FDA advises consumers who believe they have counterfeit Alli to contact the FDA's Office of Criminal Investigations at 800-551-3989 or online at www.fda.gov/OCI as soon as possible.*

Z-Trim is another entry into the fake-fat foray. Developed by the U.S. Department of Agriculture, it's made from oat hulls, which could cut down calories and bulk up fiber—and it can be used in cooking. At this writing, it doesn't appear to have any side effects, but until long-term safety is assured, I'd recommend lowering your fat intake the old-fashioned way—by cutting back on products that contain it.

As for other fake fats such as Simpless, which is a milk and egg white fat substitute used primarily in low-calorie frozen desserts, they are unstable in heat and, at least at this time, cannot be used in cooked products. Considering most of our fats come from cooked foods, the percentage of fat saved by eating products with this type of fake fat is *not* impressive. What's worse is that these fake fats can lull you into a false sense of low-fat security and get you to indulge in products you ordinarily wouldn't eat—and they don't get you to change your basic fat-eating patterns at all!

What's the difference between foods labeled "Cholesterol-Free" and those labeled "Low Cholesterol"?

Anywhere between 18 mg. and 20 mg. per typical serving. Cholesterol-free foods have 2 mg. or less of cholesterol per serving, and less than 2 g. of saturated fat per serving. (Saturated fat stimulates the production of cholesterol in the body.) "Low cholesterol" on a label means the food contains no more than 20 mg. of cholesterol per serving. Just remember that while you're watching your cholesterol, it's important to keep your eye on serving sizes as well!

VII

ANTIOXIDANTS ON PURPOSE

104. Do I Need to Take Antioxidants?

The answer is an unqualified *yes!* With every breath you take you generate free radicals, the uncontrolled oxidants that damage cells. The older you get, the fewer natural antioxidants your body produces to keep these destructive molecules in check. As they accumulate, health deteriorates and aging accelerates—leaving you more susceptible to everything from wrinkles to serious degenerative diseases.

Though we get antioxidants from food, many people have increased antioxidant needs that diet alone cannot meet. Smokers, for instance, need two to three times as much vitamin C to achieve the same antioxidant blood levels as nonsmokers. Other factors that can increase free radicals are: air pollution, chronic disease, secondhand smoke, dietary carcinogens (foods fried at high temperatures or charcoal-broiled, nitrites, cured meats), inherited susceptibility to a disease, infection, vigorous exercise, menopause, mental stress, sun exposure, and X-rays. Additionally, it's not always what foods you eat but how the food is prepared. For example, cooked carrots supply more bioavailable beta-carotene than raw ones. Your best free radical defense is to know your antioxidants and how to maximize their effectiveness in your diet and supplements.

CAUTION: *Antioxidant supplements should not be taken by anyone undergoing chemotherapy or radiation. These treatments work by creating free radicals to destroy cancer cells, and antioxidant supplements could counteract their effectiveness.*

105. What Antioxidants Can Do for You

Slow the aging process.

Lower cholesterol levels.

Decrease risk of atherosclerosis.

Help protect against heart disease and stroke.

Reduce the risk of all types of cancer.

Help slow down progression of Alzheimer's disease.

Aid in suppressing the growth of tumors.

Help the body detoxify carcinogens.

Protect eyes from macular degeneration, a disease that causes vision loss.

Aid in defending the body against damage from cigarette smoking.

Help protect against chronic obstructive pulmonary diseases (COPDs)—such as asthma, bronchitis, and emphysema.

Offer protection against environmental pollution.

106. Phytochemicals

These are natural chemical substances found in plants; health-promoting nutrients (sometimes referred to as phytonutrients) that give fruits, vegetables, grains, and legumes their color, flavor, and protection against disease. They form the plant's immune system. Potent antioxidants, they have been shown to have a protective effect against many ailments, including heart disease, diabetes, high blood pressure, osteoporosis, lung ailments, and cancer.

107. Carotenoids

Carotenoids are powerful phytochemicals that act as antioxidants and have strong anticancer properties. They are the fat-soluble pigments found in orange, yellow, red, and green fruits and vegetables that protect them from constant exposure to the sun's ultraviolet (UV) rays and other environmental carcinogens, preventing the formation of dangerous free radicals. There are at present six hundred known carotenoids, and about fifty can be found in edible fruits and vegetables. The six being touted as antioxidant stars for the twenty-first century are alpha-carotene, beta-carotene, cryptoxanthin, lycopene, lutein, and zeaxanthin.

Alpha-carotene: Converted into vitamin A as the body needs it, alpha-carotene has been shown to drastically reduce tumors in animals and may be *ten times* more powerful than beta-carotene in protecting skin, eye, liver, and lung tissue against free-radical damage.

Food and Supplement Advice: Your best food sources are cooked carrots and pumpkin. As a supplement, alpha-carotene is sold alone, but it is also included in mixed carotenoid and antioxidant formulas. My recommendation is 3–6 mg. of mixed carotenoids daily.

Beta-carotene: Converted into vitamin A only as the body needs it, leaving the remainder to act as an antioxidant. Studies have shown beta-carotene to play a significant role as a cancer preventive by inhibiting the formation of free radicals. Additionally, it has been found to help strengthen the immune system, reduce the risk of atherosclerosis, heart attack, and stroke, and protect against the formation of cataracts.

Food and Supplement Advice: Look for brightly colored fruits and vegetables, such as apricots, sweet potatoes, broccoli (even better steamed), cantaloupe, pumpkin, carrots, mangoes, peaches, and spinach. Supplements are sold separately, but beta-carotene is included in mixed carotenoid formulas as well as most multivitamins and antioxidant formulas. Beta-carotene is available in two forms: all-*trans*-and 9-*cis*-beta-carotene. The 9-*cis* form may be better absorbed by the body.

CAUTION: *If you have hypothyroidism, your body probably cannot convert alpha- or beta-carotene into vitamin A, so it's best to avoid these supplements.*

Cryptoxanthin: Can be converted into vitamin A as the body needs it. Studies comparing blood carotenoid levels of women who have cervical cancer with those of cancer-free women found that cancer-free women had significantly higher blood levels of cyptoxanthin, suggesting that cryptoxanthin may offer some protection against this form of cancer. Cryptoxanthin may be depleted by smoking. When scientists compared the blood levels of vitamin E and carotenoids in men who chewed or smoked tobacco with blood levels in those who abstained from tobacco, they found significantly lower levels of cryptoxanthin in tobacco users.

Food and Supplement Advice: For a healthy, palate-pleasing serving of cryptoxanthin, treat yourself to such fruits as peaches, papaya, tangerines, and oranges daily.

Cryptoxanthin is included in mixed carotenoid formulas. The recommended dose is 3–6 mg. daily.

Lycopene: A carotenoid that does not have any pro-vitamin A activity (meaning that it is not converted into vitamin A as the body needs it), and has significantly more antioxidant capability than beta-carotene. Lycopene is the substance that gives tomatoes, watermelon, pink grapefruit, and other fruits and vegetables their red color; and lycopene has been shown to inhibit the growth of many types of cancer cells. In fact, men who eat pizza have been found to have a reduced risk of prostate cancer because of the lycopene-rich tomato sauce. Lycopene has also been found to protect against the carcinogens in tobacco smoke and exposure to the sun's ultraviolet rays.

Food and Supplement Advice: Blood levels of lycopene decline with age. Also, lycopene is a fat-soluble pigment and not well absorbed by the body unless it is heated and combined with a small amount of fat, such as olive oil. For this reason cooked tomato sauce provides more of this carotenoid than plain tomatoes. So, if you are over fifty and not eating tomato products on a daily basis, one 6–10 mg. capsule a day with meals might be advisable.

Lutein: Another carotenoid that does not convert to vitamin A in the body but is an impressive antioxidant. Especially helpful in protecting the eyes, lutein has been found to clear away free radicals caused by harmful ultraviolet rays and slow macular degeneration, the most common cause of blindness in people age sixty-five and over.

Food and Supplement Advice: Lutein is abundant in spinach and collard greens, so if you eat plenty of those daily you probably do not need a supplement. But if you're not a fan of those particular veggies, you can find lutein in tablets and combination products (which should contain at least

6 mg. of it). If taken separately, I'd suggest one 6–20 mg. tablet a day with a meal. Medications or supplements that decrease fat absorption (like orlistat or chitosan) may reduce your body's ability to use lutein. If you're pregnant, consult your doctor before supplementing with lutein. Also, avoid lutein supplements if you're allergic to marigolds.

Zeaxanthin: This carotenoid, like lutein, also protects the eye from free radical–induced macular degeneration. (Damage to the macular, a tiny dimple on the retina responsible for fine vision, can cause blurry vision and eventually lead to loss of central vision. Though surgery may slow its progress, there is no cure for macular degeneration, which is why prevention is so important.) Zeaxanthin may also help protect against different forms of cancer by scavenging free radicals and decreasing the growth of tumor cells.

Food and Supplement Advice: Zeaxanthin is found in substantial concentrations in watercress, Swiss chard, chicory leaves, beet greens, spinach, and okra. If your diet does not frequently include these greens, a good mixed carotenoid or antioxidant supplement with 30–130 mg. zeaxanthin taken daily with meals should be considered.

108. Flavonoids

These antioxidant phytochemicals form the water-soluble colors of vegetables, fruits, grains, leaves, and bark. (Biologically active antioxidant flavonoids are bioflavonoids.) There are many types of flavonoids, and different plants contain varying concentrations of them. In fact, studies have shown that some flavonoids possess up to fifty times more antioxidant activity than vitamins C and E—and those in red grapes are more than one thousand times more powerful than vitamin E in inhibiting oxidation of human

LDL cholesterol! The following are just some of the flavonoids you should at least know a little about because they can do a lot for your health!

Catechins: These members of the polyphenol-flavonoid family have been found to inhibit the growth of antibiotic-resistant staphylococcus bacteria, which can cause life-threatening infections, as well as help people who eat a high-cholesterol diet maintain normal cholesterol levels and aid in preventing dental caries and gum disease. There is also strong evidence that they may help in reducing the rate of stomach and lung cancers, prevent DNA damage, and delay the onset of arteriosclerosis.

Food and Supplement Advice: Catechins are found in large concentrations in green tea. They are also in grapes, grape juices, and the wines made from them. Excessive ingestion of catechins can be toxic. I've found, however, that 1 or 2 cups of green tea a day appears to be both safe and beneficial.

CAUTION: *Women who are pregnant or nursing or anyone with a heart arrhythmia should limit their intake to no more than 2 cups of green tea daily. (Caffeine-free green tea extract supplements are available.)*

Resveratrol: Another important polyphenol-flavonoid family member. Studies have shown it can reduce the risk of heart disease and stroke by inhibiting the formation of blood clots and LDL, the bad cholesterol. It has also been found capable of helping to block the formation of cancer cells, being able to turn malignant cells back to normal, reducing diabetic neuropathy (nerve pain that often occurs in the legs and feet), improving memory, activating the body's *sirtuins* (enzymes that slow cellular aging), and sparking the production of the amazingly beneficial gas nitric oxide. (See section 438.)

Food and Supplement Advice: Resveratrol is a compound found in the skin and seeds of grapes. Along with catechins and anthocyanidin, the antioxidant responsible for the deep purple color in red grapes, it may account for the "French Paradox." Despite the fact that the French eat a diet of extremely high-fat, high-cholesterol food, they have one of the lowest rates of heart disease in the world. Researchers believe this is because of the red wine they drink with meals. (Resveratrol is unstable on exposure to air and can lose potency within a day of popping the cork.) If you're not a drinker, don't want the negative effects of alcohol overconsumption, and still want to reap the health benefits, there are alternatives.

Pomegranate juice is a terrific source of resveratrol (3–5 oz. daily); dark unsweetened or semisweet chocolate with at least 70 percent cocoa (1 bite-sized square daily); blueberries (1 cup fresh or frozen daily); green tea, which also contains other polyphenols (three 8-oz. cups daily); and unsweetened purple grape juice (4–16 oz. daily).

Resveratrol supplements are available. Because absorption is believed to be enhanced when combined with other natural polyphenols, a mixed-polyphenol supplement is preferable. I'd suggest taking either one 1,000 mcg. resveratrol capsule daily or two 30 mg. polyphenol capsules.

Proanthocyanidins and Anthocyanidins (PCOs): Also known as oligomeric proanthocyanidins (OPCs), these flavonoids (technically, "flavonals") are powerful vascular protectors and remarkable in their ability to connect and strengthen the body's many strands of collagen protein—particularly in soft tissues, tendons, ligaments, and bones. Because of this, they help promote good circulation to all glands and organs (crucial to preventing and overcoming disease); act therapeutically for fragile capillary conditions such as bruising, varicose veins, and hemorrhoids;

and may offer significant aid in preventing osteoporosis. Additionally, they may be beneficial to athletes and fitness buffs because they are water soluble and therefore capable of neutralizing the free radicals in tissue fluids generated by heavy exercise.

Food and Supplement Advice: PCOs or OPCs (you say "tomato"; I say "toMAHto") are derived primarily from grape-seed and pine bark extract. Pycnogenol, which is one of the few antioxidants that cross the blood-brain barrier to help protect brain and nerve tissue from oxidation, has become synonymous with pine bark benefits, though it is actually a trademarked name for the patented process of extracting flavonoids and other substances from pine bark and consists of 50–60 percent proanthocyanidins. These flavonoids are present in other fruits and vegetables, too, but because bark, stems, leaves, and skins are not high on most people's must-eat lists, they are usually discarded. Fortunately, supplements are available. My recommendation would be to take up to three 30–100 mg. PCO tablets daily *between* meals. Preferably, grape-seed and grape skin extract tablets. (Use the lower dose unless you are over sixty-five or have a compromised immune system.)

109. Phytoestrogens

This important group of chemicals found in plants can act like the hormone estrogen in the body and may offer significant health benefits, including protection against breast and prostate cancer, cardiovascular disease, osteoporosis, and brain function disorders, among others.

Most food phytoestrogens are from one of three chemical classes: the isoflavones, the lignans, or the coumestans.

Isoflavones: See section 110 below.

Lignans: An antioxidant with anticancer, antiviral, and anti-bacterial properties. The highest amount of lignan phytoestrogens is found in flaxseeds. Other good sources are sesame, poppy, and sunflower seeds; high-fiber cereal brans and beans; products made with wheat and rye flours; as well as whole-grain rice, tofu, tomato paste, and chocolate. Lignans are also plentiful in fruits such as strawberries, peaches, pears, raisins, kiwi, grapefruit, plums, oranges, and apricots (which contain the most). All cruciferous vegetables (see section 120) are excellent sources, with kale being the richest.

Coumestans: Although they don't produce as strong an estrogen effect as isoflavones, many scientists believe that coumestans in combination with isoflavones are more effective synergistically than either group alone. Found in beans, such as split peas, pinto beans, and lima beans, the highest concentrations are in alfalfa and clover sprouts. (Coumestans form during the germination phase, which is why sprouts top the list.)

110. Isoflavones

Found in soybeans and other legumes, these phytonutrients are related to flavonoids. In the body they are converted into phytoestrogens (plant estrogens), hormonelike compounds that may help block the growth of hormone-dependent—and other—cancers. They also seem to help lower total cholesterol levels and reduce high blood triglycerides, providing protection against heart disease. (They may even prevent hot flashes in menopausal women.) The best-known isoflavones are genistein and daidzein.

Genistein: Helps block the spread of cancerous tumors by preventing the growth of new blood vessels to nourish the cancer cells. May reduce the risk of breast and prostate cancers.

Food and Supplement Advice: Genistein is found exclusively in soy foods, such as soy milk, tofu, miso, and tempeh. If you're not a tofu fan, and your feeling about soy is just soy-so, it is available in pill and powdered supplement form with daidzein and other isoflavones. One soy protein shake or 2 soy concentrate supplement tablets (containing 10 mg. genistein and daidzein) is what I would recommend.

Daidzein: Works with genistein to block enzymes that promote tumor growth. May be especially beneficial to women in controlling the effects of potent estrogens that could stimulate the growth of breast cancer cells. Helps reduce blood-alcohol levels and relieve hangovers. (See section 302.)

Food and Supplement Advice: Like genistein, daidzein is found in soy products. As an antioxidant, cancer-fighting supplement, 1 soy protein shake daily or 2 soy concentrate tablets (containing genistein and other isoflavones) is recommended. Daidzein is also the isoflavone in the oriental herb kudzu (*Pueraria lobata*), which has been shown to help prevent hangovers and reduce the desire for alcohol. Kudzu supplements are available in capsules. If you'd like help getting "on the wagon"—or getting over the night before—my recommendation is three 500 mg. capsules daily before or after drinking alcohol.

111. Vitamins

The major vitamins that act as antioxidants are vitamin A, vitamin C, and vitamin E.

Vitamin A: A potent and important free radical scavenger, vitamin A—particularly its precursors alpha- and beta-carotene—destroys carcinogens and has been found to protect against many forms of cancer.

Food and Supplement Advice: See section 30.

Vitamin C: This water-soluble wonder worker could well be called the antioxidant's antioxidant because it helps protect other antioxidants in the body. It inhibits the production of cancer-causing nitrosamines, cuts the risk of many types of cancer, increases the activity of vital immune cells, prevents dangerous oxidation of LDL cholesterol, and reduces your chances of heart attack.

Food and Supplement Advice: See section 46.

Vitamin E: A fat-soluble free radical fighter that protects cell membranes and other lipid-containing tissues. It has been found to help prevent cataracts, enhance the body's immune response, protect against many types of cancer, and significantly reduce the risk of fatal heart attacks.

Food and Supplement Advice: See section 48.

112. Minerals

All minerals are antioxidants, but, unlike some vitamins, not a single one can be manufactured by the body and all must be acquired through diet. Their presence in the body in proper amounts cannot be overemphasized, since vitamins cannot function, be assimilated, without the help of minerals. The major mineral free radical scavengers are selenium and zinc.

Selenium: Synergistic with vitamin E, meaning each increases effectiveness of the other, selenium has been shown to be an important cancer preventive, particularly helpful in protecting against damage caused by radiation and chemical carcinogens. It also stimulates increased antibody response to infection; aids in the prevention of blood clots, which can cause a stroke; and may help reduce the pain and stiffness of arthritis. Additionally, it is reputed to increase the male sex drive.

Food and Supplement Advice: See section 68.

Zinc: A potent fighter of the common cold, it has been shown to enhance the immune system, increasing the level of infection-fighting T cells, particularly in older people. It may also help slow vision loss caused by macular degeneration as well as aid in protecting the prostate from enlargement and even cancer.

Food and Supplement Advice: See section 72.

113. Allium Vegetables

There are more than five hundred plants in the genus *allium*, but the antioxidant superstars are garlic (see section 136), onions, shallots, and leeks. These vegetables contain flavonoids, vitamin C, selenium, and sulfur compounds that have been shown to have potent cancer-fighting properties—particularly in helping cells dispose of carcinogens. They may also help prevent heart attack and stroke by lowering cholesterol and blood pressure and preventing blood clots. Additionally, allium vegetables benefit the liver by helping activate detoxification enzyme systems, and may be helpful, too, in the prevention of allergies and asthma.

Food and Supplement Advice: You don't have to eat raw onions or garlic to reap benefits from this group; even when cooked, they seem to have antioxidant capabilities. And if you'd rather not chance heartburn or bad breath, odorless garlic caps are available. Parsley sprigs are natural breath-fresheners, but internal breath freshening capsules made from parsley seed oil might be easier to carry around.

114. Acai Berry

Often categorized as a superfood, this dark purple berry of South America's acai palm tree has one of the highest known antioxidant activity potentials in the world. Readily absorbed by the body, it is an anti-inflammatory, antibacterial, immune system booster that's low in sugar and a good source of fiber. It also contains an A-list powerhouse of nutrients, including omega fatty acids, vitamin E, theobormine, phytosterols, and an almost perfect complex of essential amino acids. An amazing energy fruit with ten to thirty times the anthocyanidins of red wine, it may help in the treatment of colon cancer, cardiovascular diseases, and in maintaining healthy cholesterol levels, as well as enhance the body's energy, endurance, and muscle development. Last, but far from least, it has been found to be a safe and effective appetite suppressant and weight-loss supplement.

Food and Supplement Advice: Available as juice, puree, freeze-dried powder, and capsules. If purchasing, make sure the product is 100 percent pure USDA-certified organic, with no sugars added (products that contain additional ingredients might cause side effects). Keep in mind that acai berries are harvested manually in the Brazilian rain forest, which is very labor-intensive, so I'd suggest steering clear of products that are very cheap. You'll get (or rather, not get) what you pay for. Acai powder can be mixed with juices or yogurts and enjoyed as smoothies. It is advisable, though, to limit your intake to no more than 4,000 mg. of supplements or 4 ounces of puree daily.

115. Bilberry

This herb, also known as European blueberry, is a potent antioxidant. It contains anthocyanosides, which have been found to help keep capillaries strong, protect against cataracts, night blindness, and other vision problems, and improve circulation. It may also inhibit the growth of bacteria and act as an anti-inflammatory, as well as have anti-carcinogenic effects.

Food and Supplement Advice: As a supplement, bilberry is available in capsules and liquid extract. Take one 500 mg. capsule up to three times daily or mix 15–40 drops in water or juice, and drink three times daily. Bilberry works best when combined with vitamin C (up to 500 mg. vitamin C daily).

CAUTION: *Do not exceed recommended dosages! Although commercially prepared extracts are safe, bilberry leaves can be poisonous if consumed over a long period of time.*

116. Camu Camu (*Myrciaria dubia*)

Picked at the height of ripeness, flash-frozen, and then processed into a potent powder, this fruit of an Amazon rain forest bush tree contains powerful phytochemicals and more natural vitamin C than any other known botanical on the planet. An antiseptic immune system booster that can improve circulation and lower blood pressure, camu camu is effective at treating colds and also a natural antidepressant that can be used safely in combination with most prescription antidepressants and other pharmaceutical drugs.

Food and Supplement Advice: As a supplement, camu camu is available in powdered extract capsules. Recommended dosage is one to three 100 mg. capsules daily.

CAUTION: *Camu camu should not be taken during pregnancy.*

117. Cha de Bugre

A South American plant that is rich in beneficial phyto-chemicals, cha de bugre produces a red fruit that can be roasted and brewed into tea as a coffee substitute. Containing caffeine, allantoin, and allantonic acid, cha de bugre has been long known in Brazil as an energizing stimulant with diuretic properties and works as an appetite suppressant by creating a sense of being full after eating only a few bites of food. Traditionally used in wound healing, cha de bugre has also been found to regulate and support liver, kidney, colon, and heart functions; as well as to reduce cellulite, kill viruses, and reduce fever.

Food and Supplement Advice: Leaf extract powders are available as teas and in capsules. Recommended dosage is one to three 400 mg. capsules taken a half hour before meals.

118. Chokeberry (Red and Black)

Rich in their anthocyanin content, having one of the highest ORAC (measurement of antioxidant strength) values yet recorded, chokeberries—also known as aronia berries—are power players when it comes to controlling oxidative stress. Long used by Native Americans for a variety of traditional health applications, chokeberries, which can improve circulation, strengthen blood vessels, and suppress viruses, may also be beneficial for reducing the risk of colorectal cancer, cardiovascular disease, peptic ulcers, eye inflammations, and liver failure.

Food and Supplement Advice: Supplements are available as fruit extract capsules. Recommended dosage is 1 capsule daily with food and water.

119. Coenzyme-Q10 (Co-Q10, Ubiquinone)

This antioxidant nutrient is found in every living cell and is essential for providing us with the energy necessary to carry out bodily functions effectively. Without it, our cells simply won't work. As we age, levels of coenzyme-Q10 fall, which may directly relate to numerous diseases and illnesses associated with age (see section 436). Poor eating habits, stress, and infection can also affect the body's ability to provide adequate amounts. Sharing many of vitamin E's antioxidant properties, it has been shown to increase energy, improve heart function, help reverse gum disease, and improve the immune system. Additionally, a study funded by the National Institute of Neurological Disorders and Stroke (NINDS) suggested that Co-Q10 may slow the rate of deterioration in Parkinson's disease. Further studies are needed, but this is very exciting because although levodopa and other drugs can ease symptoms of the disease, none of the current treatments have been shown to slow the course of the disease. The investigators believe Co-Q10 works by improving the function of mitochondria, the "powerhouses" that produce energy in cells—especially since earlier studies have shown that the Co-Q10 levels in the mitochondria of Parkinson's disease patients were impaired.

An almost immediate boost in energy levels has been reported by many older people whose heart function has degenerated. And angina suffers have said that Co-Q10 was more effective in reducing or eliminating pain than other traditional medications. Statin drugs, taken by millions to control high cholesterol—a significant risk factor for heart disease—deplete the body's stores of Co-Q10. In other words, by taking a drug that's supposed to reduce the risk of heart disease, these millions may actually be *increasing* it. If you have to take a statin drug (Zocor, Pravachol, Lipitor, or Crestor), it would be wise to supplement with Co-Q10.

Food and Supplement Advice: Coenzyme-Q10 is found in meat, cereals, vegetables, eggs, and dairy products, but it is significantly reduced by the length of storage, processing, and methods of cooking. As a supplement, I'd suggest one 30 mg. capsule up to three times daily. The gel form of Co-Q10, with the Co-Q10 absorbed in soy oil, is the best absorbed and easiest to swallow. Oil-based supplements are more bioavailable—and therefore more potent—because Co-Q10 is a fat-soluble nutrient.

120. Cruciferous Vegetables

This group of antioxidant-rich vegetables (broccoli, brussels sprouts, cabbage, kale, etc.) contains—along with vitamin C and other flavonoids—phytochemicals called indoles and sulforaphane. Indoles inactivate estrogens that can promote the growth of tumors, particularly those in the breast. Sulforaphane has been found to stimulate cells to produce cancer-fighting enzymes. The combination of all these potent antioxidants in cruciferous vegetables has been found to help protect against many forms of cancer.

Food and Supplement Advice: Despite the nutritional benefits of cruciferous vegetables such as broccoli, kale, cauliflower, brussels sprouts, bok choy, and others, they're not high on most people's favorite foods list. Fortunately, many of the beneficial substances in these vegetables can now be obtained in supplement form. Swallowing a pill won't provide you with fiber and all the other nutrients in fresh vegetables, but it's better than passing these health benefits by altogether. I find that taking a combination supplement of mixed fruits and vegetables that contains broccoli isolates or extracts is a terrific pick-me-up between meals—and a great way to cover my nutritional bases!

121. Ginkgo Biloba

This potent antioxidant herb is best known for improving circulation. By increasing the supply of oxygen to the heart, brain, and all other body parts, it aids in mental functioning and the ability to concentrate, helps relieve leg cramps and other muscle pain, and may alleviate impotency. In fact, quite a few men have told me they think of it as nature's Viagra. It can relieve symptoms of vertigo and tinnitus (ringing in the ears), and may improve perception and social function in victims of Alzheimer's disease. Because it helps protect cells from free radical damage, it may also aid in slowing the aging process and preventing cancer.

New studies have shown that ginkgo may help in the prevention and treatment of macular degeneration and has significant value as an antidepressant in people who haven't responded to standard antidepressant treatment.

Food and Supplement Advice: Standardized ginkgo biloba is available in 40 mg. and 60 mg. strengths. You can take up to three 60 mg. capsules or tablets daily.

CAUTION: *This herb is contraindicated for anyone with a bleeding disorder. Ginkgo biloba interferes with blood clotting and should not be used by anyone taking nonsteroidal anti-inflammatory drugs (NSAIDs), such as aspirin or ibuprofen; or prescription blood thinners, such as warfarin (Coumadin). It also may affect insulin and lower blood sugar levels.*

122. Glutathione

This triple-powered antioxidant is produced in the liver from three amino acids—cysteine, glutamic acid, and glycine. It protects cells throughout the body, as well as all organ tissues, and may help prevent cancer, especially of the liver. Glutathione functions as an immune system booster, a detoxifier of heavy metals and drugs, and may also protect against radiation poisoning and the detrimental effects of cigarette smoke and alcohol abuse. It has also been used as an anti-inflammatory treatment for arthritis and allergies.

Food and Supplement Advice: Glutathione is found in fruits and vegetables, but cooking can reduce its potency. As a supplement, I'd suggest a 50 mg. capsule one or two times daily. The amino acid methionine helps protect against glutathione depletion, so a diet that includes natural food sources of methionine—such as beans, eggs, fish, garlic, lentils, soybeans, and yogurt—is a good idea. Taking an amino acid supplement containing L-cysteine and L-methionine can also boost the body's own production of glutathione.

123. Goji (aka Wolfberry or "the Happy Berry")

Used for thousands of years by herbalists in China, Tibet, and India to protect the liver, improve sexual function, increase sperm production, help eyesight, boost the immune system, and improve circulation, these antioxidant-rich berries—high in carotenoids, phytosterols, amino acids, vitamins, minerals, and essential fatty acids—may also decrease the risk of age-related macular degeneration.

Food and Supplement Advice: Goji berries can be eaten raw, brewed into teas or drunk as a juice (which is available in health-food stores).

CAUTION: *Goji berries may interact adversely with anticoagulant medications and increase risk of bleeding.*

124. Lipoic Acid

A unique defender against free radicals, frequently called the universal antioxidant, lipoic acid is a vitaminlike substance that the body produces naturally. Unlike other internally produced antioxidants that have specific jobs, lipoic acid is neither exclusively fat soluble nor water soluble, enabling it to enhance the activity of other antioxidants in the body as well as be an all-around pinch hitter. If, for example, your stores of antioxidant vitamins C or E are low, lipoic acid can fill in for them temporarily. Because of its ability to pass through the blood-brain barrier, it can also help reverse the negative effects to the brain caused by strokes. Lipoic acid also helps normalize blood sugar levels and can prevent serious complications from diabetes.

Food and Supplement Advice: As we age, our bodies stop producing lipoic acid in sufficient quantities to provide benefits. If you've passed the big 4-0, you might *not* want to pass on a supplement. Lipoic acid is available in tablets and included in antioxidant formulas. I'd suggest one or two 50 mg. tablets daily.

125. Melatonin

This antioxidant hormone is produced by the brain's pineal gland during sleep and helps maintain the body's natural biorhythms. Because of its control of our body clock (sleep-wake cycles), I've found it helpful as a treatment for jet lag as well as insomnia.

As we age, our levels of melatonin decline. Supplements may help retard the aging process, particularly by helping to prevent the oxidative damage to brain cells that contributes to a variety of illnesses, including Alzheimer's disease. Melatonin has also been found to reduce the incidence of cluster headaches and can boost immune function by activating cancer-fighting cells that help stop malignancies from spreading.

Food and Supplement Advice: Melatonin is found in foods such as tomatoes, which is why, even though it is a hormone, it can be sold as a supplement and not a drug. My recommendation for avoiding jet lag is 1–3 mg. (sublingual form) dissolved under the tongue half an hour before you want to go to sleep at your arrival destination. If taking tablets or capsules, which are not as fast-acting, I'd suggest 1–3 mg. one and a half hours before desired sleep time. For insomnia, 1–5 mg. before bedtime. (Start with 1 mg. and increase if necessary. Do not exceed 5 mg.) As a general antiaging supplement, I'd recommend 0.5–1.0 mg. (sublingual form) taken before bedtime. *Tip*: If you're in the habit of having a midnight snack, a banana would be a good one as it can boost melatonin production.

Some drugs, including over-the-counter NSAIDs, interfere with the brain's production of melatonin. In fact, just one dose of normal aspirin can reduce your melatonin production by as much as 75 percent. If you're taking these drugs, take the last dose after dinner. Other drugs that can interfere with melatonin production in the brain include benzodiazepines such as Valium and Xanax, caffeine, alcohol, cold medicines, diuretics, beta-blockers, calcium channel blockers, diet pills, and corticosteroids such as prednisone.

Because even short exposure to light can suppress the brain's production of melatonin, I'd suggest sleeping in as dark a room as possible and minimizing nighttime exposure to bright overhead lighting by keeping a night-light only in the bathroom.

CAUTION: *Melatonin may make you very sleepy and should be taken at bedtime. Do not drive or operate heavy machinery after taking it. If you are taking any medication, have a serious illness, are pregnant, trying to become pregnant or breast-feeding, are diabetic, have a hormonal imbalance from another illness, or are menopausal and on hormone replacement therapy (HRT), melatonin should not be taken without consulting your doctor. Because it may overstimulate immune function, anyone with an autoimmune disease or on immune-suppressing medication should not take melatonin!*

126. Mangosteen

A tropical fruit grown primarily in southeast Asia, mangosteen has been found to have anti-inflammatory, antimicrobial, antifungal, and antiseptic properties and is one of the most potent, natural providers of antioxidants available. The rind of this "superfruit"—which contains powerful xanthones, catechins, and tannins—has been used for centuries as a tea for medicinal purposes, treating diarrhea, irritable bowel syndrome, and skin conditions, among many others.

Food and Supplement Advice: Look for mangosteen products (capsules or juices) that use "the whole plant" in the supplement. For 500 mg. capsules, follow dosing instructions provided on individual product labels.

CAUTION: *Mangosteen xanthones may interact adversely with blood-thinning medications and increase risk of bleeding. They may also cause excess sedation when combined with other herbs or medicines.*

127. Pomegranate

The applelike fruit of the pomegranate tree has become one of the most popular antioxidant-rich superfruits in foods and supplements. Loaded with high levels of vitamin C, B, potassium, and polyphenols—including catechins and anthocyanins—its potential health benefits show reduced risk of heart disease, decreased levels of LDL cholesterol, diminished skin wrinkling, and possible inhibition of various types of cancer.

Food and Supplement Advice: Pomegranates and pomegranate juices are widely available in grocery stores. The fruit, peeled and seeded, is usually eaten raw. Supplements are available as extracts in concentrated form, the advantage being that the less-useful ingredients of the juice (mainly sugar) are removed.

128. Quercetin

A plant-derived flavanol and powerful antioxidant found in apples, onions, black tea, and red wine, quercetin is a natural antihistamine and anti-inflammatory that may help protect against heart attacks and strokes, as well as relieve symptoms of prostatitis and aid in the treatment of gout, eczemza, allergies, hives, and asthma. Quercetin has also been found to boost mitochondria—the power generators of the cell—helping to reduce fatigue and increase endurance capacity.

Food and Supplement Advice: Found mostly in dark-pigmented fruits, quercetin is also, in lesser amounts, in broccoli, a variety of leafy greens, and citrus fruits.

Flavonoids hesperidin and rutin are often combined with quercetin in supplements for increased synergistic effect. Available in pill and tablet form, the suggested dosage is 200–400 mg. three times daily.

129. Superoxide Dismutase (SOD)

An enzyme that acts as a powerful antioxidant, especially with skin tissue, revitalizing cells and reducing the rate of cell destruction. In fact, SOD injections have been shown to help in the treatment of scleroderma, a hardening of the skin. SOD helps the body utilize essential zinc, copper, and manganese but can become inactive if these minerals are not supplied. As we age, our bodies produce less and less SOD, so supplementation may prove an important factor in reducing wrinkles and slowing the aging process on all levels.

Food and Supplement Advice: Among the best natural sources of SOD are barley grass, broccoli, brussels sprouts, cabbage, and wheatgrass. SOD is destroyed in the stomach, so supplements must be enteric coated in order for them to pass through the stomach intact so that the enzyme can reach and be absorbed in the small intestine. As part of an antiaging regimen (see section 436), take 125 mcg. daily.

DID YOU KNOW?

- Blueberries, blackberries, and red cabbage are better for you if cooked.
- Onions, garlic, radishes, and leeks contain a natural antibiotic that can destroy disease germs without harming good bacteria.
- Two or more servings a week of tomato sauce can lower a man's risk of prostate cancer.

130. Any Questions About Chapter VII?

Is there any way to tell if I'm low on antioxidants?

As a matter of fact, there is. It's called an oxidative stress test and uses urine and blood samples to determine your body's free radical levels and glutathione reserves. If you're in good health with no distressing symptoms or serious concerns, I don't feel there is a need to incur the expense of a test. But if you are worried about it, your best bet is to consult a nutritionally oriented doctor. (See section 462.)

What can I take to increase the levels of my body's antioxidants naturally?

A couple of supplements come to mind. Silymarin is one that contains three bioflavonoids extracted from the milk thistle plant: silybin, silydianin, and silychristin. It is a natural antioxidant that enhances liver function (milk thistle has been used for centuries to treat liver disorders) and also increases the levels of two of the body's own most important antioxidants, glutathione and superoxide dismutase (SOD). You can take up to three 500 mg. silymarin capsules a day.

There is also an ancient Chinese tonic herb called cordyceps, traditionally used to fight fatigue and promote vitality, that can raise levels of the body's own antioxidants. I'd suggest taking two 525 mg. capsules daily with meals.

What's the best way to preserve antioxidants when cooking vegetables?

Microwaving and "griddling" (cooking on a flat metal surface with no oil) have been found to best preserve the antioxidant content of most vegetables. Boiling, frying, pressure-cooking, and baking take an antioxidant toll.

Do dogs and cats need antioxidant supplements?

Possibly even more than we do. Think about it: They're exposed to chemicals more intensively than most humans because they breathe in greater concentrations of them from floors and lawns. Their self-grooming behavior also increases their risk of toxic exposure, to say nothing of chemically treated flea collars and the unhealthy "snacks" they often pick up when out and about.

Although dogs and cats do manufacture their own vitamin C, it is not in amounts needed for disease prevention or supplying significant health benefits. Supplementing your pet's diet with this powerful antioxidant vitamin can reduce cancer risk, boost the immune system, stimulate wound repair, reduce the risk of cataracts, alleviate allergies, and aid in preventing and curing cystitis. Vitamin C is also important for proper bone formation.

Supplement dosage:

For adult dogs: 500–1,000 mg. daily

For adult cats: 50–300 mg. daily

To avoid stomach upset, sodium ascorbate or buffered vitamin C are recommended.

Specially formulated supplements for dogs and cats are available at pet stores or can be obtained from your veterinarian.

NOTE: *Loose stools or diarrhea are usually signs of too much vitamin C, so reduce dosage.*

Cats, unlike dogs and humans, cannot convert beta-carotene to vitamin A and must obtain it from retinol (an animal source). Unless you suspect a serious deficiency, a little liver (no more than 25 percent of the cat's usual meal) three or four times a week is sufficient. Dogs process vitamin A differently, allowing them to tolerate higher doses than humans, but toxic levels are the same (see section 30) and an oversupply can cause serious problems. Check with your vet before supplementing.

Vitamin E offers pets protection from environmental pollutants and stress, and can reduce a cat's risk of steatitis (a condition caused by an all-fish diet that depletes this vitamin).

Supplement dosage:

For adult dogs: 100–400 IU (depending on size) daily

For adult cats: 10–15 IU (for aging, pregnant, or lactating cats, dosage may be increased to 15–30 IU daily, divided in two doses with meals).

Selenium works with vitamin E to boost your pet's immune system, but most dogs and cats get adequate amounts in their diets from fish, red meat, organs, eggs, and chicken.

Zinc, which aids in wound healing and removing toxins from the body, also supports the immune system. Dogs and cats usually get sufficient zinc in their diets from lamb, pork, beef, liver, and brewer's yeast. (See section 72 for best natural sources.)

Is there any truth to the delicious rumor I heard about chocolate being an antioxidant booster?

If you like dark chocolate, I have sweet news—there is. According to a study reported in the *Journal of Nutrition*, researchers found that eating dark chocolate—but not milk chocolate—raises levels of antioxidants in the blood. A daily intake of 6.7 g. of dark chocolate daily significantly lowered levels of C-reactive protein in the blood and was deemed the ideal amount for a protective effect against inflammation and subsequent heart disease. So, enjoy dark chocolate to your heart's healthy content—in moderation.

Does black tea contain the same antioxidants that green tea does? And what about white and red tea?

Black tea is more processed than green tea so it has slightly less antioxidants, but it does improve coronary vessel function, reduce LDL cholesterol, and lower blood pressure, even though it has more caffeine than green tea. White tea has the highest antioxidant potency and a lower caffeine content than green or black teas. Red tea has some unique health-giving properties, namely those of superoxide dismutase (SOD), (see section 129). It also contains zinc, magnesium, and alpha hydroxy acid and is known to benefit the management of allergies, asthma, and eczema.

Interestingly, although tea is consumed in a variety of ways and varies in its chemical makeup, studies have shown that steeping these teas for about five minutes releases more than 80 percent of their catechins (the antioxidants found in tea). Instant iced tea, on the other hand, contains negligible amounts of catechins. So, for the best nutritional teatime, steep it and keep it hot.

When choosing a red wine, are there any that offer more resveratrol than others?

For more resveratrol bang from your bottle of red, chose a pinot noir. Wines from colder, damp climates— like pinot poir—have more resveratrol because it's needed to protect the grapes from mold.

Do all alcoholic beverages contain resveratrol?

If they did, alcoholics would be a lot healthier and have the antioxidant edge on the rest of us. Hard liquor is distilled, so it does not contain resveratrol or other polyphenols. Beer, on the other hand, because it's made with barley as well as hops, does contain a surprisingly wide variety of polyphenols. But there's no need to up your alcohol consumption to get their benefits. Nonalcoholic beer and red wine offer them as well.

I need to keep my grocery bills down, so what supermarket fruits and vegetables will give me the most antioxidants for my money?

The best ones, according to the U.S. Department of Agriculture, are blueberries, blackberries, cranberries, strawberries, spinach, raspberries, brussels sprouts, plums, broccoli, beets, avocados, oranges, red grapes, red bell peppers, cherries, and kiwis.

I take coenzyme-Q10. Is it okay to give to my dog who's getting on in years (she's ten)?

It's not only okay, I recommend it. Coenzyme-Q10 is a safe, nontoxic nutrient that's vital to life. Without it, your dog's cells would not work properly. As dogs age they produce less Co-Q10, so now would be a very good time to supplement. It can strengthen her heart, her immune system, and her ability to cope with stress. It is available as a powder in a capsule or in a gel capsule. (The gel capsule is more potent). For small and medium dogs I suggest 10 mg. daily. If she is one of the large or giant breeds, you can give her 30 mg. daily, mixed with food.

VIII

OTHER WONDER WORKERS

131. Probiotics: *Lactobacillus acidophilus*

Probiotics are organisms that contribute to the health of the intestinal tract. They're the beneficial bacteria that help fight illness and disease. *Lactobacillus acidophilus*, or *acidophilus* as it is commonly known, is one source of friendly intestinal bacteria. More potent as a capsule or granule supplement than yogurt, it is available as *acidophilus* culture, incubated in soy, milk, or yeast bases.

Many doctors prescribe *acidophilus* in conjunction with oral antibiotic treatment because antibiotics destroy beneficial intestinal flora, often causing diarrhea as well as an overgrowth of the fungus *Candida albicans*. This fungus can grow in the intestines, vagina, lungs, mouth (thrush), on the fingers, or under the nails. It will usually disappear after a few days' use of generous amounts of *acidophilus* culture.

Regular use of *acidophilus* culture keeps the intestines clean. It can eliminate bad breath caused by intestinal putrefaction (the sort resistant to mouthwash or breath spray), constipation, foul-smelling flatulence, and aid in the treatment of acne and other skin problems. It can also boost the immune system, which weakens as we age, and help menopausal women who are more susceptible to vaginal yeast infections because of the dryness that accompanies the drop in estrogen.

Keep in mind that lactose, complex carbohydrates, pectin, and vitamin C plus roughage (see fiber, section 137) encourage additional growth of intestinal flora. This is important since friendly bacteria can die within five days unless they are continuously supplied with some form of lactic acid or lactose.

What Probiotics Can Do for You:

Work with antibiotics by helping to prevent diarrhea, which can minimize antibiotic effectiveness, and keep the good bacteria from being destroyed with the bad.

Produce infection-fighting substances.

Probiotics increase the strength and effectiveness of good bacteria so the bad bacteria (pathogens)—the ones that can cause illness and infection—are held at bay.

Keep your intestinal tract healthy.

Help to correct bowl problems—including constipation, bloating, and gas.

May be beneficial in treatment of colitis, irritable bowel syndrome, and Crohn's disease.

May help in the prevention of colon cancer.

Produce enzymes needed to digest milk and dairy, helping calcium strengthen bones.

Aid in management of lactose intolerance.

May help fight allergies that lead to acne and eczema.

Help to inactivate toxins in the intestinal tract.

If you're buying yogurt, buy yogurt that contains inulin. Inulin is a prebiotic, meaning it is scientifically proven to increase the activity of the benefical bacteria (such as bifidobacteria) as well as help prevent the growth of harmful bacteria in the digestive tract (see section 132). Inulin—present in common fruits and vegetables such as artichokes, asparagus, onions, raisins, and bananas—is a good source of natural soluble dietary fiber, fine for diabetics because it doesn't increase the glucose or insulin level in the blood, boosts the absorption of calcium, and helps protect against bacteria that cause many food-borne illnesses, such as *E. coli,* salmonella, staphylococcus, and listeria.

As a general diet supplement: take 1 *acidophilus* vegetarian capsule daily containing 25 billion friendly bacteria of *Lactobacillus rhamnosus, helveticus, casei, plantarum,* and *lactis ssp. lactis,* along with *Pediococcus acidilactici, Bifidobacterium* in gum, and *Bifidobacterium breve.* Since stomach acid rises when you eat, you'll get more probiotic bang for your friendly bacteria by taking supplements between meals.

NOTE: *Products that list a specific strain of bacteria on labels are generally more effective than those that neglect to do so.*

132. Prebiotics

Prebiotics are nondigestible foods that help good bacteria (probiotics) grow and thrive, enabling them to restore and retain proper balance in your digestive tract. (Think of them as vitamins for probiotics.) They are derived primarily from carbohydrate fibers called oligosaccharides, which—because they are not digested—are able to remain in your digestive tract and keep beneficial bacteria healthy. Good sources of oligosaccharides are fruits, legumes, and whole grains.

Both prebiotics and probiotics are available as supplements. Adding prebiotic oligosaccharides to your probiotic will kick-start its action, keep it healthy in your system, and maximize effectiveness.

133. Bromelain

Pineapple is good for more than dessert! Bromelain, an enzyme derived from the stem of the pineapple plant, is a mixture of protein-processing enzymes that aids in digestion while enhancing the absorption of nutrients from food *and* supplements. It can also help reduce pain and swelling due to arthritis or injury, similar to nonsteroidal anti-inflammatory drugs (NSAIDs), but without their gastrointestinal side effects. (NSAIDs such as aspirin, ibuprofen, and Naprosyn inhibit prostaglandins, compounds that cause inflammation but also have a protective effect on the stomach lining.) Bromelain may also prevent abnormally high levels of fibrinogen, which can cause blood clots to form spontaneously and lead to heart attack or stroke.

As a digestive aid, I recommend one or two 500 mg. tablets after meals. As an anti-inflammatory, one to three 500 mg. tablets daily. For cardiovascular health, take one 500 mg. tablet daily.

CAUTION: *Bromelain may interact with heartbeat medications and increase the risk of bleeding when taken with blood thinners.*

134. Curcumin/Turmeric

If you eat Indian food often, you've been spicing up your health in more ways than you probably realized. Derived from turmeric, the spice that gives curry powder its distinctive yellow color, curcumin (not the same as cumin, which is also in curry powder) is a potent antioxidant shown to be particularly helpful in reducing the free radical damage inflicted on smokers by the carcinogenic chemicals in cigarettes. It also may reduce inflammation from rheumatoid arthritis. In fact, for some arthritis sufferers it has produced improvement that's comparable to phenylbutazone, a prescription nonsteroidal anti-inflammatory, with none of the unpleasant side effects of NSAIDs. Additionally, it appears to inhibit the activity of certain proteins that may trigger the growth of breast tumors and may also lower high blood cholesterol levels.

Turmeric, the spice itself, has long been used by Indian healers in the practice of ayurvedic medicine to strengthen liver function, and many alternative practitioners today prescribe curcumin to people with the common liver ailment hepatitis C. Turmeric also helps prevent the formation of blood clots that can lead to heart attack. As a supplement, one to three 500 mg. curcumin capsules daily with food is the suggested dosage. Many commercial preparations combine curcumin with bromelain, another anti-inflammatory. The two appear to work best together, and bromelain may increase the absorption of curcumin.

135. Ginseng

It is generally well accepted that ginseng is a stimulant of both mental and physical energy. The Chinese have been using it for nearly five thousand years and still revere it as a preventive and cure-all. It is a mild laxative and helps the body pass poisons through more rapidly. It may also help reduce LDL (bad) cholesterol, improve circulation, alleviate discomfort caused in menopause by increasing estrogen levels (it is a rich source of phytoestrogen), inhibit the growth of cancerous tumors, normalize blood pressure, and help cure colds. Purported to be an aphrodisiac for centuries, many women say that it does enhance their sexual desire. Because of its stimulating effect, men may find it improves their sexual performance as well. (According to a study in the *Journal of Urology*, men with erectile dysfunction given 900 mg. of Korean red ginseng three times daily for eight weeks, with a two-week break, and then the same dosage for another eight weeks, had International Index of Erectile Function scores that were significantly higher than those of men taking a placebo.)

The big nutritional plus for ginseng is that it helps you assimilate vitamins and minerals by acting as an endocrine-gland stimulant. For maximum effectiveness, it is best to take it on an empty stomach—preferably before breakfast—or at least an hour before or after eating. Vitamin C may interfere with the absorption of ginseng. If you take a vitamin C supplement, wait two hours before or after taking your ginseng to do so. (A time-release vitamin C supplement makes any counteraction less likely.)

The primary types of ginseng available are Asian ginseng (*Panax ginseng*), also called oriental, Chinese, or Korean ginseng; American ginseng (*Panax quinquefolius*); and Siberian ginseng (*Eleutherococcus senticosus*), which is not a true (*Panax*) ginseng but is enough of a relative to provide many of the same benefits—particularly increasing stamina and helping to lower cholesterol levels.

Ginseng is available in capsule form in 500–650 mg. (10-grain) doses. I don't recommend more than six 500 mg. capsules daily. It can also be purchased as a tea, powder, or liquid concentrate. It is now considered a class-A adaptogen (a nontoxic substance that increases the body's resistance to a wide variety of stress factors, whether they be physical, chemical, or biological in nature). If you use Asian or American ginseng, look for products containing 4–7 percent ginsenosides (biologically active ingredients); for Siberian ginseng, find products that contain eleutherosides equal to 1 percent of the total weight.

CAUTION: *In rare cases, ginseng may cause vaginal bleeding in menopausal women. Though not dangerous, it could be mistaken as a symptom of uterine cancer. In any event, if bleeding does occur, you should notify your doctor and don't forget to tell him that you're taking ginseng. Also, some people may develop headaches or high blood pressure from* Panax *ginseng, so it's advisable to check with your doctor before starting a ginseng regimen.*

136. Alfalfa, Garlic, Chlorophyll, and Yucca

Alfalfa has been dubbed "the great healer" by noted biologist and author Frank Bouer, who discovered that the green leaves of this remarkable legume contain *eight* essential enzymes. Also, for every 100 g., it contains 8,000 IU of vitamin A and 20,000–40,000 units of vitamin K, which protects against hemorrhaging and helps in blood clotting. It is additionally a fine source of vitamins B6 and E; rich in calcium, magnesium, potassium, and beta-carotene; and contains enough vitamin D, lime, and phosphorus to secure strong bones and teeth in growing children.

A good laxative and a natural diuretic, alfalfa is often used to treat urinary tract infections. Also, it is reputed to provide relief from rheumatoid arthritis, improve poor appetite, and has been used for treating stomach ailments and gas pains. It is available as a supplement in capsules and tablets; 3–6 daily is my recommended dosage.

CAUTION: *Alfalfa has been known to aggravate lupus and should be avoided by anyone with that disease or any other autoimmune disorder.*

Garlic contains potassium, phosphorus, a significant amount of B and C vitamins, as well as calcium, protein, and some amazing health-giving compounds that have finally become recognized by traditional doctors for their remarkable medicinal value. A natural antibiotic, once relied on so heavily by the Soviet army that it became known as "Russian penicillin," it has now been found to lower cholesterol—specifically LDL (bad) cholesterol—and also act as a natural blood thinner, helping to prevent the formation of blood clots, offering protection against heart attack and stroke.

Recent research has shown that a component of garlic oil, diallyl sulfide (DAS), may inactivate potent carcinogens and suppress the growth of cancerous tumors. Garlic has also been found effective in lowering blood pressure, cleansing the blood of excess glucose (blood sugar ranks with cholesterol as a causative factor in arteriosclerosis and heart attacks), and alleviating bronchial congestion, sore throat, and flu symptoms.

The best way to take garlic as a supplement is in the form of aged, raw, odorless capsules. These leave no after-odor on the breath. For extra breath-friendly assurance, you might want to also take an internal breath freshener made from parsley seed oil.

Chlorophyll possesses positive antibacterial action. It also appears to act as a wound-healing agent, and, while stimulating the growth of new tissue, it reduces the hazard of bacterial contamination.

Nature's deodorant, it is used in commercial air fresheners, as a topical body deodorant, and as an oral breath refresher. It is available in tablets and in liquid preparations.

Yucca extract comes from the genus of trees and shrubs belonging to the *Liliaceae* family. (The Joshua tree is a yucca.) The Indians used the yucca for many purposes and revered it as a plant that guaranteed their health and survival. Dr. John W. Yale, a botanical biochemist, extracted the steroid saponin from the plant and used the extract in a tablet for the treatment of arthritis. The treatment proved safe and effective, the average dose being 4 tablets daily, and there was no gastrointestinal irritation. Yucca extract tablets and liquid are nontoxic and available in most health-food and vitamin stores. To help reduce inflammation and joint pain caused by arthritis or rheumatism, I'd suggest 1 tablet or capsule—or 10–30 drops liquid—up to three times daily.

CAUTION: *Long-term use may slow the absorption of fat-soluble vitamins such as A, D, E, and K. If you are using yucca over an extended period of time, check with your physician to see if you need supplements of these oil-soluble vitamins.*

137. Fiber and Bran

When research appeared in the *Journal of the American Medical Association* indicating that we would all be a great deal healthier and live longer if we ate coarser diets that sent more indigestible dietary fiber through our digestive tracts, a lot of people, wisely, jumped on the fiber bandwagon, though most weren't aware (and still aren't) that all fiber is not the same and that different types perform different functions.

Soluble fiber, for instance, dissolves in water. In your intestine it binds with bile and helps carry cholesterol out of your body. It also slows down the rate your stomach empties, giving it more time to extract nutrients from food and keeps you feeling full longer.

Insoluble fiber doesn't dissolve in water, but like soluble fiber it does absorb water and promotes movement of food through your digestive system, resulting in softer, bulkier stools that help alleviate constipation.

CAUTION: *Increase your fiber intake gradually to avoid uncomfortable consequences, and remember to increase your fluid intake at the same time.*

TYPES OF FIBER YOU SHOULD KNOW ABOUT AND WHERE TO FIND THEM

Cellulose: This is found in whole wheat flour, bran, cabbage, young peas, green beans, wax beans, broccoli, brussels sprouts, cucumber skins, peppers, apples, and carrots. (Provides insoluble fiber.)

Hemicelluloses: These are found in bran, cereals, whole grains, brussels sprouts, mustard greens, and beets. (Provide insoluble and soluble fiber.)

Cellulose and hemicelluloses absorb water and can smooth functioning of the large bowel. Essentially, they "bulk" waste and move it through the colon more rapidly. This not only can prevent constipation, but may also protect against diverticulosis, spastic colon, hemorrhoids, cancer of the colon, and varicose veins.

CAUTION: *Increased fiber is contraindicated in certain bowel disorders. A physician should be consulted before starting any high-fiber diet.*

Gums: These are usually found in oatmeal and other rolled-oat products as well as in dried beans. (Provide soluble fiber.)

Pectin: This is found in apples, citrus fruits, carrots, cauliflower, cabbage, dried peas, green beans, potatoes, squash, and strawberries. (Provides soluble fiber.)

Gums and pectin primarily influence absorption in the stomach and small bowel. By binding with bile acids, they decrease fat absorption and lower cholesterol levels. They delay stomach-emptying by coating the lining of the gut, and by so doing they slow sugar absorption after a meal, which is helpful to diabetics since it reduces the amount of insulin needed at any one time.

CAUTION: *Gums and pectin can interfere with the effectiveness of certain antifungal medications containing griseofulvin, such as Grifulvin V, Grisactin, and Fulvicin.*

Lignin: This type of fiber is found in breakfast cereals, bran, older vegetables (when vegetables age, their lignin content rises, and they become less digestible), eggplant, green beans, strawberries, pears, and radishes. (Provides insoluble fiber.)

Lignin reduces the digestibility of other fibers. It also binds with bile acids to lower cholesterol and helps speed food through the gut.

CAUTION: *While it's true that most of us still don't have enough fiber in our diets, too much can cause gas, bloating, nausea, vomiting, diarrhea, and possibly interfere with the body's ability to absorb certain minerals, such as zinc, calcium, iron, magnesium, and vitamin B12, though this is easily prevented by varying your diet along with your high-fiber foods.*

WHAT FIBER CAN DO FOR YOU:

Improve blood-cholesterol levels (Soluble fiber lowers LDL, "bad" cholesterol.)

Help prevent hemorrhoids.

Aid in attaining and maintaining a healthy weight.

Reduce risk of diverticular disease.

Help manage blood sugar levels and reduce risk of diabetes.

Significantly lower high blood pressure.

May reduce risk of small-bowel cancer.

Lower risk of digestive disorders such as irritable bowel syndrome (IBS).

CAUTION: *For people already suffering from IBS, fiber can make gas and cramping worse.*

HOW MUCH IS ENOUGH? *The recommended intake of fiber for adults is 20–38 g. a day. (For men over fifty, the target intake is 30 g.; under age fifty, it's 38 g. For women over age fifty, it's 21 g.; under fifty, it's 25 g.) When increasing fiber, remember to drink at least 8 cups of fluid daily. The following chart should help you locate sources that offer the most fiber bang for your food buck.*

FINDING FIBER FAST

Serving	Food	Grams of Fiber
1 cup	All-Bran cereal	23
¾ cup	All-Bran Buds cereal	18
1 medium	Avocado	12
1 cup	Acorn squash	9
½ cup	Black beans	8
1 cup	Raspberries	8
1 cup	Blackberries	7.2
½ cup	Lima beans	7
½ cup	Kidney beans	6.9
1 large	Apple	6
1 cup	Seedless raisins	6
¾ cup	Parsnips, cooked	5.9
1 cup cooked	Whole wheat spaghetti	5.4

5 dried	Peach halves	5.3
1½ cups popped	Low-fat popcorn	5
3 medium	Figs	5
1 large	Pear	5
1 medium	Potato with skin	5
1 cup	Yams	5
⅔ cup	Corn kernels	4.2
½ cup	Peas	4
1 average	Whole wheat muffin	4
1 medium	Carrot, raw	3.7

138. Kelp

This amazing seaweed contains more vitamins (especially Bs) and valuable minerals than any other food! Because of its natural iodine content, kelp has a normalizing effect on the thyroid gland. In other words, thin people with thyroid trouble can gain weight by using kelp, and obese people can lose weight with it. In fact, one of the most widespread fads for many years has been the kelp, lecithin, vinegar, and B6 diet (see section 399). Kelp has also been used by homeopathic physicians in the treatment of obesity, poor digestion, flatulence, obstinate constipation, and to protect against effects of radiation. It is reported to be very beneficial to brain tissue, the membrane surrounding the brain, the sensory nerves, and the spinal cord.

Kelp can be eaten raw, but it is usually dried and ground into a powder, which can be used as a flavoring or a salt substitute. It is also available in tablets and as a liquid.

I see more and more kelp as a snack in strips available in natural food stores. For the best selection find a Japanese or other Asian supermarket.

139. Mushrooms

Revered for centuries in China and Japan for their flavor and unique medicinal properties, mushrooms have finally come into the health spotlight in the West. They have been shown to strengthen the immune system, inhibit tumor growth, lower cholesterol, reduce blood pressure, help prevent heart attacks, work as an effective cancer therapy in combination with chemotherapy drugs, and more.

Mushrooms are high in water and low in fat, carbohydrates, and calories (a *fresh* pound has only 125 calories). But when they are dried, they have almost as much protein as veal, ounce for ounce. Cooking also removes moisture and concentrates protein. No mushrooms should be eaten raw in quantity.

Maitake mushroom (Grifola frondosa): This basketball-size mushroom, whose name literally means "dancing mushroom" because legend has it that those who find it start dancing with joy, works as an adaptogen, meaning it helps the body adapt to stress and normalize bodily functions. It has been shown to shrink tumors, enhance chemotherapy effectiveness, reduce chemo side effects such as nausea and fatigue, lower blood pressure as well as blood sugar, and prevent the destruction of T cells by HIV, the virus that causes AIDS—with little or no side effects. (Large doses of maitake on an empty stomach should be avoided.) Taking vitamin C along with mushroom supplements provides better absorption and enhances effectiveness. Dosages will vary according to individual health needs. For basic preventive purposes, I suggest one 100 mg. tablet daily.

Reishi mushroom (Ganoderma lucidum): Known as an "elixir of immortality" and one of the most valued plants in the Chinese pharmacopoeia for more than two thousand years, the reishi mushroom has been prescribed by Asian healers for hundreds of years for people suffering from angina or chest pain. Considered an adaptogen, increasing the body's resistance to stress and general well-being, reishi has been used with success as an analgesic, a natural anti-inflammatory agent, a remedy for insomnia, and as a cancer treatment. (Compounds in reishi activate macrophages and T cells, the disease fighters that help rid the body of all foreign invaders, including cancer cells.) Reishi has also been used to treat high cholesterol, liver disorders, chronic fatigue syndrome, and altitude sickness. It is available in capsule, pill, and extract form, as well as fresh or dried for use in foods. (Soak dried mushrooms in warm water or broth for half an hour before using.) Recommended dosages increase according to the severity of individual health needs. Though there is no known toxicity, for treating serious illness a nutritionally oriented practitioner always should be consulted. To ease joint pain, reduce inflammation, or as a general immune system booster, I advise 100 mg. extract of reishi daily.

Shiitake mushroom (Lentinus edodes): Another fungal wonder worker, the shiitake contains a polysaccharide called lentinan that strengthens the immune system by increasing T-cell function. It has also been found to inhibit tumor growth, according to studies reported by scientists from Japan's National Cancer Center. It may also lower cholesterol, prevent heart disease, and have antiviral properties equal to the prescription drug amantadine—without the serious side effects. Like reishi mushrooms (see above), shiitakes are available fresh, dried, and as supplements in capsule, pill, and extract form.

140. Shark Cartilage

Purified shark cartilage, derived from the tough, elastic material that makes up the skeleton of the shark, contains a compound that inhibits the development of new blood vessels that tumors need in order to grow, basically starving them. The cartilage supplement Benefin has been shown to have a similar mechanism to the prescription drugs angistatin and endostatin in the treatment of Kaposi's sarcoma and various forms of cancer. It has also been found to boost the immune system, help reduce arthritic pain and joint inflammation, as well as help treat psoriasis, scleroderma, eczema, and a host of other skin diseases. It is available in capsules and powder forms, but read labels carefully; not all products contain 100 percent pure shark cartilage.

CAUTION: *Shark cartilage blocks the body's ability to generate new blood vessels and should not be taken by children, bodybuilders, pregnant women, women attempting to conceive, or anyone who has recently suffered a heart attack or had major surgery.*

141. Propolis

A bee-smart wonder worker rich in bioflavonoids that appears to help protect against viruses, especially in the elderly and others with weakened immune systems. A by-product of honey, propolis has been valued for its medicinal wound-healing properties for thousands of years. It has natural antibiotic, antiviral, and anti-inflammatory compounds; and, in addition, recent studies show that it may inhibit the growth of cancerous cells in the colon.

Propolis can be used both externally and internally. It has been shown to be an excellent treatment for sore throats and gum disease. Additionally, it is effective against the herpes virus; when applied to herpes lesions, it can help relieve pain, when taken orally in capsule form, it can help stimulate immune function. As a supplement, propolis is available as a salve (to be used externally), as a lozenge (good for sore throats), and in capsule form. My supplement recommendation is one 200 mg. capsule daily. (As part of an antiaging regimen, 500 mg. capsules may be taken up to three times daily.)

142. Yeast

It's known as nature's wonder food, and it does a lot to deserve its reputation. Yeast is an excellent source of protein and a superior source of the natural B-complex vitamins. It is one of the richest sources of organic iron and a gold mine of minerals, trace minerals, and amino acids. It has been known to help lower cholesterol (when combined with lecithin), help reverse gout, and ease the aches and pains of neuritis.

There are various sources of yeast:

Brewer's yeast (from hops, a by-product of beer), sometimes called nutritional yeast.

Torula yeast, grown on wood pulp used in the manufacture of paper or from blackstrap molasses.

Whey, a by-product of milk and cheese (best-tasting and most potent nonyeast product).

Liquid yeast from Switzerland and Germany, fed on herbs, honey malt, and oranges or grapefruit.

Avoid live baker's yeast! Live yeast cells deplete the B vitamins in the intestines and rob your body of all vitamins. In nutritional yeast, these live cells are heat-killed, thus preventing that depletion.

Yeast has all the major B vitamins (except B12), which can be especially bred into it. It contains sixteen amino acids, fourteen or more minerals, and seventeen vitamins (except for A, E, and C). It can be considered a whole food.

Because yeast, like other protein foods, is high in phosphorus, it is advisable when taking it to add extra calcium to the diet. Phosphorus, though a coworker of calcium, can take calcium out of the body, leaving a deficiency. The remedy is simple: Increase your calcium (calcium lactate assimilates well in the body). *B-complex vitamins should be taken together with yeast to be more effective. Together they work like a powerhouse.*

Yeast can be stirred into liquid, juice, or water and taken between meals. Many people who feel fatigued take a tablespoon or more in liquid form and feel a return of energy within minutes, and the good effects last for several hours. Yeast can also be used as a reducing food. Stir into liquid and drink just before a meal. It takes the edge off a large appetite and saves you a lot in calories.

CAUTION: *Be aware that virtually all commercial yeast is produced using some form of genetic modification.*

143. The Soy Phenomenon

The biggest wonder about this wonder food is why more of us aren't eating it! For centuries, the Chinese and Japanese have been eating a diet high in soy foods and reaping impressive longevity benefits as well as much lower rates of death from cancer and heart disease than Americans. In fact, researchers now believe that adding as little as 2 ounces of soy food to your daily balanced diet can be a powerful protective weapon against disease!

Soy is high in fiber and rich in phytoestrogens, particularly the two important isoflavones, genistein and daidzein. (See section 110.) It is also one of the few plant foods that is a complete protein containing the proper balance of the eight essential amino acids. (See section 75.) The US government recognizes it as a protein alternative equivalent to meat, and, according to the *American Journal of Clinical Nutrition*, "except for premature infants, soy protein can serve as a sole protein source in the human body." As with other vegetable proteins, the nutritional value of soy is enhanced by eating it with a grain such as rice or pasta.

SOY ADVANTAGES OVER ANIMAL PROTEIN

- Lower in fat
- No cholesterol
- High in phytochemicals
- Good source of fiber
- Good source of minerals such as calcium, iron, magnesium, phosphorus, and the B vitamins thiamin, riboflavin, and niacin.

NOTE: *Soybeans—with the exception of tempeh, a fermented whole soybean product—are a poor source of vitamin B12. Vegetarians should take supplementary vitamin B12.*

POTENTIAL SOY BENEFITS

- Antioxidants present in soy foods may protect against many forms of cancer as well as premature aging.
- May slow down or prevent kidney damage in people with impaired kidney function.
- Can help lower cholesterol levels.

- Help retain bone density and prevent osteoporosis.
- Lower risk of colon and rectal cancers.
- Aid in boosting the immune system.
- Can help lower blood pressure in menopausal woman.
- Help stave off colds.
- May alleviate hot flashes in menopausal women.

SOY FOODS AND PRODUCTS TO CHOOSE AND CHOOSE FROM

Soy nuts: These are deep-fried or dry-roasted soybeans, often salted or flavored with seasoning. An excellent source of protein, fiber, and isoflavones. In a recent study of 61 menopausal women (12 with high blood pressure and 49 with normal blood pressure) Dr. Francine Welty found that women with high blood pressure who consumed one-half cup of roasted low-sodium soy nuts for eight weeks lowered their systolic blood pressure by 10 percent and their diastolic blood pressure by 7 percent. The women with normal blood pressure lowered theirs by half that. Keep in mind, though, like other nuts, soy nuts are high in fat and calories.

Soy sprouts: Whole soybeans that have been sprouted for up to six days. Good source of protein and fiber. Easy to add to vegetable dishes.

Fresh green soybeans: These are the bean and fuzzy green pod. Unlike dried soybeans, they are eaten young, steamed like fresh vegetables, and a good source of protein, fiber, and isoflavones. A popular Japanese snack known as *edamame*, soybean in the pod, is also served in many natural-food restaurants in the United States.

Soy milk: Lactose-free, soy milk is made by soaking and grinding whole soybeans with water. It is also made by adding water to whole, full-fat soy flour. It is a great source of isoflavones, protein, B vitamins, and minerals. (Only fortified soy milk, however, contains as much calcium, vitamin D, or B12 as regular milk.)

Tofu: A white, cheeselike cake made from soy milk. (Also called bean curd.) Available in many different forms, it can literally soak up any flavor that is added to it. In fact, it's so versatile it can be used as a cheese as well as a meat substitute. Firm tofu (cotton tofu) is higher in protein, fat, and calcium than other forms; it's best in cooked dishes when you want it to retain its shape and consistency. Soft tofu (silken tofu) is creamier and good puréed or blended. Yakidofu is firm tofu that's been lightly broiled, and koyodofu is freeze-dried tofu that must be reconstituted before being used in cooking. Powdered instant tofu mix is also available.

Natto: Fermented soybeans, a traditional Japanese staple for more than one thousand years (especially as a breakfast food), has been found to help prevent heart attacks, cancer, strokes, osteoporosis, intestinal disease caused by pathogens, and more. It is easy to make and inexpensive, but you need to acquire a taste for it. Unfortunately, that might not be so easy. Natto is stringy, gooey, and smells awful—but it does have remarkably bountiful health benefits.

Miso: A versatile, fermented bean paste that can be used as a condiment, made into soup, or used as a base for salad dressings and sauces. It is low in fat, but high in sodium, and can keep in the refrigerator for up to a year.

CAUTION: *It's advisable to avoid miso if you have high blood pressure or are sodium sensitive.*

Soy sauce: One of the world's most popular condiments, this salty sauce—made from a fermented mixture of soybeans, wheat, and *aspergillus* spores—does not contain isoflavones, but some studies suggest it does have other anticarcinogenic compounds. Though low-sodium soy sauce is available, at 605 mg. per tablespoon it isn't "no-sodium sauce"; I'd suggest you pass on it if you have high blood pressure or are sodium sensitive.

Soy protein isolate (or isolated soy protein): Sold as a plain or flavored powder that contains at least 90 percent protein. Frequently found in meal-replacement bars, infant formulas, and "muscle-building" protein powders, it is a powerful cholesterol-lowering agent, and can be used as a fat-reducing meat extender in baking, sprinkled on cereal, or blended with fruit or juice for a non-dairy shake. If you can't find soy protein isolate, look for a protein powder that has soy protein isolate as the first or second ingredient. (*NOTE*: Products labeled "soy protein" could merely refer to soy flour, which is lower in protein than isolated soy protein and often higher in fat. Read labels carefully.)

Soy flour: A terrific source of isoflavones, soy flour contains no less than 50 percent protein. Made from the "meat" of the roasted soybean, full-fat soy flour can be very full in fat, so look for defatted or low-fat flour, which is actually a more concentrated source of protein. Though it is good for microwave baking because it helps retain moisture, keep in mind that soy flour is gluten-free, which means it cannot be used as a substitute for wheat or rye flour in yeast-raised breads. (In non-yeast-raised products, you can substitute 20 percent of the total flour with the heavier soy flour.)

Texturized soy protein: Made from soy flour, texturized soy protein (TSP) is low in fat and calories and high in protein, isoflavones, calcium, iron, and zinc. It can be used to replace part or all of the meat in ground beef dishes such as meat loaf, chili, or hamburgers, but must be rehydrated before use in recipes.

Soybean oil: Though it does not contain isoflavones, soy oil—unlike most other vegetable oils—is rich in omega-3 and omega-6 fatty acids similar to those found in marine fish oils. (See section 100.) It also contains linoleic acid, which is essential for life but cannot be produced by the body. Nonetheless, like all oils, it should be used sparingly.

Soy supplements: Tablets rich in the isoflavones genistein and daidzein are available. The recommended daily dose is two 10 mg. tablets for men and four 10 mg. tablets for women.

CAUTION: *Eating huge amounts of soy foods may interfere with thyroid function, triggering goiter (enlargement of the thyroid) and hypothyroidism.*

BEST FOODS AND SUPPLEMENTS FOR 2020'S CONDITIONS

144. Healthy Skin

1. Fatty fish such as cod, mackerel, albacore tuna, wild salmon, sardines, and anchovies—rich in omega-3s, which decrease inflammation that can cause redness and acne
2. Avocados—essential to keep your skin flexible and moisturized
3. Walnuts—rich in essential fatty acids, which decrease inflammation
4. Sunflower seeds—excellent source of vitamin E, an antioxidant for healthy skin

5. Red or yellow red peppers—excellent source of vitamin C and beta-carotene. Beta-carotene converts to vitamin A, which protects your skin from harmful sun damage

6. Sweet potatoes—a good source of beta-carotene, a natural sunblock

7. Broccoli—a good source of zinc, vitamins A and C. All are important for healthy skin

8. Tomatoes—a source of vitamin C, which is important for collagen production

9. Soy—can reduce wrinkles and improve skin flexibility

10. Dark chocolate—rich in antioxidants, which help the skin to be thicker and more hydrated

11. Green tea—protects your skin from the damage of aging by neutralizing harmful oxidative stress

12. Red wine—contains resveratrol, which reduces the effect of dryness, wrinkles, and aging to your skin

13. Hyaluronic acid—lost during sun exposure, which weakens skin structures and leads to age-related dryness and wrinkles

14. Collagen—same as hyaluronic acid

145. Super Foods and Fruits

1. Mangosteen—boosts immunity, regulates blood pressure and heart health, works as an anti-inflammatory, boosts skin care, helps digestion problems such as upset stomach, and has weight management effects

2. Goji berries—protect vision; decrease risk of certain cancers; promote healthy skin; stabilize blood sugar; improve depression, anxiety, and sleep; and prevent liver damage

3. Acai berries—rich in antioxidants and boost brain function

4. Blueberries ("brain berries")—enhance heart health; maintain brain function; sustain healthy blood sugar levels (when already within normal range); support smooth, firm skin; improve movement and coordination

5. Cranberries—are high in fiber and antioxidants, are anti-inflammatory, support gut health, support immunity, support urinary tract health

6. Acerola berries—are rich in vitamin C and are a potent antioxidant

7. Apples—are high in fiber, are heart healthy, lower the risk of diabetes, promote gut health, can help fight asthma

8. Bananas—are a good source of vitamin C and potassium, improve digestive health, are highly filling, improve insulin sensitivity

9. Walnuts—contain antioxidants, offer immune function support, are a good source of omega-3 and vitamin E, promote healthy gut, support weight control, help manage type 2 diabetes, lower blood pressure

10. Fucoidan (edible nutrient in seaweed)—slows blood clotting, boosts immune system, fights against infections, regulates inflammation, assists digestion, is anti-aging and an antioxidant, assists weight loss by boosting your metabolism

11. Resveratrol—An anti-aging nutrient and antioxidant, lowers blood pressure, lengthens life span in animals, offers brain protection, decreases joint pain, increases blood flow

12. Pine bark extract—boosts antioxidant strains, improves erectile dysfunction, balances blood sugar, fights off

the common cold, boosts brain function, reduces inflammation

13. RNA—offers memory and digestive health support, is anti-aging, assists injury management

14. Pomegranate—blocks inflammation; decreases the risk of the formation, growth, and spread of cancer; is heart healthy

146. Brain and Memory Supplements

1. Butterbur—helps relax the constrictions of cerebral blood vessels, reduces pain from migraines, fights insomnia, stimulates appetite, reduces pain from urinary tract infections, calms stomach upset, eases symptoms of hay fever

2. Blueberries—help inhibit age-related decline in overall cognitive function

3. Choline—improves memory and cognition, boosts metabolism, improves cystic fibrosis symptoms. Other benefits: is heart healthy, reduces pregnancy complications

4. Dopamine—encourages mental activity by suppressing cerebral artery dilation for healthy brain blood flow

5. Huperzine A—maintains healthy levels of acetylcholine, enhances memory learning, reduces inflammation, boosts energy

6. Inositol—can reduce anxiety, promotes normal hormone levels, promotes female fertility, promotes healthy mood, other benefits: supports regular menstruation, heart healthy

7. Lithium—promotes brain health and prevents depression, prevents age-related cognitive decline, and supports memory health. A 300 mg. capsule can

be obtained by prescription only, but lithium carbonate is available over the counter in 30 mg. capsule strength. Lithium was also an ingredient in the original recipe for the soft drink 7UP!

8. Magnesium—supports high blood pressure treatment by aiding blood vessel relaxation and dilation; prevents headaches; prevents clots from forming inside blood vessels; tempers the secretion of aldosterone, which causes the kidneys to retain sodium and water, affecting blood pressure; reduces the level of catecholamines released in response to stressors, thereby relaxing the fight-or-flight stress response and preventing vasoconstriction, which raises blood pressure; protects against the aging and hardening of the arteries; protects the blood vessel lining against permeability that allows more LDL cholesterol into the vessel wall; protects against metabolic syndrome and type 2 diabetes, thereby also protecting against atherosclerosis; supports healthy memory and youthful cognitive function

9. Phosphatidyl serine—supports brain cellular structure and function; helps your brain use its fuel efficiently by facilitating glucose metabolism and stimulating the production of acetylcholine, an essential neurotransmitter

10. Pregnenolone—increases energy and endurance, is anti-stress. Other benefits: improves immunity, promotes healthy skin

11. Sage leaf extract—supports attention and memory; promotes positive mood and cognitive performance; promotes healthy modulation of neurotransmitters such as GABA, dopamine, and serotonin

12. Vinpocetine—promotes cognitive function, supports oxygen and nutrient delivery to the brain, prevents motion sickness

147. Heart Health Update

1. Nitric oxide—widens blood vessels and keeps them flexible, is essential in small amounts. Low nitric oxide can cause erectile dysfunction
2. Vitamin D3—reduces arterial stiffness, which contributes to heart attacks, strokes, and cognitive decline; restores healthy balance between two compounds key to endothelial function—nitric oxide and peroxynitrite—thereby reducing overall risk for heart disease; restores the normal ratio of endothelial cells

148. Bone Health Update

1. Vitamin K—supports healthy bones and joints, is necessary for proper blood coagulation, helps avoid calcium deposits in the arteries and blood vessels
2. Boron—builds strong bones, treats osteoporosis, aids in building muscle, increases testosterone levels, increases thinking skills, increases muscle coordination
3. Magnesium—prevents heart attacks, regulates the severity of angina pain, promotes a healthier cardiovascular system, keeps cholesterol levels under control
4. Zinc—stimulates the activity of about 300 enzymes, fortifies your immune system, maintains healthy vision, lessens symptoms of the common cold, is an antidepressant, is anti-acne, decreases risk of diabetes
5. Silicon—treats weak bones; is anti-stroke; is heart healthy; supports healthy hair, skin, and nails
6. Bone broth—builds healthy bones
7. Manganese—improves bone health in combination with other nutrients; works as a cofactor in

manganese sod, a potent antioxidant; is beneficial in treating osteoporosis, arthritis, PMS, diabetes, and epilepsy

8. Threonine—supports a healthy immune system by helping in the production of collagen, supports liver and bone health, provides connective tissue support, is essential for the production of collagen

149. Digestive Enzymes for Gut Health

As we age, our digestive tract loses the ability to tolerate the effect of too many calories, especially fried fast foods that are rich in hydrogenated vegetable oils and other saturated fats.

1. Proteinase—breaks down protein
2. Lactase—breaks down milk sugar from dairy products
3. Lipase—breaks down fats
4. Cellulase—breaks down fiber, which prevents digestive gas
5. Amylase—breaks down carbohydrates and sugars
6. Bromelain (the pineapple enzyme)—improves digestion and absorption of protein and fat
7. Probiotics—help restore balance to your gut, which prevents constipation

150. Hormonal Balance Supplements

1. DHEA—promotes healthy mood, sexual function, and well-being; helps support and maintain lean muscle mass; encourages healthy immune function; is heart healthy

2. Broccoli—promotes liver health, estrogen metabolism, and hormone health

3. Watercress and cabbage—promote healthy estrogen metabolism and cell division

4. Pregnenolone—supports youthful hormone levels, maintains mental focus, maintains memory health

151. Nature's Most Powerful Antibiotics

1. Apple cider vinegar
2. Garlic
3. Ginger
4. Horseradish root
5. Habanero peppers
6. Oregano oil
7. Echinacea
8. Curcumin
9. Raw honey
10. Onions

152. Prostate Health Supplements

Promote healthy sex and function of the prostate, help maintain prostate specific antigen (PSA) levels that already exist, promote healthy prostate cell division, support healthy urination, support healthy inflammation response, and encourage healthy prostate hormone metabolism.

1. Lycopene
2. Boron
3. Saw palmetto
4. Boswellia extract
5. Pollen extract

6. Pygeum
7. Pumpkin seeds
8. Phospholipids
9. Flax seed
10. Stinging nettle root

153. Protection from Blood Clots

1. Olive oil decreases production of pro-inflammatory and pro-thrombiotic factors.
2. Tea EGCG decreases plaque formation.
3. Quercetin inhibits collagen-induced platelet aggregation.
4. Fish oil decreases platelet accumulation and aggregation.
5. Curcumin decreases fat peroxidation and plasma fibrinogens, which can hasten hardening of your arteries.
6. Pine bark extract contain polyphenols with anti-inflammatory and free radical scavenger properties.
7. Pomegranate juice drunk over two weeks reduces platelet aggregation.

154. Circulation Supplements

1. Nattokinase enzyme (natto) has an anti-clotting effect.
2. Pine bark extract—supports healthy blood flow and vascular function, promotes your body's natural clotting process, helps maintain healthy blood pressure
3. Gotu kola helps maintain arterial plaque stability
4. Olive leaf extract—supports optimal heart health, inhibits inflammation to support vascular system health

155. Supplements for Energy Management

1. NAD creates ADP, which is the compound your body uses for fuel.
2. PQQ—super-charges cell energy production, promotes the growth of new cellular mitochondria, encourages youthful cellular energy levels, provide powerful antioxidant protection, supports heart and cognitive health

156. Supplements for Healthy Eyes

1. Lutein, zeaxanthin, and meso-zeanthin—help maintain healthy pigment density, help your eyes defend against blue light from digital devices, help against the effects of light glare.
2. Astaxanthin fights eye fatigue.
3. Black currant berry helps older eyes see better at night.
4. Maqui berry promotes healthy tear production and supports healthy eye function.
5. Pine bark extract promotes healthy circulation that helps maintain already healthy ocular pressure.

157. Blood Sugar Management

Maqui berry and clove extract help maintain already healthy blood sugar levels after you eat, encourage healthy blood sugar production in the liver, and promote healthy insulin response and hemoglobin A1c levels.

158. Foods and Nutrients for Healthy Lungs and Better Breathing

1. Bananas, avocados, and oranges are excellent sources of vitamin C.

2. Sweet potatoes are a source of vitamin A and potassium.
3. Vitamin D3
4. Omega-3 fatty acids
5. Mushrooms (maitake, morel, chanterelle, shiitake) are a source of vitamin D.
6. Thyme is anti-cough.
7. Apples, onions, grapes, citrus fruits, cherries, and capers all are sources of quercetin.
8. Ginger is important for lung health.
9. Garlic is a detoxifier.
10. Horseradish opens the sinuses.

159. Sports Activity Supplements

1. Tart cherry extract (anthocyanins)—contains potent antioxidants, promotes rapid muscle recovery and faster relief from minor discomfort and stiffness that come with exercise, promotes healthy blood flow, and inhibits peripheral muscle fatigue
2. Whey protein isolate, l-glutamine, and creatine—help build lean muscle, support against protein breakdown, and promote immune system health and longevity
3. Branch chain amino acids (BCAA)—build lean muscle mass and promote healthy immune function

160. Most Popular Supplements of the 2020s

1. Curcumin (turmeric)—is anti-inflammatory and heart healthy, reduces symptoms of osteoporosis, decreases risk of type 2 diabetes and Alzheimer's, is antidepressant, helps treat rheumatoid arthritis, improves skin

health, is antioxidant and anti-aging, and prevents eye degeneration

2. Astaxanthin—is antioxidant, heart healthy, and eye healthy; helps prevent Alzheimer's and Parkinson's; is anti-inflammatory; and can help against plaque buildup in arteries in the heart

3. Vitamin D3—supports lung function and heart health, can protect against cancer and type 2 diabetes, helps prevent obesity, prevents hair loss, prevents respiratory tract infections and autoimmune disease, prevents belly fat in women and liver/abdominal fat in men, helps calcium absorption, promotes healthy bones and teeth, and regulates insulin levels

4. AMPK—supports weight loss, particularly by decreasing belly fat, increases insulin sensitivity, reduces cholesterol, reduces chronic inflammation, regulates energy usage and maintains homeostasis, supports healthy aging, and improves endurance in physical performance

5. Methylsulfonylmethane (MSM)—promotes healthy hair, skin, and nails; enhances hair growth, appearance, and condition; reduces fine lines and wrinkles; supports good joint health and mobility and reduces pain and stiffness; promotes muscle growth and speeds recovery from workout fatigue; supports immune health; and is anti-inflammatory.

6. Cinnamon—is anti-inflammatory and rich in antioxidants, lowers the risk of heart disease, improves sensitivity to insulin, lowers blood sugar, and is antidiabetic

7. Asparagine—may play a role in deadly triple-negative breast cancer; is important for production of the body's proteins, enzymes, and muscle tissue; and balances nervous system function.

8. Taurine—maintains healthy energy supply, increases growth of new brain cells, decreases oxidative stress, and decreases inflammation

9. N-acetyl-l-cysteine—is essential in making glutathione, one of the body's most powerful antioxidants; aids in detoxification process, thereby reducing kidney and liver damage; helps regulate glutamate, an important neurotransmitter; boosts brain health and helps maintain good mental state and mood; relieves symptoms of respiratory conditions; may improve fertility in men and women; decreases inflammation in fat cells and may stabilize blood sugar; prevents oxidative damage and may protect against heart disease; and works as an immune booster.

10. Krill oil—is an excellent source of omega-3; lowers LDL (bad) cholesterol; can raise HDL (good) cholesterol; and can treat high blood pressure, osteoarthritis, depression, and PMS

11. New Zealand green lipped mussel—can help treat asthma, exercise-induced muscle soreness, ADHD, osteoarthritis, and rheumatoid arthritis

12. Gamma tocopherol—is heart healthy; decreases cancer risk; is an antioxidant and anti-inflammatory; is hair-and-skin healthy, anti-aging, and brain-protecting; and improves gut health

13. Delta tocopherol—protects brain from radical oxygen molecules, reduces cancer risk, improves gut health, and improves hair and skin health

Just because herbs are natural doesn't mean that they can be used indiscriminately. Before trying any herbal remedy, be sure you know what it does, how to prepare and use it—and what cautions or side effects you should be aware of.

As a rule, few medical problems occur from ingesting herbal remedies, but the potential for an allergic or toxic response is always there.

IMPORTANT: *If you are now taking any drugs, or have any medical problems, it's wise to consult a nutritionally oriented physician who is aware of herb-drug interactions, as well as any potentially dangerous side effects.*

161. Aloe Vera

The aloe vera plant contains a wound-healing substance called aloe vera gel, a mixture of antibiotic, astringent, and coagulating agents.

Taken internally, it works as a mild laxative. One tablespoon taken at regular intervals (preferably on an empty stomach), totaling a pint a day, can help in the treatment of stomach ulcers.

External uses of aloe vera gel are many.

- It acts as an immediate and effective wound healer, aiding in the treatment of burns, insect stings, and poison ivy. Split a leaf and apply pulp directly to the injured area, or soak cloth with aloe vera gel and bind on.
- Aloe vera gel ointments, creams, and lotions can prevent blistering and peeling from sunburn.
- It can help soften corns and calluses on the feet.
- Applied to the face and throat, it can soften skin and hold aging lines in check.
- It can alleviate the pain and itching of hemorrhoids and bleeding piles.
- It can be used as an effective hair conditioner.

CAUTION: *As an ointment it can cause hives, rashes, itching, and other allergic reactions in sensitive individuals—and can be extremely dangerous if taken internally by pregnant women.*

162. Amla (Indian Gooseberry)

If you've been looking for a way to increase the effectiveness of your vitamin C, look into amla. Rich in polyphenols and flavanoids, it has been found to help in the treatment of respiratory and intestinal problems, including asthma, gout, constipation, and colitis, among others. Pilot studies have also found it to lower cholesterol levels in men and to be effective against such age-related disorders as osteoporosis, heart palpitations, and deteriorating vision.

As a supplement, amla powder—which has a bit of a spicy taste—can be added to a variety of recipes, from soups and salads to gravies and pasta. The suggested dose is 2 tsp. a day.

163. Anise (Seed)

This is a natural diuretic and gastric stimulant and is often used to relieve flatulence. It's also been used in home remedies as a treatment for dry cough and has been known to stimulate milk production in nursing mothers.

As a supplement, crush seeds into a powder. Add 1 tsp. to a cup of boiling water and drink three times daily.

164. Arnica

Commonly called leopard's bane, the daisylike flower heads of this summer-flowering plant have been used in homeopathic remedies for hundreds of years to reduce inflammation and pain. Arnica stimulates the activity of white blood cells, dispersing trapped fluids from injured tissue. As an external ointment it is rubbed on the affected area and provides healing and pain relief for bruises, sprains, burns, eczema, muscle strains, and acne. It has antibacterial and anti-inflammatory qualities that can reduce swelling and improve wound healing—but it should *not* be applied to broken or bleeding skin.

Arnica is also available as sublingual pellets, frequently recommended by homeopathic physicians to be taken pre- and postsurgery to minimize bruising. The usual dose is 4 pellets under the tongue the night before, the morning of the surgery, and the morning after.

CAUTION: *Arnica is known to stimulate blood circulation and can raise blood pressure.*

165. Artichoke

The heart of this popular vegetable—the flower of the plant—tastes great when baked, steamed, marinated, or combined in recipes with other veggies. But the artichoke is much more than a culinary treat. Reputed to be an aphrodisiac (although never scientifically proven), artichokes have been found to lower cholesterol levels after being eaten. In fact, an anticholesterol drug, cynara, is derived from this herb. Additionally, artichokes have been shown to increase bile production of the liver and work as a good diuretic.

166. Ashwagandha

The roots of this shrub, found in North America and in India, have been used for centuries in ayurvedic medicine for their anti-inflammatory, antitumor, antistress, antioxidant properties. Recent lab studies have borne out ashwagandha's reputation as an antidepressant and memory booster.

The root extract is available as a supplement in 450 mg. strengths, and a dosage of 1 capsule two to three times daily has been found to be effective in relieving stress and healing broken bones.

CAUTION: *This herb is not recommended for children, pregnant or breast-feeding women, or anyone taking other medications unless directed to do so by a physician.*

167. Astragalus

This herb has been found to alleviate fatigue, lessen the frequency of colds, and help provide support for the respiratory system, which often falls under attack from influenza. An all-around immune system booster, it improves resistance to viruses and bacterial infections while also accelerating healing. It may also prevent the spread of malignant cancer cells to healthy tissue. It works best with zinc and vitamins A and C.

As a supplement, take 1–3 (400 mg.) capsules daily.

CAUTION: *If you are undergoing chemotherapy, do not take astragalus—or any other medication—without first consulting your doctor.*

168. Basil

Sweet basil is a plant that can be used as a poultice to draw poison from the skin. It is frequently used to alleviate bee stings and to draw underskin pimples to a head.

169. Bilberry

An herb that has been a folk remedy for poor vision and night blindness for years, bilberry works by accelerating the regeneration of retinol—visual—purple, a substance required for good eyesight. It has also been found to help prevent eye damage and in some cases reduce the severity of myopia. Additionally, bilberries have been used for varicose veins, hemorrhoid conditions, and venous insufficiency of the lower limbs, as well as overall vascular support.

Supplements are available in capsule and extract form. Recommended dosage is 1 capsule one to three times daily, or mix 15 to 40 drops of extract in water or juice, and drink three times daily.

CAUTION: *The leaves of this herb can be poisonous if consumed over a long period of time. Although the prepared extract is safe, do not exceed the recommended dosage.*

170. Black Cohosh

A natural, hormone replacement therapy (HRT) alternative and one of the most popular herbs for relief of hot flashes and other menopausal symptoms. It is also used to induce menstruation, relieve menstrual cramps, promote labor, and ease delivery. Persistent coughs, swelling and soreness due to rheumatism have also benefited from black cohosh. Combined with skullcap, wood betony, passionflower, and valerian, it works as a natural tranquilizer.

Supplements are available in capsule and extract form. Recommended dosage is 1 capsule one to three times daily. If using an extract, follow directions on bottle.

CAUTION: *Black cohosh may not be safe for women who have breast cancer or undetected breast tumors. Use of black cohosh is also not recommended for women undergoing chemotherapy, as it has been found to increase the toxicity of chemotherapy drugs doxorubicin (Adriamycin) and docetaxel (Taxotere). That it makes these drugs more potent may or may not be a good thing, but while there's doubt, I would suggest avoiding it. Do not use black cohosh during pregnancy until in labor and then only under a doctor's supervision. Large doses can cause symptoms of poisoning.*

171. Black Currant

An effective anti-inflammatory herb and a rich source of antioxidants and vitamins, black currant's oil-rich seeds contain significant amounts of essential fatty acids (EFAs), including gamma-linolenic acid (GLA). The oil can help increase circulation, reduce muscle stiffness in rheumatoid arthritis sufferers, and lessen the severity of premenstrual cramps and breast tenderness. It has also been found to help with dry skin disorders.

Supplements of black currant seed oil are available in capsule form. Recommended dosage is one to three 500 mg. capsules daily.

172. Blessed Thistle

Often used as an appetite stimulant and in the treatment of digestive problems, it can reduce fevers and break up congestion.

Supplements are available in capsule and extract form. Recommended dosage is 1–3 capsules daily, or mix 10–20 drops in juice or water and drink once a day.

CAUTION: *In high doses, this can cause burns of the mouth and esophagus, as well as diarrhea. It may also reduce effectiveness of antacids and is not recommended for anyone with stomach ulcers, acid reflux, or a hiatal hernia.*

173. Boswellia

Found to have anti-inflammatory and antiarthritic properties, this ayurvedic herb derived from the resin of Indian frankincense acts much like NSAIDs (nonsteroidal anti-inflammatory agents) to treat pain. But unlike NSAIDs such as aspirin and ibuprofen, boswellia extract can be used for significant periods of time without causing stomach upset.

As a supplement, the recommended dosage is one 300 mg. capsule three times a day with food.

174. Butcher's Broom

Used to improve circulation and reduce edema in legs or feet, butcher's broom is particularly helpful to people who are on the feet all day and as a result experience swelling at night. This herb also contains steroidal-type compounds that can constrict veins and reduce inflammation, making it helpful in easing the pain and swelling of arthritis and rheumatism. Many people find that butcher's broom, taken orally or used as an ointment, significantly reduces the discomfort caused by hemorrhoids.

Supplements are available in capsule and extract form. Recommended dosage is 1–3 capsules daily, or mix 10–20 drops in juice or water and drink once a day.

175. Calendula

An aromatic annual plant of the Asteraceae family with antiseptic, anti-inflammatory, and antioxidant properties known for promoting healing. Found to quickly seal the edges of minor cuts and help prevent the formation of scar tissue, it is frequently used in the homeopathic treatment of scrapes, cuts, muscle strains, abscesses, and other skin ulcerations.

In addition to its topical uses, calendula has also been used as a mouthwash for gum and tooth infections. As a tea, it has been used to treat bladder infections.

CAUTION: *Calendula salve (or any fat-based preparations) should not be applied to wounds that are oozing or weeping. On recently stitched wounds, it's advisable to wait until the stitches have been removed and scabs have formed before applying calendula ointments. Although nontoxic, it should not be taken internally during pregnancy.*

176. Camphora (*Camphoroa officinarum, Cinnamomum camphora, Laurus camphora*)

Obtained from the leaves of the Cinnamomum camphora tree (and other evergreens in that family), this herb has been used for centuries as a culinary spice as well as a medicine. One of the five most popular homeopathic herbs, camphora, which is said to increase energy, is used therapeutically for the relief of general coldness (particularly of extremities), cramps, anxiety, minor physical trauma, and recovery from flu symptoms.

CAUTION: *Camphora is not recommended for use by anyone with asthma or allergies.*

177. Cat's Claw (Una de Gato)

Used by herbal healers in South and Central America for centuries to strengthen the immune system, cat's claw contains a natural anti-inflammatory agent found helpful as a treatment for arthritis. Compounds from the plant also have anticancer properties and have been found helpful by some HIV-positive patients in increasing their T-cell count.

Supplements are available in capsule form. Recommended dosage is 1–3 capsules daily.

CAUTION: *Excessive intake may cause diarrhea.*

178. Cayenne or Capsicum

Cayenne, also known as capsicum, is more than a spice, it's an overall digestive aid. It actually helps relieve gas! Cayenne also has a beneficial effect on blood fats, reducing triglycerides and low-density lipoproteins (LDL), or "bad" cholesterol. (See section 93.) Additionally, capsicum, the compound that gives cayenne its kick, has been found to trigger the release of endorphins, brain chemicals that can cause a mild euphoria and relieve pain. As a tea, it's great for alleviating the discomfort of colds and chills. As an ointment, it's been found to reduce the stiffness and inflammation of rheumatism and arthritis.

Supplements are available as capsules. Recommended dosage is 1–3 capsules daily.

CAUTION: *Do not exceed recommended dosage. High dosages taken internally may cause gastroenteritis and kidney damage. Cayenne should not be used by anyone with gastrointestinal problems. The ointment can be irritating to hemorrhoids and should never be applied to broken skin.*

179. Chamomile

This plant has antispasmodic and gastric-stimulant prop-erties, and is usually taken internally for migraines, gastric cramps, and anxiety. Externally it's used as a treatment for wounds, skin ulcers, and conjuctivitis.

Supplements are available in capsule and extract form. Recommended dosage is one capsule one to three times daily, or mix 10–20 drops of extract in water and drink one to three times daily. As a tea, which is much tastier, drink a cup a day and enjoy it.

CAUTION: *May cause severe allergic reactions—including fatal shock—in individuals with hay fever, or those sensitive to ragweed, asters, and related plants.*

180. Chasteberry (Vitex)

The fruit of the Mediterranean chasteberry tree (also known as Vitex or chaste tree) remains extremely popular in Europe where it is used to treat bloating, mood swings, and other symptoms of PMS, as well as the unpleasant side effects associated with menopause, such as hot flashes and vaginal dryness. With all the new information about the risks in taking the popular hormone-replacement ther-apy Prempro, chasteberry is a terrific natural alternative. Reputed to be a hormone balancer, and possibly helpful in the treatment of infertility, it has also been used success-fully in treating fibroid tumors.

As a supplement, I suggest taking 1 capsule up to three times daily (400 mg. per day). Or mix 10–30 drops of extract in liquid and drink up to three times daily.

181. Comfrey (aka *Symphytum officinalis*)

Because this herb contains allantoin, a cell proliferent that accelerates the natural replacement of body cells, it has been used to treat a wide variety of ailments, from bronchial problems to broken bones. It assists in cartilage repair, healing of joints, relieving neuralgia, and is reputed to have teeth-building properties in children. When used in teas, comfrey has been found to alleviate stomach ailments, coughs, diarrhea, arthritis pain, and liver and gallbladder conditions. As an external salve, comfrey ointments are effective in soothing skin irritations and promoting wound healing.

CAUTION: *Whether called symphytum or comfrey, this herb by any name still contains pyrrolizidine alkaloids, compounds known to cause liver disease if taken over a long period of time. Opinions differ as to its safety, but because of this uncertainty, I don't recommend that it be taken internally. There are other, much safer herbs that can be used instead, such as peppermint and ginger. I'd also suggest that the salves being marketed to nursing mothers with chafed nipples be avoided since comfrey should not be ingested by infants.*

182. Cranberry

Cranberry sauce is a favorite side dish for turkey, but the cranberry is also one of the best natural weapons against cystitis and urinary tract infections and routinely recommended as a preventive by doctors. Safe for pregnant and lactating women, it is cited in the United States Pharmacopeia official listing of drugs as an effective remedy for these problems. Cranberry extract capsules, in a 50:1 concentration of 4,200 mg., can suppress overactive urinary and bladder function by preventing the bacteria from sticking to the walls of the bladder.

Supplements are available as capsules. The recommended dosage is 1 capsule one to three times daily. Commercial cranberry juice cocktails are highly sweetened and processed and not recommended. Real cranberry juice is effective but extremely tart. You might find a cranberry-apple juice combination at a health-food store that would work, provided it doesn't contain added sugar.

183. Devil's Claw

An anti-inflammatory found to promote flexibility in joints, reducing pain caused by arthritis and rheumatism. European studies of the root of this herb have compared its anti-inflammatory action to the drugs cortisone and phenylbutazone.

Supplements are available as capsules. Recommended dosage is 1 capsule one to three times daily.

CAUTION: *Should not be taken during pregnancy.*

184. Dong Quai

An herb shown to be effective in alleviating menopausal hot flashes, as well as vaginal dryness and depression, and often used as a natural alternative to hormone replacement therapy. Chinese women have used this herb for centuries to regulate the menstrual cycle and reduce painful menstrual cramps caused by uterine contractions. It's used frequently to treat premenstrual syndrome (PMS) and to help women resume normal menstruation after going off the pill. It potentiates the effectiveness of female (as well as male) sex hormones and helps the body to maximize utilization of existing hormones. For instance, during menopause, it assists the transition of estrogen production from the ovaries to the adrenal glands.

Supplements are available as capsules. Recommended dosage is 1 capsule one to three times daily.

CAUTION: *Do not use dong quai during pregnancy. It should also not be used if you are still menstruating or typically have a heavy flow unless directed to do so by a nutritionally oriented doctor.*

Do not use dong quai if you are using the blood thinner warfarin (Coumadin), as it may increase the risk of bleeding.

Some people using dong quai may develop photosensitivity.

185. Echinacea

This herb has been found to protect healthy cells from viral and bacterial attack by stimulating activity of the immune system in general and T cells—which attack pathogens and toxins—in particular. The immunity-enhancing effect may take several weeks to build up. Echinacea is also helpful in lessening the severity of colds and flu, and in speeding recovery.

Supplements are available in a variety of forms. Use as instructed on labels.

CAUTION: *People with autoimmune disorders, such as lupus and AIDS, should take echinacea under a healthcare professional's supervision.*

186. Elderberry

The cooked berry of the elderberry tree, made into a tea, is used to relieve symptoms of coughs and colds. (Elderberry tea can be found in most health-food stores.) As an ointment it's been found to alleviate dry skin problems.

CAUTION: *Never eat raw elderberry seeds; they are toxic. Store-bought elderberry teas and salves are safe.*

187. Ephedra

Known as *ma huang* in China, it has been used as a remedy for asthma, colds, and other respiratory ailments. Ephedra contains ephedrine and pseudoephedrine, two alkaloids used in many over-the-counter cold and allergy medications. It speeds up metabolism and has been used for weight loss and bodybuilding, but has never been proven safe or effective for either.

CAUTION: *Ephedra can have an amphetaminelike effect, causing rapid heartbeat, a dangerous rise in blood pressure, and lead to heart attacks, strokes, and death. In fact, it has, at this writing, been linked to 155 deaths. In December 2003, the FDA banned sales of all ephedra dietary supplements in the United States.*

188. Evening Primrose Oil

As a dietary supplement, evening primrose oil can help lower blood cholesterol, lower blood pressure, help in weight reduction, relieve premenstrual pain, improve eczema, aid in the treatment of moderate cases of rheumatoid arthritis, slow progression of multiple sclerosis, help hyperactive children, improve acne (when taken with zinc), and help build stronger fingernails. It has also been found to aid in the reduction of menopausal hot flashes.

The active ingredient in evening primrose oil is gamma linoleic acid (GLA), which is needed for the body to produce hormonelike compounds called prostaglandins (PGs), vital for good health. In other words, a deficiency of the former can result in impaired production of the latter and adversely affect your physical well-being.

Supplements are available as capsules. Recommended dosage is 250 mg. one to three times daily. For PMS, I advise taking the supplement two to three days before symptoms usually appear until the onset of menstruation.

CAUTION: *Do not use if you are taking antipsychotic medicines, as evening primrose oil may increase the risk of seizures.*

189. Eyebright

An herb used as a general tonic for eye health that's been found to aid in reducing eyestrain and eye inflammations. It is also helpful in relieving runny, itchy eyes due to colds or allergies.

Supplements are available as capsules and extracts. Recommended dosage is 1 eyebright capsule one to three times daily. If using the extract, I suggest mixing 15–40 drops in liquid and taking it every three to four hours. Eyewash products containing eyebright (*euphrasia*), usually with other herbs, are available at health-food stores. Use an eyecup and rinse eye three to four times daily.

190. Fennel

Fennel seeds have been found to be very effective for digestive problems, generally providing quick and effective relief from gassiness, cramps, and acid indigestion. Their phytonutrient content is believed to inhibit spasms in smooth muscles in the intestinal tract.

The seeds taste like licorice, and chewed after meals they act as an herbal mouth freshener. Because a little goes a long way, chewing ¼–½ teaspoon after eating is all that's necessary. (*NOTE*: Fennel seeds may be yellowish or green. The yellow seeds are usually used in cooking. The greener ones are naturally sweeter and much better as an oral digestive and mouth freshener.)

191. Fenugreek

Long used as a medicinal plant, fenugreek acts as an expectorant for coughs and colds. As a gargle, it can relieve sore throat. Pulverized seeds have been found to reduce blood sugar and may be helpful to diabetics. As an external poultice, pulverized seeds can aid in soothing skin irritations and may help reduce swollen glands and other inflammations.

Supplements are available as capsules and pulverized seeds. The recommended dosage is 1 fenugreek capsule one to three times daily. To make a gargle, mix 1 tbsp. of pulverized seed in 8 ounces of hot water and steep for ten minutes. Strain. Gargle every three to four hours to relieve a sore throat. To use as a poultice, mix enough pulverized seeds in 8 ounces of warm water to make a thick paste and apply directly to affected areas.

192. Feverfew

Herbalists have been using feverfew to treat headaches since the seventeenth century. It has been found to be of great help to migraine sufferers, reducing the severity of symptoms (nausea, vomiting, and head pain) as well as the number of headaches. The British medical journal *Lancet* reported that extracts of feverfew inhibited the release of serotonin and prostaglandin, two inflammatory substances thought to contribute to the onset of migraine headaches.

Supplements are available in capsule form. I suggest migraine sufferers take 1 feverfew capsule one to three times daily. It frequently takes several months for improvement to be noticed.

CAUTION: *Do not take in conjunction with Imitrex or other migraine medications. The combination can raise blood pressure and heart rate to dangerous levels. Feverfew has also been known to cause mouth ulcers in some individuals. If this happens, discontinue use immediately.*

193. Flaxseed Oil

A rich source of essential fatty acids (alpha-linolenic acid and omega-3 and omega-6 essential fatty acids in just the right proportions), flaxseed is also an excellent source of vitamins, minerals, soluble and insoluble fiber, as well as lignans (phytochemicals that have antioxidant, antiviral, antibacterial, and anticancer properties). Additionally, it is a gentle natural laxative that may help soothe irritable bowel disorders; and because it contains lecithin, it can help stabilize glucose levels and enhance cardiovasular health.

Flaxseed oil supplements are available in capsule form. The recommended dosage is 1 capsule a.m. and p.m.

NOTE: *Flaxseed oil has a short shelf life and should be refrigerated (never heated). If you're going to use flaxseeds, be sure to grind them before adding to foods; otherwise, they won't be absorbed.*

CAUTION: *Precaution is advised if you're at risk for developing hormone-dependent cancers.*

194. Fo-Ti

A Chinese herb that is used as a rejuvenating tonic for maintaining strength and vigor. It is claimed by some that it can prevent hair from going gray. It is also used to increase fertility. Because it has been shown in animal tests to evidence antitumor properties, it may help in preventing some cancers. And it may promote heart health by preventing blood clots and reducing blood pressue.

Supplements are available in capsule form. The recommended dosage is 1 Fo-Ti capsule one to three times daily.

195. Garcinia Cambogia

The fruit of this plant has been found to modulate blood fat levels, which can increase metabolism and potentially aid in weight loss. It may also help to suppress appetite by increasing production of glycogen in the liver and small intestine, signaling the brain that the stomach is satisfied.

Supplements are available. The recommended dosage is 500 mg. three times a day, a half hour before meals.

CAUTION: *Because garcinia lowers blood sugar, it may interact adversely with diabetic and hypoglycemic medications. It may also alter the effects of antihyperlipidemic medications and necessitate a prescription change. If you are* *on these medications, consult your physician before taking garcinia.*

196. Gotu Kola

A tropical plant native to India and widely used in oriental and Indian ayurvedic medicine, gotu kola has been found to help circulation by strengthening veins and capillaries, improving the flow of blood throughout the body. It has been used successfully to treat pain and swelling due to phlebitis as well as leg cramps and tingling in the legs. Having a calming effect on the body, gotu kola may alleviate depression and may also help improve memory.

Gotu kola supports connective-tissue health and is believed to aid in healing skin sores and wounds by stimulating the production of keratin. This may help decrease scarring during wound healing and stretch marks after pregnancy. Additionally, a study of women treated with gotu kola after childbirth, reported in a French medical journal, found that they healed more rapidly than women given standard treatment. And, despite its name, gotu kola bears no relationship to cola beverages and contains no caffeine.

Supplements are available. The recommended dosage is 50 mg. one to three times daily.

CAUTION: *This herb should not be taken during pregnancy or by anyone with an overactive thyroid. Always tell your doctor, pharmacist, or other healthcare provider of any supplements you're taking to avoid potential interactions or side effects.*

197. Grape-Seed Extract

One of the most exciting antioxidants on the herbal scene. Grape-seed extract is a potent free radical scavenger, rich in flavanoids, and believed to be more powerful than vitamin E and vitamin C. It helps improve circulation by inhibiting the destruction of collagen needed by cell membranes. It may also have a heart-healthy, aspirinlike effect in slowing the formation of blood clots.

Proanthocyanidins, the active components of grape seed, may also protect the eyes and aid in the prevention and treatment of glaucoma, macular degeneration, and other vision-related disorders. There are also indications that these active components may protect the body against the damaging effects of radiation and some types of chemotherapy.

Supplements are available. The recommended dosage is 50 mg. twice daily.

CAUTION: *Because of its potential for delaying blood clotting, you should stop taking this supplement at least two weeks before any surgery or dental work. Do not take grape-seed extract if you are taking anticoagulants, antiplatelet medications, or have a bleeding disorder.*

198. Green Tea Extract

Green tea, also known as Chinese tea, is more lightly processed than black tea and has a different, delicate flavor. But aside from its satisfying taste, it's a terrifically rich source of polyphenols—those compounds that continue to show great promise as potent cancer fighters. People who regularly drink green tea have lower rates of stomach, lung, esophageal, pancreatic, and colon cancer than those who don't.

Green tea polyphenols stimulate the production of important antioxidants and detoxifying enzymes that block cancerous changes. Found in many skin creams sold at natural-food stores, green tea also helps heal sun-damaged skin. Additionally, it can help prevent abnormal blood clotting, lower high blood pressure, and raise the levels of good (HDL) cholesterol. But wait, there's more. It may promote weight loss by increasing fat oxidation and inhibiting enzymes that process carbohydrates and fats. And when sipped as a beverage, green tea prevents bacteria from sticking to your teeth, helping to prevent cavities. What better teatime could you ask for?

To get the full beneficial effects of green tea, you'd need to drink between 5 and 10 cups daily. And, although green tea has less caffeine than coffee (see section 372), more than 5 cups is enough to make you really jittery. There are some decaffeinated brands, but they are not widely available. Fortunately, there are caffeine-free supplements in tablet form. One green tea extract tablet is the equivalent of 1½ cups of green tea.

199. Gugulipid

This extract, from the mukul myrrh tree and used in ayurvedic medicine, is recognized in India as a cholesterol-lowering drug. In addition to lowering high blood cholesterol levels and high blood triglyceride levels, this herb also raises the levels of HDL, the good cholesterol, without the unpleasant side effects of many prescription cholesterol-lowering drugs.

Supplements are available. The recommended dosage is one 25 mg. gugulipid capsule with meals three times daily.

200. Hawthorn

Rich in bioflavonoids, compounds that are essential for vitamin C function and help strengthen blood vessels, hawthorn enhances cardiovascular health. Working as a vasodilator, it increases the flow of blood and oxygen to the heart. It also lowers blood pressure, reducing the strain on the heart to pump blood throughout the body. And it works as a diuretic, helping the body get rid of excess salt and water. Additionally, the berries from the hawthorn tree have long been used to treat digestive problems and insomnia.

Supplements are available. The recommended dosage is 1 capsule one to three times daily.

CAUTION: *Hawthorn should never be taken with Lanoxin (digoxin), the medication prescribed for most heart ailments. The mix can lower heart rate too much, bringing on possible heart failure. Be aware that although most hawthorn preparations are safe, this herb also comes in a highly concentrated form that should not be used without medical supervision.*

201. Horse Chestnut

Traditionally used as a remedy to bring down a fever and relieve cold symptoms, extracts of horse chestnut seed have been shown to be successful in soothing the discomfort of hemorrhoids and helpful in reducing the swelling of varicose veins. Horse chestnut extract has also been used as a sunscreen. In Germany, prescriptions for oral, standardized horse chestnut seed extract are widely written to treat edema when there is venous insufficiency and the lower extremities cannot return blood to the heart, causing varicose veins and pain and swelling in the legs.

Supplements are available. Oral supplements should be taken a half hour before or one hour after meals. The recommended dosage is 300 mg. standardized extract twice daily. For topical application, apply a 2 percent gel gently to the affected areas once or twice daily.

CAUTION: *Horse chestnut can change the rate at which food and medications go through the digestive tract, possibly altering the absorption and changing the dose needed for effectiveness. Also, be aware that this herb affects the blood's clotting ability and should not be used if you are taking anticoagulants unless under the direct supervision of your physician.*

202. Juniper (Berries)

These are often used as a stomach tonic and can act as appetite and digestion enhancers, as well as a diuretic and a disinfectant of the urinary tract.

CAUTION: *Excessive ingestion of the berries, or beverages and tonics containing them, can cause hallucinations.*

203. Kava

This plant, grown in the Polynesian and South Sea Islands, has slight hypnotic properties. It promotes relaxation, can be gently stimulating to the genital area, and small amounts may produce a mild euphoria. It is traditionally used by herbalists as a remedy for nervousness and insomnia. A mild diuretic, it helps reduce water retention and relieve cramping due to muscle spasms. Many women have found it helpful in relieving the discomfort of PMS and controlling symptoms of depression and anxiety in menopause.

Supplements are available. The recommended dosage is 100 mg. three times daily. For insomnia, I'd suggest 200 mg. at bedtime. As a tea, ½ cup twice daily.

CAUTION: *Long-term use can cause liver damage and therefore kava should not be taken by anyone with liver problems. Additionally, kava is not recommended for people with Parkinson's disease. Be aware, too, that this herb may cause drowsiness and also increases the effects of alcohol. It may also add to the effects of SSRI antidepressants and cause the effects of anesthesia to last longer, which is why some practitioners recommend stopping usage two to three weeks before surgery.*

204. Kudzu

An ancient Chinese herb, now growing wild throughout the southeastern United States, that is being touted as the antidote to the common hangover. It contains a pair of important phytochemicals, daidzin and daidzein, which help reduce blood alcohol levels. Taken immediately before or after drinking, kudzu supplements can virtually eliminate the headache and queasiness so familiar to drinkers the morning after.

Supplements are available. The recommended dosage is one to three 500 mg. capsules daily before or after drinking alcohol.

205. Licorice

An effective restorer of membrane and tissue function, it is also a hormone balancer, an intestinal secretion stimulant, a respiratory stimulant, and a laxative.

CAUTION: *High blood pressure and cardiac arrhythmias are possible side effects of licorice. Additionally, it may cause water retention and should be avoided by women who suffer from PMS. (American-manufactured licorice, the sort used in candy, is a synthetic flavoring and does not have these potential side effects—of course, it also doesn't offer any of the benefits.)*

206. Meadowsweet

Meadowsweet, a Native American herb high in salicylic acid, has been found to effectively calm inflammation in the stomach without medication. Easy to prepare as a tea (2 tsp. of the dried herb steeped for twenty minutes in a cup of hot water and drunk once a day), this natural heartburn and GERD remedy generally spells relief within a day or two.

207. Papaya

A natural antacid, papaya juice or tablets can be taken freely without any fear of rebounding. And dried papaya slices are also an excellent way to take advantage of this herb's benefits. Additionally, papaya may be the only fruit in your supermarket with more omega-3 than omega-6. (See section 101.)

208. Parsley (Seeds and Leaves)

A diuretic and gastric stimulant, parsley is used medicinally to treat coughs, asthma, amenorrhea, dysmenorrhea, and conjunctivitis. Rubbed on the scalp, parsley oil may stimulate hair growth. Best of all, it works wonders as nature's breath freshener. Try it after eating onion or garlic, and you'll be surprised how easy it is to pass on those big-and-chalky breath mints.

I recommend eating parsley raw. As a tonic, steep the chopped leaves and stems in hot water and drink a cup daily.

CAUTION: *Pregnant women should not take parsley juice or oil.*

209. Passionflower

The extract from this common vine is one of nature's best tranquilizers. It relieves muscle tension and spasms, as well as other manifestations of extreme anxiety. Passionflower is especially good for nervous insomnia, the kind that keeps you lying awake in bed worrying throughout the night.

As a supplement, mix 15–60 drops of extract in liquid and take as needed daily. For a calming tea, use 1 tsp. of dried herbs per cup and drink twice daily or before bedtime. The most common dosage is 100 mg. twice daily.

CAUTION: *This herb may cause sleepiness in some people and should not be used before driving or operating machinery. It may also enhance the effects of alcohol, as well as antianxiety medications, barbiturates, and antidepressants, necessitating a change in dosage for those medications.*

210. Pennyroyal

This herb, often referred to as "lung mint," is used as an inhalant in treating colds; it's also used as a tea for curing headaches, menstrual cramps, and pain, including bloating and breast tenderness. Pennyroyal oil makes an excellent natural bug repellent for pets. Part your pet's fur and put a few drops directly on your dog or cat's skin.

As a daily supplement, mix 20–60 drops of extract in liquid, or 1 tbsp. dried herb in 8 ounces of warm water, for relief of symptoms.

CAUTION: *Pennyroyal can induce abortion and should therefore NEVER be used during pregnancy.*

211. Peppermint

An antispasmodic, tonic, and stimulant, peppermint has been used to treat nervousness, insomnia, cramps, dizziness, and coughs. (For headaches, you might want to try a strong cup of peppermint tea, then lie down for fifteen to twenty minutes. It usually works as effectively as aspirin— and there are no side effects.) It aids in digestion, relaxing the stomach muscles and promoting burping, relieves nausea, and is excellent at alleviating heartburn.

As a supplement, peppermint teas are widely available. A cup daily is recommended.

CAUTION: *Although peppermint in drop form has been used for centuries for colic in infants and in liquid form for older children, check with your pediatrician before giving this or any other herb to your child.*

212. Pokeweed

This is a root that's used primarily to treat arthritis pain. It's also an ingredient in creams that help fight fungal infections.

213. Pygeum

For general prostate health, this herb, derived from the bark of an African evergreen, can help in preventing benign prostatic hypertrophy (BPH). This condition, where the prostate becomes enlarged, pressing against the urethra and interfering with urination, causes symptoms that are often severe enough to require corrective surgery. But pygeum, combined with saw palmetto (see section 217), has been found to be very effective as a treatment for BPH as well as preventing early symptoms from becoming more serious.

Supplements are available. I recommend taking up to three 500 mg. capsules daily with a full glass of water.

214. Reishi Mushroom

Derived from the cap and stem of the mushroom, reishi mushroom is used as an immune stimulant by patients with HIV or cancer and may also alleviate chemotherapy-induced nausea. It is known for boosting the immune system—helping to protect against viral infections, including swine flu and avian flu, and treating lung, heart, and kidney diseases, as well as high blood pressure, high cholesterol, and even irritable bowel (IBS) and chronic fatigue syndrome (CFS). The most common adverse reactions are dry nose and throat and upset stomach.

Supplements are available in a variety of forms. I recommend taking two 600 mg. capsules twice daily with meals.

CAUTION: *Reishi should be avoided by anyone on antihypertensive medication as it can cause blood pressure to drop too low. It also interacts with anticoagulants, slowing blood clotting and increasing the risk of bleeding.*

215. Rosemary

Not just a savory spice anymore. Recent research shows that the whole rosemary herb may be an up-and-coming cancer fighter. It has been found to act as an antioxidant and an anti-inflammatory, to prevent carcinogens from binding to DNA, and to stimulate liver detoxification of carcinogens. Used externally in an ointment, rosemary leaves may soothe rheumatism aches, sprains, wounds, bruises, and eczema. Taken internally, in the proper preparation, it can relieve flatulence, colic, and upset stomach.

CAUTION: *Rosemary can be toxic in large quantities.*

216. St. John's Wort (aka Hypericum)

Called nature's Prozac, St. John's wort has been around for centuries to heal wounds. It contains hypericin, a natural mood-booster that also has germicidal and anti-inflammatory properties, and hyperforin, another compound that may inhibit the breakdown of mood-elevating seratonin. It also contains melatonin (see section 125). Considered a nutraceutical, this herb is also a muscle relaxer used to alleviate menstrual cramps, and is a good expectorant as well. Externally, it is an antiseptic and a painkiller.

As a treatment for depression, St. John's wort may take up to three weeks to produce any mood-elevating effects. There is, however, a form of St. John's wort with a polyphenol extract, also taken from the plant, and 1 tablet per day has been found to produce results in just two to three days. It is also available over-the-counter as dried leaves, flowers, tinctures, extract, oil, ointment, capsules, and prepared tea, but I would not recommend it for long-term use without the supervision of an herbalist or other medical professional.

CAUTION: *St. John's wort may interfere with the actions of certain chemotherapy drugs. In high doses it may cause sensitivity to light and could seriously exacerbate sunburn. It should be used with caution by anyone taking 5-HTP (see section 81), which has a similar effect on the body. Do not combine with prescribed antidepressants. (NOTE: Contrary to earlier reports, this herb's antidepressant action is not due to monoamine oxidase [MAO] inhibition, which means it is safe for users to enjoy tyramine-rich foods such as wine, cheese, and chocolate—in moderation, of course. That should perk up spirits right there.)*

217. Saw Palmetto (Berries)

Saw palmetto berries are helpful in the treatment of chronic cystitis and in the prevention of genitourinary tract infections in men and women. Most important, it has been shown to be quite effective in treating benign prostate enlargement, a condition that causes excessive urination in men.

As a supplement, I suggest 30–60 drops of saw palmetto extract taken mixed in liquid daily, or 160 mg. tablets twice daily with food.

CAUTION: *Any man experiencing pain or swelling of the prostate, or who is having difficulty in urination, or passing blood in the urine, should be examined by his physician.*

218. Sea Buckthorn (*Hippophae rhamnoides*)

Keep your nutritional radar on alert for this superfruit. Sea buckthorn berries are the only plant source of all the omega fatty acids and contain more than 190 biochemicals. Also known as seaberry, siberian pineapple, and alpine sandthorn, sea buckthorn has been found to be one of nature's most amazing medicinal plants and is believed to have potent anti-viral, antibacterial, and healing properties. Sea buckthorn oil has been successfully used to treat such skin problems as rosacea, eczema, and acne. It has also been found helpful in the treatment of such gastrointestinal problems as acid reflux (GERD), peptic ulcers, colitis, and diverticulitis.

As a supplement, sea buckthorn is available as an oil and as a powder. The recommended dosage for the oil is ½– 1 tsp. two to three times daily taken on an empty stomach at least half an hour before meals. As a powder the recommended dose is ½ tsp. twice daily.

219. Stinging Nettle

The root of this prickly plant, which reportedly has diuretic properties enabling the body to get rid of toxins, has been found to be quite helpful in the treatment of benign prostate enlargement, with indications that it may also aid in the treatment of arthritis, gout, and eczema. Additionally, the leaves of the plant—freeze-dried—may help alleviate the symptoms of hay fever.

As a supplement, I suggest 30–60 drops of the extract taken mixed in liquid one to three times daily. In capsule form the standard dosage for the root is 250 mg. twice daily, and for the dried leaves it's 600 mg. twice daily as needed.

220. Tea Tree Oil

The oil from the leaves of this Australian tree has been used for years as a topical antiseptic for cuts and burns. It also has antifungal properties and may be helpful as a body wash in fending off methicillin-resistant *Staphylococcus aureus* (MRSA), problematic in hospitals and nursing homes where patients often have compromised immune systems. Additionally, it has been shown to help in the treatment of *Candida* (see section 340), athlete's foot, some vaginal bacterial infections, and, as an oral antiseptic rinse, it can aid in the treatment of strep throat.

As an oral supplement, add 5–10 drops to a cup of water, gargle, and spit out. Apply ointments and salves to affected areas as needed.

CAUTION: *Skin products containing tea tree oil may dry the skin and worsen dryness caused by treatments such as Retin-A, benzoyl peroxide, salicylic acid, or Accutane taken by mouth.*

221. Thyme

A natural antiseptic deodorant, thyme—applied externally in compresses—can be an effective liniment for wounds; internally it can act as an antidiarrhetic and relieve gastritis cramps, as well as soothe bronchitis and laryngitis.

222. Triphala

This ayurvedic detoxifying herb contains a combination of three "fruits" (amalaki, bibhitaki, and haritaki), all of which are rich sources of antioxidants with anti-inflammatory, anticancer, and immunity-boosting properties. A bowel-regulating cleanser that treats the entire digestive system—helping to alleviate constipation, hemorrhoids, diarrhea, indigestion, and bloating—triphala also purifies the blood, removes toxins from the liver, and helps reduce serum cholesterol as well as high blood pressure. More a bowel tonic than a laxative, and often used as a food supplement, it is safe to use on a daily basis.

As a supplement, the recommended dose is two to four 500 mg. tablets right before bedtime.

223. Umckalaobo

Hard to pronounce but remarkably effective in treating respiratory infections, this South African herb has powerful antiviral and antibacterial properties. Most often used for treating bronchitis as well as tonsillitis, umckalaobo can be obtained in the form of syrup, drops, chewable tablets, or spray. Taken at the onset of symptoms, it generally brings relief within a day or two.

224. Valerian

A "natural Valium" that produces a relaxing effect on the body and is often used to treat anxiety, muscle tension, and insomnia. Unlike prescription drugs, valerian is not addictive and has few unpleasant side effects. It may also relieve gas pains and menstrual cramps.

As a supplement, I'd suggest taking 200 mg. one to three times daily to relieve symptoms. If you prefer the tincture, mix 10 drops in liquid and drink one to three times daily.

CAUTION: *Extremely high doses may cause weakened heartbeat and paralysis. Valerian may enhance the effects of sedatives, antidepressants, barbiturates, and antianxiety medications, necessitating a change in dosage, and should not be taken without first consulting your physician or a healthcare professional.*

225. White Willow Bark

A derivative of white willow bark called salicum was used for centuries as an anti-inflammatory and an analgesic for reducing the pain and swelling in arthritic joints. Based on studies of salicum, researchers eventually derived a synthetic drug called acetylsalicylic acid—better known today as aspirin. We all know that aspirin is considered a wonder drug, but not all of us have the stomach to handle it. And this is where white willow bark comes in. It has aspirin-like benefits, but does not cause stomach irritation. In fact, white willow contains tannins that are actually good for the digestive system.

As a supplement, take 2 capsules every two to three hours as needed. But be aware of the cautions below before you do.

CAUTION: *Children under the age of sixteen should NOT be given willow bark. The danger of their developing Reye's syndrome (a rare but potentially serious illness associated with children taking aspirin) is still a real possibility. Because salicylites are not recommended during pregnancy, this herb is not recommended for pregnant or breast-feeding women. Anyone with asthma, gout, diabetes, hemophelia, or stomach ulcers should also avoid willow bark. Overdoses of this herb may cause stomach and kidney inflammation, and—now hear this—could be what's causing tinnitus, that inexplicable ringing in your ears.*

226. Wild Yam

A plant source of the female hormone progesterone, wild yam is used for menstrual disorders, threatened miscarriage, as well as to relieve hot flashes, vaginal dryness, and other symptoms of menopause. It also contains saponins that have an anti-inflammatory effect and may help in treating the pain and stiffness of rheumatoid arthritis. Because the wild yam (*Dioscoria villosa*) produces chemicals from which oral contraceptives are synthesized, its extract has been used by Native Americans and many herbalists as a contraceptive. (I do not advise using this or any other herb to prevent conception unless it is under the supervision of a qualified practitioner.)

Although frequently assumed to be a natural replacement for progesterone, Dr. John R. Lee, author of *What Your Doctor May Not Tell You About Menopause: The Breakthrough Book on Natural Progesterone*, states, "There is no evidence that the body converts diosgenin (found in wild yams) to hormones." But diosgenin does have beneficial effects and has been used for centuries as an adaptogen.

CAUTION: *Do not use wild yam root if you are pregnant or taking birth control pills. Also, be aware that supplements derived from Mexican yam (*Dioscorea mexicana*) or wild yam (*Dioscorea villosa*) do not contain progesterone, or any other hormones. These products are frequently billed as progesterone "precursors," which is not true.*

227. Yohimbe Bark

The herb yohimbe is one of the few so-called aphrodisiacs that have been shown to help treat male impotence. Unfortunately, it is also quite dangerous because it contains yohimbine, which is sold by prescription and should be used only under the supervision of a physician. This weaker form, yohimbe bark, is available without prescription, although it is not as effective. (The usual dose is 1–3 capsules daily.)

CAUTION: *Yohimbe can lower blood pressure and should not be used by people with hypotension. Because of its potential serious side effects, it should not be used by anyone with a medical problem unless under the supervision of a physician.*

228. Herbs That Can Interfere with Your Rx Drugs

Antibiotics
Dong quai: may increase your skin's sensitivity to sun
St. John's wort: can weaken effectiveness
Anticoagulants (blood thinners)
Bromelain: may increase risk of bleeding
Dong quai: may increase risk of uncontrolled bleeding
Evening primrose oil: may cause additive effects
Garlic supplements: may cause spontaneous, heavy bleeding
Ginkgo biloba: may cause uncontrolled bleeding
Horse chestnut: may increase risk of bleeding
Willow bark: may increase potency of your drug and increase risk of bleeding
Antidepressants
Ginkgo biloba: may increase levels in the blood
Antipsychotic Medications
Kava: can cause liver damage and coma
Beta-Blockers
Willow bark: may decrease effectiveness
Birth Control Pills
St. John's wort: can weaken effectiveness

Calcium Channel Blockers
Celery seed: may amplify hyperglycemic side effects
Diuretics
Kava: may have additive effects
Willow bark: may decrease effectiveness
Heart Medications
St. John's wort: can cause dangerous interaction
Immunosuppressant Medications
Echinacea: may interfere with effectiveness
Garlic supplements: may decrease effectiveness
Methotrexate and Phenytoin (Dilantin)
Willow Bark: may increase potency in body to toxic levels
Nonsteroidal anti-inflammatory drugs (NSAIDs)
Horse chestnut: may increase risk of bleeding
Willow bark: can increase risk of stomach bleeding
Sedatives and Sleeping Pills
Kava: can cause liver damage and coma
Tranquilizers
Bromelain: may increase amount of drowsiness
Chamomile: may increase amount of drowsiness
Echinacea: may cause liver damage

229. Dangerous Herbs

The following herbs can be hazardous to your health and should not be brewed in teas or used in other fashion without the direction and supervision of a naturopathic doctor or other nutritionally oriented health professional.

NOTE: *Since many herbs have several common names, the botanical name of the plant is given in italics.*

Arnica, Wolf's Bane, Leopard's Bane, Mountain Tobacco (*Arnica montana*)

Arnica, which is helpful in the treatment of bruises, traumas, and pain, is safe to use as directed as a sublingual, homeopathic remedy (which contains only minute amounts of active ingredients in tiny pellets) or as a commercially prepared external salve.

Arnica is an irritant and can produce violent toxic gastroenteritis, intense muscular weakness, nervous disorders, and death.

Belladonna, Deadly Nightshade (*Atropa belladonna*)
Poisonous. Contains toxic alkaloids.

Bittersweet, Dulcamara, Woody or Climbing Nightshade (*Solanum dulcamara*)
Poisonous.

Bloodroot, Sanguinaria, Red Puccoon (*Sanguinaris canadensis*)
Contains the poisonous alkaloid sanguinarine, among others.

Broom Tops, Scoparius, Spartium, Irish Broom, Scotch Broom, Broom (*Cytisus scoparius*)
Contains toxic sparteine and other harmful alkaloids.

Buckeyes, Aesculus, Horse Chestnut (*Aesculus hippocastanum*)
A poisonous plant that contains a toxic coumarin substance.

Calamus, Sweet Flag, Sweet Root, Sweet Cane, Sweet Cinnamon (not to be confused with the bark used as a popular spice) (*Acorus calamus*)
Oil of calamus is a carcinogen (a cancer-causing agent).

Heliotrope (*Heliotropium europaeum*)
This plant is poisonous and also contains alkaloids that cause liver damage. (It should not be confused with garden heliotrope, whose botanical name is *Valeriana officinalis*, and safe.)

Hemlock, Conium, Spotted Hemlock, Spotted Parsley, St. Bennet's Herb, Spotted Cowbane, Fool's Parsley (*Conium maculatum*)
Contains poisonous alkaloids. It's often mistaken for water hemlock (*Cicuta maculata*) and hemlock spruce (*Tsuga canadensis*).

Henbane, Hyoscyamus, Hog's Bean, Poison Tobacco, Devil's Eye (*Hyoscyamus niger*)
Poisonous. Contains dangerously toxic alkaloids.

Jalap Root, Jalap, Ture Jalap, Vera Cruz Jalap, High John Root, John Conqueror, St. John the Conqueror Root (*Exagonium purga, Ipomoea jalapa,* and *Ipomoea purga*)
This is a twining Mexican vine known by many different names, but it can be extremely dangerous. The drug is a potent cathartic, and its extreme purgative action can result in life-threatening excessive bowel movements.

Jimson Weed, Datura, Stramonium, Apple of Peru, Jamestown Weed, Thornapple, Tolguacha (*Datura stramonium*)
This is a poisonous plant that contains stropine, hyoscyamine, and scopolamine, drugs that are illegal (for good reason) for nonprescription use.

Lobelia, Indian Tobacco, Wild Tobacco, Asthma Weed, Emetic Weed (*Lobelia inflata*)
A poisonous plant that is often unwisely used as an emetic. Overdoses of extracts from the plant's leaves or fruit

produce severe vomiting, sweating, paralysis, rapid but feeble pulse, and—more often than not—collapse, coma, and death.

Mandrake, Mandragora, European Mandrake (*Mandragora officinarum*)

A poisonous narcotic similar to belladonna.

May Apple, Mandrake, Podophyllum, American Mandrake, Devil's Apple, Umbrella Plant, Vegetable Calomel, Wild Lemon, Vegetable Mercury (*Podophyllum pelatum*)

A poisonous plant with complex toxic constituents.

Mistletoe, Viscum, American Mistletoe (*Phoradendron flavescens* and *Viscum flavescens*)

Contains toxic amines. Consider it poisonous.

Mistletoe, Viscum, European Mistletoe (*Viscum album*)

This branch of mistletoe definitely contains toxic amines and is considered poisonous.

Mistletoe, Viscum, Juniper Mistletoe (*Phoradendron juniperinum*)

This particular mistletoe may or may not be poisonous, but too little is known about it for any wise person to use it for anything but holding up at Christmas time and kissing beneath.

Morning Glory (*Ipomoea purpurea*)

The seeds of this particular morning glory do contain amides of lysergic acid, but with a potency much less than that of LSD. Anyone planning to take a "trip" on them will be in for an unpleasant and potentially dangerous surprise, since the seeds also contain a very unhealthy purgative resin.

Periwinkle, Vinca, Greater Periwinkle, Lesser Periwinkle (*Vinca major* and *Vinca minor*), Creeping Myrtle

Keep these in your garden and out of your system. They contain toxic alkaloids that can cause adverse neurological actions and injure the liver and kidneys.

Sassafras

A "blood purifier" that's carcinogenic and can damage the liver.

Spindle Tree (*Euonymus europaeus*)

An extremely violent purgative.

Tonka Bean, Tonco Bean, Tonquin Bean (*Dipteryx Odorata, Coumarouna odorata, Dipteryx oppositifolia,* and *Coumarouna oppositifolia*)

The active constituent of these seeds is coumarin, which the FDA has prohibited marketing as a food or food additive, after having been found to cause extensive liver damage, slowing of growth, and testicular atrophy when used in the diet of experimental animals. (Check the labels on your OTC medicines!)

Wahoo Bark, Euonymus, Burning Bush (*Euonymus atropurpureus*)

Often used as a laxative, but though its poisonous qualities have not been thoroughly identified, it's best to play it safe and keep away from it.

White Snakeroot, Snakeroot, Richweed (*Eupatorium rugosum, E. ogeratoides, and E. urticaefolium*)

This poisonous plant contains a toxic, unsaturated alcohol. It causes "trembles" in livestock and can engender milk sickness in humans who ingest milk, butter, and possibly meat from animals who have eaten this plant.

Wormwood, Absinthium, Absinth, Madderwort, Wermuth, Mugwort, Mingwort, Warmot, Magenkraut, Herba Absinthii (*Artemisia absinthium*)

Oil of wormwood is an active narcotic poison. It is used to flavor an alcoholic liqueur—*absinthe*—which is now illegal in America because its use can damage the nervous system.

Yohimbe (*Corynanthe yohimbi* and *Pausinystalia yohimbe*)

Not an herb to play around with. It contains the toxic alkaloid yohimbine.

230. Homeopathy Basics

The key to homeopathy is the "Law of Similars" or that like cures like, a principle often used in conventional medicine for allergy treatments. Symptoms are signs that the body is trying to reestablish its own natural balance. Homeopathic treatment uses the same natural substances that cause certain symptoms if given to a healthy individual in large quantities to stimulate a sick person's body to get better if given in extremely tiny amounts. For example, when you peel an onion, your eyes itch and water and you often get a runny nose, much like when you have a cold. Well, when you have a cold, the homeopathic remedy would be a much-diluted, minute dose of red onion (*Allium cepa*) to help the body heal itself.

Homeopathic medicines are prepared from natural plant, mineral, and animal substances. The fact that medically active substances in these medicines are diluted to such infinitesimally small amounts makes them nontoxic, with no known adverse side effects. They're safe for adults and children when taken as directed for self-limiting conditions, such as the flu, minor bruises, allergies, PMS, hot flashes, motion sickness, and the like.

The manufacture of homeopathic medicines is regulated in this country by the FDA, which provides guidelines for their labeling and sale. Available as tablets, liquids, suppositories, and ointments, the most popular form is the tiny beadlike pellet. Most homeopathic medicines are taken sublingually (under the tongue) because the large number of capillaries in the mouth get them into the bloodstream quickly.

THE RIGHT WAY TO TAKE AND HANDLE HOMEOPATHIC MEDICINES

- Keep medicine tightly capped, away from light, in a dry place.
- Do not expose to aromatic substances such as perfumes, camphor, or menthol, which can neutralize them.
- Before taking medicine, make sure your mouth is clean of any flavors—especially coffee or mint, which can interfere with the effects of homeopathic remedies. (It's best to avoid mint-flavored toothpaste entirely while on a regimen.)
- Do not touch the pellets. Spill the remedy into the cap, then drop it on the tongue and let it dissolve.
- Don't brush your teeth, drink, or eat anything for at least a half hour to give the remedy a chance to work.

COMMON COMPLAINTS AND THEIR
HOMEOPATHIC REMEDIES

Symptom	Remedy
Anxiety	*Argentum nitricum* (Silver nitrate)
	Camphora officinarum (Camphora)
Bruises	*Arnica montana* (Mountain daisy)
Burns	*Calcarea sulphurica* (Calcium sulphate)
Colds (with sneezing and watery eyes)	*Allium cepa* (Red onion)
Conjunctivitis	*Euphrasia officinalis* (Eyebright)
Constipation	*Graphites* (Black lead-plumbago)
Cough (bronchitis)	*Antimonium tartaricum* (Tartar emetic)
Cough (dry)	Phosphorus
Cuts and scrapes	*Calendula officinalis* (Calendula)
Depression	*Hypericum* (St. John's wort)
Diarrhea (with cramps)	*Veratrum album* (White hellebore)
Fever (colds and flu)	*Belladonna* (Deadly nightshade)
	Camphora officinarum (Camphora)
Flu (aches and stiffness)	*Eupatorium perfoliatum* (Boneset)
Hangover	*Nux vomica* (Poison nut)
Hemorrhoids	*Hamamelis virginiana* (Witch hazel)
Hot flashes	*Lachesis mutus* (Bushmaster snake)

Insect bites	*Ledum palustre* (Wild rosemary)
Insomnia (stress-induced)	*Coffea cruda* (Unroasted coffee)
Joint pain	*Calcarea fluorica* (Calcium fluoride)
	Symphytum officinale (Symphytum)
Menstrual cramps	*Caulophyllum thalictroides* (Blue cohosh)
Motion sickness	*Cocculus indicus* (Indian cockle)
Mouth sores	*Borax* (Sodium borate)
Nasal congestion	*Pulsatilla* (Wind flower)
Nausea	*Ipecacuanah* (Ipecac)
PMS	*Sepia* (Cuttlefish ink)
Poison ivy	*Rhus toxicodendron* (Poison ivy)
Sinusitis	*Kali bichromicum* (Potassium bichromate)
Skin eruptions (with itching)	*Sulphur* (Brimstone)
Urinary problems (burning /itching)	*Cantharis* (Spanish fly)
Varicose veins	*Calcarea fluorica* (Calcium fluoride)
Warts	*Thuja occidentalis* (Arbor vitae)

231. Aromatherapy, Essential Oils, and Tinctures

Aromatherapy is the use of essential oils from plants—and some animal extracts—for psychological and physical well-being. It is a holistic practice that incorporates mind, body, pleasure, and healing, and has been used for centuries throughout the world to treat conditions ranging from minor physical blemishes to near-fatal illness.

Although aromatherapists utilize many different parts of plants (leaves, flower petals, bark, roots), it is the essential oils, the highly concentrated essences derived from these parts, that are used in treatments. These oils contain powerful vitamins and enzymes, and because they are so concentrated, they are used only in tiny doses and work best when diluted. They may be diluted in a humidifier or bathwater, inhaled from a bottle, or combined with other oils and applied directly to the skin.

POSSIBLE HEALTH BENEFITS

Help cure acne
Help slow aging
Improve concentration
Relieve anxiety
Repel insects
Improve stamina
Promote healthy skin, nails, hair

Alleviate arthritis pain
Relieve migraines
Draw wastes directly out of the skin
Stimulate the immune system
Alleviate water retention
Aid in relief of menopausal symptoms
Help cure viral and bacterial infections

Stimulate drainage of the lymph glands to aid in disintegration of cellulite

COMMON ESSENTIAL OILS AND THEIR USES

Basil—aid in mental alertness
Cinnamon—energy, sexual stimulant
Chamomile—sedative/stress reliever
Geranium—hormonal balance for women
Juniper—diuretic, improve circulation
Lavender—all skin ailments, muscle pain, stress reliever
Neroli—calm anxiety, improve skin
Patchouli—anti-inflammatory for skin
Rosewood—antidepressant
Sandalwood—immunity booster, aphrodisiac
Tea tree—antifungal, antiviral, antiacne
Ylan-ylan—relaxant, lower blood pressure, stabilize mood swings

CAUTIONS: *Essential oils should not be taken internally. Some essential oils should be avoided during pregnancy as well as by individuals with asthma, epilepsy, or other medical health conditions. Check with a naturopath, a reputable holistic physician, or a nutritionally oriented doctor about the safety of each ingredient before using any essential oil.*

Keep essential oils away from children; even in small amounts, many oils can be toxic.

Essential oils, as a rule, should not be used undiluted on the skin.

TINCTURES

Tinctures are a convenient way to ingest herbs. In 1-ounce dropper bottles, with glass droppers, they're easy to carry anywhere, allowing you to take the herbs anytime. While herbs in capsule form are also convenient, their essential components are not as readily available or as easily assimilated. Tinctures begin to be absorbed immediately upon entering your mouth; capsules are digested in the stomach.

When using a tincture, be sure to try a few drops first to make sure you're not allergic to it. After that, you can increase the dosage according to your needs. Very often you will need 3–4 dropperfuls for a desired feeling.

Be sure you know what the herb will do before you take it. (See sections 145–229 for cautions and possible drug-herb interactions.) In general, anyone taking hormones, thyroid medications, anticholinergics, or antibiotics should check with a healthcare professional before combining them with herbs.

Most naturopathic doctors and herbalists feel that herbs work best when taken regularly in small doses over a period of time. Dosages for children are one-third to one-half the adult dosage, but I'd recommend you check with an herbalist or naturopath before giving any herbs to children.

Store tinctures in a cool, dark place. Their alcohol content acts as a preservative. When kept away from heat, sunlight, and exposure to air, tinctures can keep their freshness for more than a year.

SOME COMMON TINCTURES AND THEIR HERBS

Brain stimulating tinctures: ginkgo biloba, gotu kola, blessed thistle, Siberian ginseng

Calming tinctures: catnip, chamomile, comfrey, elderberry, evening primrose, hyssop, jasmine flowers, juniper berries, lemon balm, mullein, passionflower, rose flowers, slippery elm, vervain, violet

Cleansing tinctures: burdock root, buckthorn root, chaparral leaf, dandelion root, nettle, milk thistle, gingerroot

General tonic tinctures: blackberry leaves, comfrey, dandelion, ginseng, jasmine flower, nettle, patchouli, rasberry leaves

Stimulating tinctures: basil, bay, calendula flowers, citronella, fennel, lavender flowers, lemon verbena, mint, rosemary, sage, savory, thyme

Tinctures for muscles and joints: bay, juniper berries, mugwort, oregano, sage

---

DID YOU KNOW?

- Avoiding black coffee may help prevent cancer of the esophagus.
- Store-bought milk with synthetic vitamin D can rob your body of magnesium.

- Brushing your teeth within an hour of drinking soda can cause layers of tooth enamel to deteriorate.
- Goldenrod extract can relieve nasal congestion.
- Oral contraceptives can interfere with the availability of vitamins B6, B12, folic acid, and vitamin C.
- Daily vitamin C supplements can reduce your risk of developing cataracts.
- Taking antibiotics with green tea can make them nearly twice as effective.

232. Any Questions About Chapter VIII?

What is dysbiosis?

Dysbiosis is a bacterial imbalance in the intestinal tract—usually caused by antibiotics, poor diet, or stress—that results in an unwanted increase of bad bacteria and yeast. It has been implicated in disorders such as yeast infections, irritable bowel syndrome, and rheumatoid arthritis. Including prebiotics and probiotics in your diet can usually reverse the condition and is definitely the best way to avoid it.

What's the difference between red and white ginseng?

The red is considered to be of superior quality. The natural color of the ginseng root is white. When it is simply cleaned and dried, it retains its natural color. Red ginseng, on the other hand, is the result of being steamed with a solution of herbs. Adulteration and dilution of ginseng products are not uncommon, so be sure you buy from a reputable company and look for standardized, guaranteed-potency products.

The label on my yogurt says it contains fiber. How can manufacturers get away with that?

They're not getting away with anything. These days fiber is showing up in products you'd least expect. (Would you believe grape juice?) The reason is that scientists have created a new class of fiber, "functional fiber," molecules that can be added to numerous processed foods. You don't have to see or feel fiber for it to be present—or for it to provide all its nutritional benefits.

I'm a thirty-eight-year-old woman. I take vitamins and exercise, but I want better muscle tone. I've heard about creatine, but I'm not sure what it is or what it does. Is it right for me?

It might be; it's already a favorite of bodybuilders and athletes. Creatine monohydrate is a synthetic version of an amino acid found naturally in the body, primarily in skeletal muscles. It is essential for the production of adenosine triphosphate (ATP), the fuel for motion involving muscle contraction. When ATP is depleted, you become fatigued. By increasing your creatine levels, you produce more ATP fuel for longer intense workouts, which leads to increased fat-burning muscle mass. Because creatine pulls water into your muscle cells (which increases protein synthesis), you will probably gain weight quickly. But keep in mind that muscle weighs more than fat, and if you take advantage of the creatine energy boost and intensify your workouts, you'll lose fat and reduce blood lipid levels, helping to protect you against heart disease.

Creatine occurs naturally in meats and fish, but serious athletes use it up faster than it can be replenished through diet. If, though, you're involved in endurance sports such as long-distance running or swimming, creatine can be counterproductive since the extra muscle mass might slow you down. Creatine is available as a powder or as chewable wafers. One tablespoon of the powder (5,000 mg.) mixed with juice or water should give your muscles a boost. Look for supplements that promise 99 percent creatine. Cheaper brands may have only about 60 percent. (*NOTE*: Studies have shown that some individuals who try creatine are unable to absorb the extra amounts into their muscles and, as a result, experience no improvement in muscle mass or athletic performance. Taking it in conjunction with a beta-alanine supplement may rectify this, but if you don't notice *any* improvement in two or three weeks, creatine, as well as beta-alanine, is probably not the supplement for you.)

CAUTION: *Taking large doses of creatine while engaged in a regimen of intense exercise can cause kidney dysfunction. If this occurs, increase your intake of fluids to dilute the supplement and eliminate it. Creatine should not be used by children unless recommended by a physician.*

I'm trying to reduce my cholesterol by upping my intake of soy foods. How many isoflavones should I be getting on a daily basis and am I getting enough—or too much—from tofu?

Most researchers feel that staying in the 30–50 mg. isoflavone range is enough to reap health benefits. For your reference, a cup of tofu, or tempeh, contains about 70 mg., a cup of soy milk 30 mg., and ½ cup roasted soy nuts about 120 mg. Asians—and many vegetarians in this country who use soy products as diet mainstays—consume in the neighborhood of 100 mg. of isoflavones per day, according to Dr. Stephen Barnes, a leading soy researcher and professor of pharmacology and toxicology at the University of Alabama. Staying within this range is advisable since long-term intakes at much higher levels have not been studied.

What's the scoop on spirulina? Is it some sort of wonder drug?

It's not a drug at all. Spirulina is a natural, easily assimilated complete protein. (It's known as spirulina plankton or blue-green algae.) It's nature's highest source of chlorophyll pigment, rich in such chelated minerals as iron, calcium, zinc, potassium, and magnesium, a fine source of vitamin A and B-complex vitamins, and it contains phenylalanine, which acts on the brain's appetite center to decrease hunger pangs—while also keeping your blood sugar at the proper level.

And if you'd like to slim down, this is a wonderful aid for weight reduction. Take three 500 mg. tablets a half hour before meals. Once the dosage begins to work, decrease to 2 or 1 tablet before meals.

I've been told about an algae (not spirulina) that's supposed to have amazing health and healing properties. Have you heard of it and can you tell me what it is?

I have, and it's chlorella. Chlorella (the emerald alga) has been touted as the perfect whole food. Aside from being a complete protein and containing all the B vitamins, vitamin C, vitamin E, and the major minerals (with zinc and iron in amounts large enough to be considered supplementary), it has been found to improve the immune system, improve digestion, detoxify the body, accelerate healing, protect against radiation, aid in the prevention of degenerative diseases, help in the treatment of *Candida albicans,* relieve arthritis pain, and, because of its nutritional content, aid in the success of numerous weight-loss programs.

It is available in tablets, powder, and water-soluble extracts (which contain the highest concentrations of chlorella growth factor [CGF]). Be aware, though, that although chlorella products are widely available, they differ depending on the particular strain of chlorella used.

The average dosage is 5–8 tablets three times daily. I'd suggest starting with only 1 tablet three times daily and working up, just to make sure you have no allergic reactions. Possible adverse reactions include gas, bloating, bowel irregularity, nausea, green stools, and mild skin breakouts or eczema. (These reactions, unless severe, are not unusual and should clear up in a few days. If not, discontinue supplementation and consult a nutritionally oriented doctor. See section 462.)

Dr. David Steenblock, author of *Chlorella: Natural Medicinal Algae*, has found that for detoxification purposes, chlorella is best taken on an empty stomach; however, because it is a food, it can also be taken with other foods as well as medications.

I know that bran is good for me. I just don't know which bran is best.

It depends on what you're looking for nutritionally. The following bran name guide may help:

Barley bran is high in soluble fiber and helpful in lowering cholesterol.

Corn bran is high in insoluble fiber and may be helpful in reducing the risk of colon cancer.

Oat bran is high in soluble fiber and helpful in lowering cholesterol. (In fact, studies have shown that just 2 oz. daily can help reduce cholesterol levels by 7–10 percent!)

Rice bran is high in soluble fiber and may be helpful in lowering cholesterol. (It's similar to oat bran in nutritional benefits, but less of it is needed to produce the same results. Two tbsp. of rice bran will give you as much soluble fiber as one-half cup oat bran.)

Wheat bran is high in insoluble fiber and may be helpful in reducing the risk of colon cancer. (For natural sources of these types of fiber—and cautions—see section 137.)

Could you tell me about royal jelly? How is it different from propolis?

Propolis is a by-product of honey. Royal jelly is the bees' "milk," a nutrient-dense white secretion produced by worker bees. All bee larvae eat this concentrated superfood for the first three days of life, but after that only the designated queen bee does. It is her only food—and she grows to be 50 percent larger than her sister bees, lives up to forty times longer, and is highly fertile! Royal jelly contains all the essential amino acids, as well as vitamins A, C, D, E, 9 B-complex vitamins (including vitamin B12, cyanocobalamin), and the minerals calcium, copper, iron, phosphorus, potassium, silicone, and sulfur. A complete protein, it is also a mild, natural antibiotic and has a stimulating effect on the adrenal glands, which affect metabolism, mood, appetite, and sex drive. It can help you increase energy, and naturopathic doctors often recommend it for treating symptoms of menopause and to improve sexual performance in men. Additionally, many women believe that it definitely helps reduce the appearance of fine lines and wrinkles. As an energizer, I recommend taking one or two 500 mg. capsules daily.

Is there a downside to the phytates in soybeans? I've heard they can impair nutrient absorption.

There has been some controversy over the high content of phytates in soybeans because phytates do bind to essential minerals such as calcium, iron, and zinc in the digestive tract and prevent them from being absorbed. Soaking and fermenting—as used in making miso, natto, shoyu, tamari, and tempeh (but not tofu, soy milk, texturized soy protein, or soy protein isolate)—significantly reduce the phytate content. But a high phytate content might not be a bad thing. Phytates have been shown in some animal studies to stop the growth of cancerous tumors by binding with the minerals that may feed them. Keep in mind that the more processed the soybeans, the less amount of usable soy isoflavones you're getting. (Also keep in mind that soy sauce and soy oil have *no* nutritional value.)

I've heard about a Chinese herb called jujube. Can you tell me something about it?

It's known in China as Da T' Sao or wild Chinese jujube (botanical name *Zizyphus spinosa*), and is a godsend for women going through menopause and anyone suffering from insomnia, anxiety, or depression. It works as a natural antidepressant, sedative, and hypnotic. It's also a body toner, helping speed recovery time after workouts, and has been shown to have antioxidant properties that may protect against heart disease. Additionally, it can reduce high serum transaminase levels in people with hepatitis. As for dosage, 150 mg. of a standardized herbal extract can be taken once or twice daily.

Does dill have any nutritive or health-giving properties?

It does indeed. It can improve appetite and digestion and also act as a diuretic. Furthermore, chewing the seeds can help eliminate bad breath.

Is it true that flaxseed is a laxative?

It can act as one. The seeds are bulk formers. Flaxseed

can be eaten raw or cooked (it's great in soups), and 1 tbsp. daily has been found to prevent constipation in adults. Flaxseed oil is also one of the richest sources of omega-3 fatty acids, helpful in reducing cholesterol and alleviating arthritis pain.

My husband has liver problems and hates doctors. I've been told about a plant extract called milk thistle. Can you tell me something about it?

I can tell you that it appears to be one of the most potent, natural liver-protecting substances there is. The fruit of milk thistle contains silymarin, a remarkable flavonoid with antioxidant as well as anti-inflammatory properties that has been found to help in the treatment of chronic hepatitis, cirrhosis, and a variety of other liver diseases. Silymarin may also protect the liver from a broad range of toxins, including overindulgence in alcohol and side effects from prescription drugs, aiding the body in detoxification while helping it regenerate healthy liver cells. Supplements are available as liquids, tincture, and pills; some forms can be brewed as tea. I'd suggest, though, that your husband consult a healthcare professional before starting a milk thistle supplement regimen to make sure it won't inhibit the metabolism of any drugs or medications he might already be taking.

What are adaptogens? And are they available as supplements?

Adaptogens are a rare group of plants that seem to be able to use their properties within the body—where the body actually needs them—to help protect it from physical, emotional, and environmental stresses (including radiation and chemical poisons).

Among other reported benefits of adaptogens are

increased immunity defenses, enhanced energy, accelerated healing from respiratory infections, improved nerve functions, blood-pressure and blood-sugar normalizing effects.

One of the most highly touted for its health benefits is suma (*Pfaffia paniculata martius kuntze*), often called Brazilian ginseng.

Although unrelated to ginseng, suma (a member of the amaranth family) has been found to contain numerous vitamins, minerals, amino acids, and other healing elements, including germanium (an immune cell activator), allantoin (a wound healer), and sitosterol and stigmasterol (two vegetable hormones that have been found to reduce blood cholesterol and increase—when needed—the body's natural estrogen).

Supplements are available in pill form and as teas.

What is germanium? Is it an herb or a mineral—and what are its natural sources?

Germanium is what is known as a trace element (Ge-132). According to Dr. Parris M. Kidd, director of the Germanium Institute of North America, it has the ability to restore and stimulate immune function, supplement tissue oxygen (important for diets high in unsaturated fats, which—although cholesterol-lowering—deplete oxygen), help inhibit tumor development, and alleviate major diseases.

It is found in trace amounts in garlic, ginseng, chlorella, pearl barley, and comfrey.

An herbalist friend of mine said that goldenrod extract was good for nasal congestion. How can this be when so many people are allergic to it?

People are not allergic to it because goldenrod does not

cause allergies. The real allergy culprit is ragweed, fuzzy stalks that grow alongside goldenrod. Ragweed spores are lightweight, wind-borne barbs that cause those sniffles and itchy eyes. Your herbalist friend is right. In nature you'll often find the remedy grows right next to the cause. A few drops of goldenrod extract under the tongue has been found to relieve nasal congestion.

What can you tell me about an herb called Pau d'arco?

In my opinion, its uses in alternative therapies are just beginning. Pau d'arco (*Tabebuia impetiginosa*) has been found to be quite effective in inhibiting the growth of *Candida albicans* (see section 340). It is also effective in treating allergies where symptoms of bronchial asthma, eczema, and sinus congestion exist. And last but far from least, it is systemically helpful after long-term antibiotic therapy, immunosuppressant therapy, and steroidal anti-inflammatory therapy.

For best results, pau d'arco should be taken in conjunction with vitamins A and C, potassium, magnesium, and digestive enzymes.

Am I better off taking a liquid herbal or a tincture?

Liquids are generally formulated in a weakly acidic solution, allowing the supplement to enter the stomach in a soluble acidic state that can enhance absorption. A tincture, where herbs are usually suspended in alcohol or cider vinegar along with water, provides a weaker but still effective concentration. Both are absorbed quickly by the digestive system. Many people feel that quality tinctures offer more potent herbal concentrates, but it depends on the manufacturer. I'd suggest that you make your choice based on the formulation that most suits your needs.

I'd like to use tinctures, but I don't want the alcohol taste. Is there a way around this?

You can evaporate the alcohol by putting the tincture in hot water.

What can you tell me about the supplement HupA?

Some very good things. Huperzine A (or HupA) is extracted from club moss, a rare plant grown in China that's been used for centuries to treat various neurological disorders. It's been shown to enhance memory and may help alleviate symptoms associated with Alzheimer's disease. It's available as soft gels and tablets, but should not be taken by pregnant women or anyone with high blood pressure.

Does bitter melon help in lowering blood sugar, and how much is safe to take?

More studies are necessary, but the preliminary research indicates that this bitter-tasting tropical fruit can not only lower blood sugar but possibly even raise HDL ("good") cholesterol levels as well. A little goes a long way. Available in natural-food stores as a liquid extract, taking ¼ to ½ teaspoon up to three times daily is safe. Exceeding this dosage may cause diarrhea, headache, abdominal pain, or fever. It is not recommended if you are hypoglycemic, pregnant, or taking diabetes medication.

Fresh bitter melon is available at many Asian grocery stores. Noted Texas herbalist Robert Rister recommends making it into a smoothie by seeding, slicing, and cutting the melon into thin slices and then steaming or boiling it until tender. When soft enough to cut with a spoon, puree in a blender with equal amounts of water for two minutes.

I've heard about a natural supplement being used in the treatment of diabetes that can also be an effective diet aid. Do you know about it? I believe it's used in ayurvedic medicine.

It has been used for thousands of years in ayurvedic medicine to treat diabetes. It is *Gymnema sylvestre* ("sugar destroyer"), a woody climbing plant native to the forests of India. The roots and leaves of the plant have traditionally been used to treat a wide variety of conditions (from poisoning and fever to bronchial asthma and coughs), but primarily to treat blood-sugar disorders by controlling blood sugar levels. And this is where it can help as a diet aid.

When the gymnema leaf is placed directly on your tongue, it eliminates the sensation of sweetness, even if you were to put a sugar candy in your mouth immediately afterward. For anyone with a weakness for sweets and a waistline that shows it, taking 400 mg. of a standardized *Gymnema sylvestre* supplement could help.

CAUTION: *If you are in treatment for diabetes, are taking medications to control your blood sugar, or are hypoglycemic, consult your physician or healthcare provider before taking* Gymnema.

IX

How to Find Out What Vitamins You Really Need

233. What Is a Balanced Diet and Are You Eating It?

A balanced diet is something easily found in books and rarely on the table. Though nutrients are widely scattered all through our food supply, soil depletion, storage, food processing, and cooking destroy many of them. Still, there are enough left to make balancing meals important. After all, supplements cannot work without food, and the better the food you eat, the more effective your supplements will be. Unfortunately, no possible "balanced" diet is likely to meet nutritional needs today.

Nevertheless, to know whether or not you are balancing your meals, you should become familiar with the basic food groups and the recommended number of portions that should be eaten from them each day. Serving sizes are given—and they are probably less than you think—but they should be individually determined; smaller amounts for less-active people, larger amounts for teenagers and people who do physically strenuous work. Keep in mind that as you get older your metabolic rate slows and your energy needs decrease.

Based on the new USDA guidelines, suggested servings per day of grains, breads, cereals, vegetables, and fruits have been significantly increased while servings of dairy and meat products have been decreased. They are now as follows:

GRAIN GROUP

Whole or enriched grains, breads, hot or cold cereals, pasta, rice
    6–11 servings per day
    1 serving = 1 slice of bread or ½ cup of rice

VEGETABLE GROUP

Dark green, leafy, yellow, or orange vegetables
    3–5 servings per day
    1 serving = 1 cup raw, leafy vegetables (4 large leaves) or 6 oz. vegetable juice

FRUIT GROUP

Citrus fruits, tomatoes, or others rich in vitamin C
    2–4 servings per day
    1 serving = 1 medium fruit or 6 oz. fresh fruit juice

DAIRY GROUP

Milk, cheese, yogurt, foods made from milk
    2–3 servings per day
    1 serving = 1 cup yogurt or milk or 1 oz. cheese

MEAT GROUP

Beef, veal, pork, lamb, fish, poultry, liver, eggs, meat substitutes, dry beans, nuts

2–3 servings per day

1 serving = 3–4 oz. animal protein, roughly the size of a deck of cards, or ¼ cup nuts

FATS, OILS, SWEETS

Use sparingly.

The recommended servings, as outlined by the National Research Council, are designed to supply 1,200 calories. You are expected to adjust the size of the servings to suit your own individual growth, weight, and energy needs.

234. How to Test for Deficiencies

If you're wondering whether or not you need vitamin or mineral supplementation, your best bet would be to contact a nutritionally oriented doctor (see section 462). Other than that, there are a variety of indicator tests that should tell you enough to point you in the right supplement direction.

Dr. John M. Ellis has devised a quick early-warning test for B6 (pyridoxine) deficiency. Extend your hand, palm up, then try to bend the two joints in your four fingers (not the knuckles of your hand), until your fingertips reach your palm. (This is not a fist, only two joints are bent.) Do this with both hands. If it is difficult, if finger joints don't allow tips to reach your palm, a pyridoxine deficiency is likely.

Betty Lee Morales, the late well-known nutritionist, stated that urine is a fair indicator of the B vitamins in your body. Since B vitamins are water soluble and lost each day through excretion, when your body demands more, your urine will be light in color. When the urine is dark, your B demands are less. (*NOTE*: Urine that is dark yellow may indicate a need for fluids—see section 73—although many drugs, illnesses, and foods also alter urine color. This should be taken into consideration.)

Hair analyses, where a tablespoon of hair clipped from the back of the neck is sent to a laboratory to check for abnormally high toxic-mineral levels, have become a subject of controversy regarding their reliability. Hair analysts say that hair can serve as a permanent record of nutrient consumption and toxic exposure, since substances entering the hair stay there until the hair falls out. Their detractors, on the other hand, say that there are too many factors besides what we eat and drink that can influence the content of hair (dyes, shampoos, colorings, waving lotions, pool chemicals, etc.) to provide a reliable analysis.

As of this writing, the controversy has not been fully resolved either way. So my advice, once again, is to check with a nutritionally oriented doctor (see section 462) before investing in an analysis on your own.

Probably the best indicator of any vitamin or mineral deficiency is your body—and the way that it's feeling.

235. Possible Warning Signs

A body in need of vitamins usually lets you know about it sooner or later. It's unlikely that any of us will come down with scurvy before realizing we need vitamin C, but more often than not our bodies are giving us clues that we just don't recognize. With the price of medical insurance rising daily, paying attention to your nutritional warning system is about the best and cheapest insurance around. Here are a few common symptoms that you might be ignoring—and shouldn't. Where I've written "Are You Eating

Enough?" I'm not implying that you should be down-ing huge portions of these foods, just suggesting that their absence in your diet could be a good reason to use supplements.

The supplements recommended are not intended as medical advice, only as a guide in working with your doctor.

NOTE: *MVP stands for Mindell Vitamin Program (or Most Valuable Player in the nutrition game). It consists of:*

- One all-natural high-potency multiple vitamin and amino acid–chelated mineral complex (with digestive enzymes for better absorption)
- One broad-spectrum antioxidant formula (containing alpha- and beta-carotene, lutein, lycopene, vitamin C, vitamin E (mixed tocopherols), selenium, ginkgo biloba, coenzyme-Q10, bilberry, L-glutathione, cysteine, soy isoflavones [genistein and daidzein], grape-seed extract, and green tea extract)
- A probiotic capsule with 25 billion organisms per serving
- One 200 mg. vegetable capsule of curcumin (anti-inflammatory)
- MSM 1,000 mg. capsule (anti-inflammatory)

The above MVP can be taken once or twice daily with food.

NEW DELIVERY SYSTEM FOR DIETARY SUPPLEMENTS

Liposome delivery system advantage: Liposomes are double-layered "bubbles," or spheres, that surround the nutrients, helping them to pass through the harsh environment of your digestive system intact for better absorption and use by your body. The advantage is maximized results with minimum waste. The nutrients arrive intact to your cells for a much higher rate of absorption.

Liposome delivery system benefits include:

- Highest bioavailability and absorption of any oral (by mouth) delivery system of nutrients compared to the bioavailability of traditionally based supplements. The results are typically 4.5 times stronger per serving size. Bioavailability is defined as the proportion of a substance that enters the circulation when the substance is introduced into your body, and so the proportion that is able to hold active effect. By utilizing enzymes, this delivery system optimizes the delivery of key nutrients within your body by helping replace lost enzymes that have been destroyed by drying. This helps ensure that the liposome-delivery-system nutrients are absorbed and utilized faster and more efficiently.
- Micronized encapsulation protects against the harsh environment of your gastrointestinal tract and increases transmucosal (oral) uptake and absorption.
- Increases intracellular delivery
- Can hold hydrophilic (water-loving) and hydrophilic (water-hating) compounds
- Ideal for those for whom swallowing tablets or capsules in not possible

Possible Deficiency—
ARE YOU EATING ENOUGH?

SYMPTOM: *Appetite Loss*

Protein	Meat, fish, eggs, dairy products, soybeans, peanuts
Vitamin A	Fish, liver, egg yolks, green leafy or yellow vegetables
Vitamin B1	Brewer's yeast, whole grains, meat (pork or liver), nuts, legumes, potatoes
Vitamin C	Citrus fruits, tomatoes, potatoes, cabbage, green peppers
Biotin	Brewer's yeast, nuts, beef liver, beef kidney, unpolished rice
Phosphorus	Milk, cheese, meat, poultry, fish, cereals, nuts, legumes
Sodium	Beef, pork, sardines, cheese, green olives, corn bread, sauerkraut
Zinc	Vegetables, whole grains, wheat bran, wheat germ, pumpkin seeds, sunflower seeds

RECOMMENDED SUPPLEMENT:

> 1 B complex, 50 mg., taken with each meal
> 1 B12, 200 mcg. with breakfast
> 1 organic iron complex tablet (containing vitamin C, copper, liver, manganese, and zinc to help assimilate iron)

SYMPTOM: *Bad Breath*

Niacin	Liver, meat, fish, whole grains, legumes

RECOMMENDED SUPPLEMENT:

> 1–2 tbsp. *acidophilus* liquid (flavored) one to three times daily

1 chlorophyll tablet or capsule three
times daily
1 amino acid–chelated zinc 50 mg. tab daily
1–3 multiple digestive enzyme capsules at
the beginning of each meal

SYMPTOM: *Body Odor*
B12   Yeast, liver, beef, eggs, kidney
Zinc   Vegetables, whole grains, wheat bran,
               wheat germ, pumpkin seeds, sunflower
               seeds
RECOMMENDED SUPPLEMENT:
               1–2 tbsp. *acidophilus* liquid (flavored) one
               to three times daily
               1 chlorophyll tablet or capsule three times
               daily
               1 chelated zinc 15–50 mg. tab daily
               1–2 multiple digestive enzyme tabs one to
               three times daily

SYMPTOM: *Bruising Easily* (when slight or minor injuries produce bluish, purplish discoloration of skin)
Vitamin C   Citrus fruits, tomatoes, potatoes, cabbage,
               green peppers
Bioflavonoids Orange, lemon, lime, tangerine, peas
RECOMMENDED SUPPLEMENT:
               1–2 C complex, 500 mg. with
               bioflavonoids, rutin, and hesperidin A.M.
               and P.M. with meals

SYMPTOM: *High Cholesterol*
B-complex inositol
               Yeast, brewer's yeast, dried lima beans,
               raisins, cantaloupe

RECOMMENDED SUPPLEMENT:

> 1 tbsp. lecithin granules sprinkled on salad or in soy shake
> 1 omega-3 fatty acid cap, 1,000 mg. daily
> 1 scoop flavored soy protein (25 gm.) in 1–1½ cups nonfat soy milk
> 1–3 tablets of combination niacin (flush-free) 200 mg., policosanol 60 mg., soy phytosterols 10 mg. (beta-sitosterol, campesterol, stigmasterol), gugulipid guggulsterone extract 2.5 percent taken at bedtime.
> (Most cholesterol produced in your body is manufactured while you sleep.)

SYMPTOM: *Constipation*

B complex — Whole grains, legumes, bran, green leafy vegetables

RECOMMENDED SUPPLEMENT:

> 8–10 glasses of water daily
> 300 million CFU microencapsulated lactobacillus cells
> 3 tbsp. bran or 4 fiber complex tablets daily
> 25 mg. triphala standardized extract
> 5 mg. aloe vera whole-leaf extract
> 75 mg. butternut bark
> 915 mg. multiple green food complex
> Chicory and Jerusalem artichoke fructo-oligosaccharides
> Larch tree arabinogalactan 500 mg.
> Mandarin-oligosaccharides and mushroom extract

SYMPTOM: *Diarrhea*

Vitamin K	Yogurt, alfalfa, soybean oil, fish liver oils, kelp
Niacin	Liver, lean meat, brewer's yeast, wheat germ, peanuts, dried nutritional yeast, white meat of poultry, avocado, fish, legumes, whole grain
Vitamin F	Vegetable oils, peanuts, sunflower seeds, walnuts

RECOMMENDED SUPPLEMENT:

4 fiber complex tablets containing 2 grams of fiber daily

Cut-up carrots, whole grains (not whole wheat), garlic, raspberry leaf tea and chamomile tea

SYMPTOM: *Dizziness*

Manganese	Nuts, green leafy vegetables, peas, beets, egg yolks
B2 (Riboflavin)	Milk, liver, kidney, yeast, cheese, fish, eggs

RECOMMENDED SUPPLEMENT:

50–100 mg. "no-flush" niacin three times a day

200 IU dry vitamin E one to three times a day

60 mg. standardized ginkgo biloba tablets one to three times a day

SYMPTOM: *Ear Noises*

Manganese	Nuts, green leafy vegetables, peas, beets, egg yolks
Potassium	Bananas, watercress, all leafy green vegetables, citrus fruits, sunflower seeds

RECOMMENDED SUPPLEMENT:

> 50–100 mg. "no-flush" niacin three times a
> day
> 400 IU dry vitamin E one to three times a
> day
> 50 mg. zinc daily

SYMPTOM: *Eye Problems* (night blindness, inability to
adjust to darkness, bloodshot eyes, inflammations, burning
sensations, sties)

Vitamin A	Fish, liver, egg yolks, butter, cream, green leafy or yellow vegetables
B2 (Riboflavin)	Milk, liver, kidney, yeast, cheese, fish, eggs

RECOMMENDED SUPPLEMENT:

> 50 mg. B complex, 1 in A.M. and P.M. with
> food
> 500 mg. vitamin C with bioflavonoids,
> rutin, and hesperidin, 1 in A.M. and P.M.
> 400 IU vitamin E (dry), 1 in A.M. and P.M.
> 1 broad-spectrum antioxidant (mixed
> carotenoids and beta-carotene, selenium,
> n-acetylcysteine, and quercetin), plus
> 200 mg. taurine, 80 mg. bilberry
> standardized extract, eyebright, ginkgo
> biloba leaf extract, green tea leaf, 100
> mg. grape seed, and 3 mg. lutein taken
> twice daily with food

SYMPTOM: *Fatigue* (lassitude, weakness, no inclination
for physical activity)

Zinc	Vegetables, whole-grain products, brewer's yeast, wheat bran, wheat germ, pumpkin and sunflower seeds

Carbohydrates	Cellulose
Protein	Meat, fish, eggs, dairy products, soybeans, peanuts
Vitamin A	Fish, liver, egg yolks, butter, cream, green leafy or yellow vegetables
Vitamin B complex	Yeast, brewer's yeast, dried lima beans, raisins, cantaloupe
PABA	
Iron	Wheat germ, soybean flour, beef, kidney, liver, beans, clams, peaches, and molasses
Iodine	Seafoods, dairy products, kelp
Vitamin C	Citrus fruits, tomatoes, potatoes, cabbage, green peppers
Vitamin D	Fish liver oils, butter, egg yolks, liver, sunshine

RECOMMENDED SUPPLEMENT:

1 B complex, 100 mg. two times daily
One 2,000 mcg. B12 A.M. and P.M.
1 DMG (dimethylglycine) 50–100 mg. with meals
Coenzyme-Q10, 30–100 mg. daily
MVP, 1 A.M. and P.M. with meals
1 dropper (1 ml.) of adaptogen formula containing siberian ginseng, ginger root, ashwagandha root, schizandra seed, ginseng root, rhodiola root, pantocene, American ginseng root, green tea, hawthorn leaf and flower, grape seed and skin taken two to three times daily between meals.
Eliminate all caffeinated beverages
Drink an energy drink with L-phenylalanine with or before each meal.

SYMPTOM: *Gastrointestinal Problems* (gastritis, gastric ulcers, gallbladder, digestive disturbances)

Vitamin B1 (thiamin)	Brewer's yeast, whole grains, meat (pork or liver), nuts, legumes, potatoes
Vitamin B2 (riboflavin)	Milk, liver, kidney, yeast, cheese, fish, eggs
Folic acid (folacin)	Fresh green leafy vegetables, fruit, organ meats, liver, dried nutritional yeast
PABA	Yeast, brewer's yeast, dried lima beans, raisins, cantaloupe
Vitamin C	Citrus fruits, tomatoes, potatoes, cabbage, green peppers
Chlorine	Kelp, rye flour, ripe olives, sea greens
Pantothenic acid	Yeast, brewer's yeast, dried lima beans, raisins, cantaloupe

RECOMMENDED SUPPLEMENT:

10,000 IU beta-carotene one to two times daily

100 mg. B complex, 1 A.M. and P.M.

Multiple minerals, 1 A.M. and P.M.

Betaine HC1 500 mg. a half hour before meals with glass of water

Multiple digestive enzyme a half hour after meals with glass of water

Fresh-squeezed cabbage juice, 1 glass after meals

1 scoop prebiotic mix (containing inulin from chicory root, cluster bean, larch bark and L-glutamine) dissolved in filtered water, drink one to three times daily

SYMPTOM: *Hair Problems*

        1. DANDRUFF (loose flakes—dry or yellow and greasy—which fall from scalp)

Vitamin B12 (cyanocobalamin)	Liver, beef, pork, organ meats, eggs, milk and milk products
Vitamin F	Vegetable oils, peanuts, sunflower seeds, walnuts
Vitamin B6	Dried nutritional yeast, liver, organ meats, legumes, whole-grain cereals, fish
Selenium	Bran, germ of cereals, broccoli, onions, tomatoes, and tuna

RECOMMENDED SUPPLEMENT:

        100 mcg. selenium twice daily

        1 MVP A.M. and P.M. with food

        1 omega-3 capsule, 1,000 mg., with each meal

        1 MSM 1,000 mg. with vitamin C complex., with each meal

SYMPTOM: *Hair Problems*

        2. DULL, DRY, BRITTLE, OR GRAYING HAIR

Vitamin A complex	
PABA	Yeast, brewer's yeast, dried lima beans, raisins, cantaloupe
Vitamin F	Vegetable oils, peanuts, sunflower seeds, walnuts
Iodine	Seafoods, iodized salt, dairy products

RECOMMENDED SUPPLEMENT:

        1 omega-3 capsule, 1,000 mg. with each meal

        3 lecithin caps with each meal

        1 MVP A.M. and P.M. with food

1 MSM 1,000 mg. with vitamin C complex, with each meal

SYMPTOM: *Hair Problems*

3. LOSS OF HAIR

Biotin	Brewer's yeast, nuts, beef liver, kidney, unpolished rice
Inositol	Unrefined molasses and liver, lecithin, unprocessed whole grains, citrus fruits, brewer's yeast
Chlorine	Sodium chloride (table salt)
B complex with C and folic acid	Yeast, brewer's yeast, dried lima beans, raisins, cantaloupe, citrus fruits, green peppers, tomatoes, cabbage, potatoes, fresh green leafy vegetables, fruit, organ meats, liver, dried nutritional yeast

RECOMMENDED SUPPLEMENT:

1,000 mg. choline and inositol daily
Cysteine 1 g. daily
Biotin 3,000 mcg. daily
B complex 150 mg. A.M. and P.M. with meals
Saw palmetto berry standardized extract 160 mg. daily
Beta-sitosterol complex 30 mg. daily

SYMPTOM: *Heart Palpitation*

Vitamin B12 (cobalamin, cyanocobalamin) — Yeast, liver, beef, eggs, kidney

RECOMMENDED SUPPLEMENT:

1 MVP A.M. and P.M. with meals
50 mg. vitamin B complex A.M. and P.M. with meals

500 mg. calcium and 250 mg. magnesium
tablet daily
Coenzyme Q-10 60 mg. daily
Hawthorn flower and leaf standardized
extract 200 mg. daily
Aged garlic 200 mg. with parsley seed oil
one to three times daily

SYMPTOM: *High Blood Pressure*
Choline   Egg yolks, beef brain, heart, green leafy
                 vegetables, yeast, liver, wheat germ
RECOMMENDED SUPPLEMENT:
                 1 MVP A.M. and P.M. with meals
                 Start with 200 IU vitamin E and work up
                 to higher strengths.
                 Coenzyme-Q10 30 mg. daily
                 500 mg. calcium and 250 mg. magnesium
                 tab three times daily (take 1 a half hour
                 before bedtime)
                 1 odorless garlic capsule three times
                 daily
                 3 celery stalks daily

SYMPTOM: *Infections* (high susceptibility)
Vitamin A
(carotene)   Fish, liver, egg yolks, butter, cream, green
                 leafy or yellow vegetables
Pantothenic acid
                 Yeast, brewer's yeast, dried lima beans,
                 raisins, cantaloupe
RECOMMENDED SUPPLEMENT:
                 1–2 tbsp. *acidophilus* three times daily
                 Vitamin A up to 10,000 IU every other
                 day for duration of infection

Standardized American feverfew, 25 mg.
two to three times daily
Standardized echinachea root, 25 mg. two
to three times daily
1 scoop prebiotic mix (containing inulin
from chicory root, cluster bean, larch bark
and L-glutamine) dissolved in filtered
water, drink one to three times daily
1 MVP A.M. and P.M. (2–5 g. vitamin C
for duration of infection)

SYMPTOM: *Insomnia*

Potassium	Bananas, watercress, all leafy green vegetables, citrus fruits, sunflower seeds
B complex	Yeast, brewer's yeast, dried lima beans, raisins, cantaloupe
Biotin	Brewer's yeast, nuts, beef liver, kidney, unpolished rice
Calcium	Milk and milk products, meat, fish, eggs, cereal products, beans, fruit, vegetables

RECOMMENDED SUPPLEMENT:

1–5 mg. melatonin at bedtime
Vitamin B6 100 mg., calcium and
magnesium tablet at bedtime
St. John's wort complex, 300 mg., 1–2
tablets at bedtime
1 MVP A.M. and P.M.

SYMPTOM: *Loss of Smell*

Vitamin A	Fish, liver, egg yolks, butter, cream, green leafy or yellow vegetables
Zinc	Vegetables, whole grains, wheat bran, wheat germ, pumpkin and sunflower seeds

RECOMMENDED SUPPLEMENT:

> 50 mg. amino acid–chelated zinc three times daily (cut back to 1–2 daily when condition improves)
>
> Standardized herbal extract of ginkgo biloba, 60 mg. two to three times daily

SYMPTOM: *Memory Loss*

B1 (thiamin) Brewer's yeast, whole grains, meat (pork or liver), nuts, legumes, potatoes

RECOMMENDED SUPPLEMENT:

> One memory support tablet containing: B1 3mg.; folacin, 200 mcg.; pantothenic acid, 25 mg.; B12, 12 mcg.; zinc citrate, 5 mg.; bacopa moniera, 100 mg.; fo-ti root; gingerroot; gotu kola leaf; siberian ginseng 15 mg.; phosphatydylcholine and phophatidylserine, 50 mg.; DMAE, 75 mg.; standardized ginkgo biloba leaf extract, 60 mg.; L-Glutamine, 50 mg.; vinpocetine, 5 mg.; wild blueberry extract, 100 mg.; huperzine A (club moss), 100 mg. taken three times daily with food

SYMPTOM: *Menstrual Problems*

B12 Yeast, liver, beef, eggs, kidney

RECOMMENDED SUPPLEMENT:

> 7–10 days before period:
>
> 1 MVP A.M. and P.M. with meals
>
> 100 mg. B6 three times daily
>
> 100 mg. B complex (time release) A.M. and P.M.
>
> Evening primrose oil, 500 mg. three times daily

> 500 mg. magnesium and half as much
> calcium once daily
> Black cohosh standardized extract, 40 mg.
> once daily
> Wild jujube seed extract, 150 mg. once daily
> CBD, 50 mg. daily

SYMPTOM: *Mouth Sores and Cracks*

Vitamin B12 (riboflavin)	Milk, liver, kidney, yeast, cheese, fish, eggs
Vitamin B6 (pyridoxine)	Dried nutritional yeast, liver, organ meats, legumes, whole-grain cereals, fish

RECOMMENDED SUPPLEMENT:

> 50 mg. B complex three times daily with
> meals
> 1 MVP A.M. and P.M.

SYMPTOM: *Muscle Cramps* (general muscle weakness, tenderness in calf, night cramps, charley horse)

Vitamin B1 (thiamin)	Brewer's yeast, whole grains, meat (pork or liver), nuts, legumes, potatoes
Vitamin B6 (pyridoxine)	Dried nutritional yeast, liver, organ meats, legumes, whole-grain cereals, fish
Biotin	Brewer's yeast, nuts, beef liver, kidney, unpolished rice
Chlorine	Sodium chloride (table salt)
Sodium	Beef, pork, sardines, cheese, green olives, corn bread, sauerkraut
Vitamin D (calciferol)	Fish liver oils, butter, egg yolks, liver, sunshine

RECOMMENDED SUPPLEMENT:

> 400 IU vitamin E (dry) three times daily
> Amino acid–chelated calcium and
> magnesium, 3 tabs three times daily

SYMPTOM: *Nervousness*

Vitamin B6 (pyridoxine)	Dried nutritional yeast, liver, organ meats, legumes, whole-grain cereals, fish
Vitamin B12 (cyanocobalamin)	Yeast, liver, beef, eggs, kidney
Niacin (nicotinic acid, niacinamide)	Liver, meat, fish, whole grains, legumes
PABA	Yeast, brewer's yeast, dried lima beans, raisins, cantaloupe
Magnesium	Green leafy vegetables, nuts, cereals, grains, seafoods

RECOMMENDED SUPPLEMENT:

B complex one to three times daily (50 mg. of all B vitamins)

1 St. John's wort complex two to three times daily

3 amino acid–chelated calcium and magnesium tabs three times daily

1 MVP A.M. and P.M. with meals

SYMPTOM: *Nosebleeds*

Vitamin C	Citrus fruits, tomatoes, potatoes, cabbage, green peppers
Vitamin K	Yogurt, alfalfa, soybean oil, fish liver oils, kelp
Bioflavonoids	Orange, lemon, lime, tangerine peels

RECOMMENDED SUPPLEMENT:

1,000 mg. vitamin C with 50 mg. rutin, hesperidin, and 500 mg. bioflavonoids (time release) A.M. and P.M.

SYMPTOM: *Slowed Growth*

Fat	Meat, butter

Protein	Meat, fish, eggs, dairy products, soybeans, peanuts
Vitamin B2 (riboflavin)	Milk, liver, kidney, yeast, cheese, fish, eggs
Folic acid	Fresh green leafy vegetables, fruit, organ meats, liver, dried nutritional yeast
Zinc	Vegetables, whole grains, wheat bran, wheat germ, pumpkin and sunflower seeds
Cobalt	Liver, kidney, pancreas, and spleen (organ meats)

RECOMMENDED SUPPLEMENT:

1 MVP A.M. and P.M. with meals

SYMPTOM: *Skin Problems*

1. ACNE (face blemishes, thickened skin, blackheads, whiteheads, red spots)

| Water-solubilized vitamin A | Fish, liver, egg yolks, butter, cream, green leafy or yellow vegetables |
| Vitamin B complex | Yeast, brewer's yeast, dried lima beans, raisins, cantaloupe |

RECOMMENDED SUPPLEMENT:

1 multiple vitamin-mineral (low in iodine) daily

1–2 400 IU vitamin E (dry) daily

10,000 IU beta-carotene, 1–2 tabs daily six days a week

50 mg. amino acid–chelated zinc once daily with food

1–2 tbsp. *acidophilus* liquid three times daily or 3–6 caps three times daily

(Iodine worsens acne, so eliminate all processed foods—high in iodized salt—from your diet.)

1 MSM (methylsulfonylmethane) 1,000 mg.
tablet two to three times daily with food
MSM therapeutic lotion can be applied to
affected areas two to three times daily as well
Astaxanthin, 4 mg. daily
CBD, 50 mg. daily

2. DERMATITIS (skin inflammation)

Vitamin B2 (riboflavin)	Milk, liver, kidney, yeast, cheese, fish, eggs
Vitamin B6 (Pyridoxine)	Dried nutritional yeast, liver, organ meats, legumes, whole-grain cereals, fish
Biotin	Brewer's yeast, nuts, beef liver, kidney, unpolished rice
Niacin (nicotinic acid, niacinamide)	Liver, meat, fish, whole grains, legumes

RECOMMENDED SUPPLEMENT:

1 multiple vitamin-mineral (low in iodine)
daily
1–2 400 IU vitamin E (dry) daily
10,000 IU beta-carotene 1–2 tabs daily six
days a week
50 mg. amino acid–chelated zinc once
daily with food
1–2 tbsp. *acidophilus* liquid three times
daily or 3–6 caps three times daily
500 mg. evening primrose oil two to three
times daily
1 MSM 1,000 mg. tablet two to three
times daily with food
MSM therapeutic lotion can be applied to
affected areas two to three times daily as well

3. ECZEMA (rough, dry, scaly skin, redness and swelling, small blisters)

Fat	Meat, butter
Vitamin A (carotene)	Fish, liver, egg yolks, butter, cream, green leafy or yellow vegetables
Vitamin B complex Inositol	Yeast, brewer's yeast, dried lima beans, raisins, cantaloupe
Copper	Organ meats, oysters, nuts, dried legumes, whole-grain cereals
Iodine	Seafoods, iodized salt, dairy products

RECOMMENDED SUPPLEMENT:

1 multiple vitamin-mineral (low in iodine) daily

1 MSM 1,000 mg. tablet two to three times daily with food

1–2 400 IU vitamin E (dry) daily

10,000 IU beta-carotene, 1–2 tabs daily six days a week

50 mg. amino acid–chelated zinc once daily with food

1–2 tbsp. *acidophilus* liquid three times daily or 3–6 caps three times daily

MSM therapeutic lotion applied externally two to three times daily

SYMPTOM: *Slow-healing Wounds and Fractures*

Vitamin C	Citrus fruits, tomatoes, potatoes, cabbage, green peppers

RECOMMENDED SUPPLEMENT:

50 mg. zinc once daily

400 IU dry vitamin E three times daily

1 MVP A.M. and P.M. with meals

SYMPTOM: *Softening of Bones and Teeth*

| Vitamin D (calciferol) | Fish liver oils, butter, egg yolks, liver, sunshine |
| Calcium | Milk and milk products, meat, fish, eggs, cereal products, beans, fruit, vegetables |

RECOMMENDED SUPPLEMENT:

1,000–1,500 mg. calcium, 500 mg. magnesium divided over two meals daily
Vitamin D, 2,000 IU daily with largest meal.
Vitamin K, 80 mcg. daily
Boron, 300 mcg. daily
Soy isoflavones, 40–80 mg. daily

SYMPTOM: *Tremors*

| Magnesium | Green leafy vegetables, nuts, cereals, grains, seafoods |

RECOMMENDED SUPPLEMENT:

B complex and 50 mg. B6 three times daily
1,000 mg. calcium, 500 mg. magnesium divided over three meals daily
1 St. John's wort complex two to three times daily
CBD, 50 mg. daily

SYMPTOM: *Vaginal Itching*

| Vitamin B2 | Milk, liver, kidney, yeast, cheese, fish, eggs |

RECOMMENDED SUPPLEMENT:

2 tbsp. *acidophilus* three times daily or 3–6 caps three to four times daily
(*Acidophilus* or mild vinegar douche can also help.)

SYMPTOM: *Water Retention*

| Vitamin B6 | Dried nutritional yeast, liver, organ meats, legumes, whole-grain cereals, fish |

RECOMMENDED SUPPLEMENT:

> 100 mg. B6 three times daily
>
> Potassium 99 mg. 3–6 tabs daily

SYMPTOM: *White Spots on Nails*

Zinc   Vegetables, whole grains, wheat bran, wheat germ, pumpkin and sunflower seeds

RECOMMENDED SUPPLEMENT:

> 15 mg. amino acid–chelated zinc three times daily
>
> MSM tab, 1,000 mg. twice daily
>
> MVP A.M. and P.M. with meals

236. Cravings—What They Might Mean

Cravings, which can sometimes mean allergies, are more often nature's way of letting you know that you're not getting enough of certain vitamins or minerals. Frequently these specific hungers develop because your overall diet is inadequate.

Some of the most common cravings are:

Peanut butter: This is definitely among the top ten, and it's not at all surprising. Peanut butter is a rich source of B vitamins. If you find yourself dipping into the jar often, it might be because you're under stress and your ordinary B intake has become insufficient. Since 50 g. of peanut butter—a third of a cup—is 284 calories, you'll find it easier on your waistline to take a B-complex supplement if you do not want to gain weight.

Bananas: When you catch yourself reaching for this fruit again and again, it could be because your body needs potassium. One medium banana has 555 mg. People taking diuretics or cortisone (which rob the body of needed potassium) often crave bananas.

Cheese: If you're more a cheese luster than a cheese lover, there's a good chance that your real hunger is for calcium and phosphorus. (If it's processed cheese that you've been snacking on, you've been getting aluminum and salt, too, without knowing it.) For one thing, you might try eating more broccoli. That's high in calcium and phosphorus, and a lot lower in calories than cheese.

Apples: An apple a day doesn't necessarily keep the doctor away, but it offers a lot of good things that you might be missing in other foods—calcium, magnesium, phosphorus, potassium—and is an excellent source of cholesterol-lowering pectin! If you have a tendency to eat a lot of saturated fat, it could account for your apple cravings.

Butter: Most often vegetarians crave butter because of their own low saturated-fat intake. Salted butter, on the other hand, might be craved for the salt alone.

Cola: The craving for cola is most often a sugar hunger and an addiction to caffeine. The beverage has no nutritive value.

Nuts: If you're a little nutty about nuts, you probably could use more protein, B vitamins, or fat in your diet. If it's salted nuts you favor, you could be craving the sodium and not the nuts. You'll find that people under stress tend to eat more nuts than relaxed individuals.

Ice cream: High as ice cream is in calcium, most people crave it for its sugar content. Hypoglycemics and diabetics have great hungers for it, as do people seeking to recapture the security of childhood.

Pickles: If you're pregnant and want pickles, you're probably after the salt. And if you're not pregnant and crave pickles, the reason is most likely the same. (Pickles also contain a substantial amount of potassium.)

Bacon: Cravings for bacon are usually because of its fat.

People on restricted diets are most susceptible to greasy binges. Unfortunately, saturated fat is not bacon's only drawback. Bacon is very high in carcinogenic nitrites. If you do indulge in bacon, be sure you're ingesting enough vitamins C, A, D, and E to counteract the nitrites.

Eggs: Aside from the protein (2 eggs give you 13 g.), sulfur, amino acids, and selenium, egg lovers might also be seeking the yolk's fat content or, paradoxically, its cholesterol-and-fat-dissolving choline.

Cantaloupe: Just because you like its taste might not be the only reason you crave this melon. Cantaloupe is high in potassium and vitamin A. In fact, a quarter of a melon has 3,400 IU vitamin A. Since the melon also offers vitamin C, calcium, magnesium, phosphorus, biotin, and inositol, it's not a bad craving to give in to. There's only about 60 calories in half a melon.

Olives: Whether you crave them green or black, you're likely to be after the salt. People with underactive thyroids are most often the first to reach for them.

Salt: No guesswork here, it's the sodium you're after. Cravers quite possibly have a thyroid iodine deficiency or low sodium Addison's disease. Hypertensives often crave salt, and shouldn't.

Onions: Cravings for spicy foods can sometimes indicate problems in the lungs or sinuses.

Chocolate: Definitely one of the foremost cravings, if not *the* foremost. Chocoholics are addicted to the caffeine as well as the sugar. (There are 5–10 mg. of caffeine in a cup of cocoa.) If you want to kick the chocolate habit, try carob instead. (Carob, also called St. John's bread, is made from the edible pods of the Mediterranean carob tree.)

Milk: If you're still craving milk as an adult, you might need a calcium supplement. Then again, it might be the amino acids—such as tryptophan, leucine, and lysine—that your body needs. Nervous people often seek out the tryptophan in milk, since it has a very soothing effect.

Chinese food: Of course it's delicious, but often it's the monosodium glutamate in the food that fosters the craving. People with salt deficiencies usually go all out for Chinese food. (MSG can cause a histamine reaction in some individuals. Headaches and flushing may occur. Most Chinese restaurants will prepare your food without MSG if you request it.)

Mayonnaise: Since this is a fatty food, it is often craved by vegetarians and people who have eliminated other fats from their diet.

Tart fruits: A persistent craving for tart fruits can often indicate problems with the gallbladder or liver.

Paint and dirt: Children have a tendency to eat paint and dirt. Frequently this is an indication of a calcium or vitamin-D deficiency. A hard reevaluation of your child's diet is essential, and a visit to your pediatrician is recommended. This craving for nonfood items is known as pica. It's a condition also experienced by pregnant women, who should be aware that ingesting such substances can harm fetal development.

237. Getting the Most Vitamins from Your Food

Eating the right foods doesn't necessarily mean that you're getting the vitamins they contain. Food processing, storing, and cooking can easily undermine the best nutritious intentions. To get the most from what you eat (not to mention what you spend), keep the following tips in mind:

- Wash but don't soak fresh vegetables if you hope to benefit from the B vitamins and C they contain.
- Forgo convenience and make your salads when you're ready to eat them. Fruits and vegetables cut up and left to stand lose vitamins.
- Use a sharp knife when cutting or shredding fresh vegetables, because vitamins A and C are diminished when vegetable tissues are bruised.
- If you don't plan to eat your fresh fruit or vegetables for a few days, you're better off buying flash-frozen ones. The vitamin content of good frozen green beans will be higher than those fresh ones you've kept in your refrigerator for a week.
- Store frozen meat at 0 degrees F. or lower immediately after purchase to prevent loss of quality and bacterial growth.
- Don't thaw your frozen vegetables before cooking.
- Broccoli leaves have a higher vitamin A value than the flower buds or stalks.
- There are more vitamins in converted and parboiled rice than in polished rice, and brown rice is more nutritious than white.
- Frozen foods that you can boil in their bags offer more vitamins than the ordinary kind, and all frozen foods are preferable to canned ones.
- Cooking in copper pots can destroy vitamin C, folic acid, and vitamin E.
- Stainless steel, glass, and enamel are the best utensils for retaining nutrients while cooking. (Iron pots can give you the benefit of that mineral, but they will shortchange you on vitamin C.)
- The shortest cooking time and the smallest amount of water are the least destructive to nutrients.

- Cut longer-cooking vegetables in large pieces for minimum surface exposure to water and heat.
- Rinse canned vegetables to eliminate excess salt.
- Milk in glass containers can lose riboflavin, as well as vitamins A and D, unless kept out of the light. (Breads exposed to light can also lose these nutrients.)
- Well-browned, crusty, or toasted baked goods have less thiamin than others.
- Bake and boil potatoes in their skins to get the most vitamins from them.
- Use cooking water from vegetables to make soups, juices from meats for gravies, and syrups from canned fruits to make desserts.
- Refrain from using any baking soda when cooking vegetables if you want to benefit from their thiamin and vitamin C.
- Store vegetables and fruits in the refrigerator as soon as you bring them home from the market.

DID YOU KNOW?

- Broccoli sprayed in the market with a fine mist of water keeps almost *twice* as much of its vitamin C as unsprayed broccoli.
- Outer leaves of lettuce have more calcium, iron, and vitamin A than inner leaves.
- Men who eat three servings a week of cruciferous vegetables reduce the risk of prostate cancer by 41 percent.
- Vegetarians who consume nuts five or more times a week have a lower risk of heart disease than those consuming nuts less than once a week.

238. Any Questions About Chapter IX?

I feed my children what I think is a pretty well-balanced diet. But they're teenagers and when they're out they often have burgers, hot dogs, shakes, and that sort of junk food. Are these really bad for them?

Well, ounce for ounce, munch for munch, and sip for sip, the bad far outweighs the good. For instance, a fast-food burger can supply 44 percent of a teenage boy's requirement for protein. But when you consider that a Big Mac, for example, is also supplying 600 calories, 33 g. of fat, 8 g. of sugar, and 1,050 mg. of sodium, you have to admit that's an awfully high nutritional price to pay for protein. No one needs all that salt (see section 426). And, unfortunately, a salad like McDonald's Crispy Chicken California Cobb is not much better nutritionally; it contains 21 g. of fat and 1,130 mg. of sodium.

If they have to have a burger, try Beyond Meat, Impossible Burger, or another of the recent meatless burger brands made from vegetable ingredients with no animal source.

As for hot dogs, there's very little good to say about them. They're a high-fat, low-protein meat, and usually contain sodium or potassium nitrite. Nitrites combine with substances called amines, commonly found in foods, and form nitrosamines, which have been found to be carcinogenic (cancer-causing). Try turkey or chicken hot dogs to decrease the fat content. The label should say no preservatives, and no artificial colors or flavors.

Shakes, which do contain milk or a milk product, also contain 8–14 tsp. of sugar and 276 to 685 mg. of salt. Your kids could blend one up at home for half the price, calories, sugar, and salt—and double the nutritional value. Passing this information along to your children might be a good way to get them to pass up those fast-food places.

I've been told that I'm developing colon polyps. Are there vitamins you can recommend to slow their growth and help reduce the risk of colon or rectal cancer?

I can and I will. I only wish more people knew that colon and rectal cancers—which are virtually epidemic in the United States—are largely preventable and due in most cases to environmental factors, particularly diet. It's a known fact that people who eat a high-fat diet are at greater risk of developing colon or rectal cancer than people whose diet is rich in fiber and different types of fruits and vegetables. Studies have found that folic acid may help reduce the risk of rectal cancer. In fact, one study suggested that just ½ cup of spinach per day could supply enough folic acid to reduce the risk. But if you're not the Popeye type, I'd recommend two 400 mcg. folate tablets or capsules daily. I'd also suggest 500 mg. calcium with 250 mg. magnesium twice daily. (Make sure you're also getting 800 to 1000 IU of vitamin D to promote the absorption of calcium.) Also, because protease inhibitors are compounds that block an enzyme that promotes tumor growth and phytic acid is an antioxidant and chelator that binds with certain metals that may promote tumor growth, I'd recommend drinking a soy shake daily. Both protease inhibitors and phytic acid are abundant in soy foods. (See section 143 for more about soy.)

Very often I experience a sort of hot, burning feeling on my tongue and lips. It doesn't seem to be related to any foods I've eaten. Could it indicate a vitamin deficiency?

It's very possible. The feeling of having a burning tongue or lips has in many instances been linked to a vitamin B1 (Thiamin) deficiency. I'd suggest increasing your intake of whole wheat, oatmeal, bran, vegetables, and brewer's yeast, along with taking a balanced vitamin B complex, 50 mg., twice a day with food—and the MVP. (See section 246.)

My mother has a craving for ice. Not just on hot days, but all the time. She chews cubes as if they were candy. Could this sort of craving have anything to do with a dietary deficiency?

If your mother is often tired, her craving for ice might indicate an iron deficiency (which can cause a low-grade anemia). You might try encouraging her to add more iron-rich foods to her diet (liver, dried peaches, red meat, oysters, asparagus, oatmeal) and to take an organic iron supplement, 50–100 mg. daily.

I'm forty-two years old and am developing yellowish growths around my eyes. Is there some vitamin or nutrient that's missing from my diet that could be causing this?

More likely those growths are cholesterol deposits, which can occur when the body is trying to rid itself of excess cholesterol. This sort of condition tends to run in families and could possibly indicate that you're in the high-risk heart disease percentile. See section 94 for how to reduce cholesterol. Also, increase your intake of vitamin B, chromium, and zinc, in foods and supplements.

How long does orange juice retain its vitamin C?

For commercial orange juice, the vitamin C life span is about one week from the time you've opened the container. For fresh-squeezed juice kept refrigerated in a sealed container, the life span of vitamin C is about three weeks.

Do you lose more or fewer nutrients by microwaving food?
As a rule, fewer. Microwaving requires minimum cooking time and minimum water.

X

READ THE LABEL

239. The Importance of Understanding What's on Labels

All too often people buy supplements and never even look at the labels. They ask a clerk for a multivitamin and take what they are given, not realizing that they might be getting shortchanged on the vitamin content. All multivitamins differ in amounts included, and the most expensive tablet is not necessarily the best. The only way to be sure you're getting the B6, folacin, or C that you need is to read the small print on the label. Also, if you have any allergies, it's wise to check what else you might be getting with your supplement (see section 25).

If there are words on the label that you don't understand, ask the pharmacist or vitamin clerk to explain them. If she can't, buy your supplements where someone can. Above all, remember to check the dosage you're getting. If you've been instructed to take vitamin E four times a day, it's unlikely that you want 400 IU. Vitamins and minerals come in different strengths. Be sure you're getting what you ask for—and need. Not understanding labels can often negate a lot of vitamin benefits.

The U.S. Food and Drug Administration (FDA) rules now in effect should make understanding labels a lot easier. They require vitamins, minerals, herbs, and amino acids to be labeled as dietary supplements. As such, these products must feature a Supplement Facts panel with information similar to the Nutrition Facts panels that appear on processed foods.

The Supplement Facts panel must include an appropriate serving/dosage size and information about 14 nutrients when present at significant levels, including vitamins A and C, sodium, calcium, and iron. Dietary ingredients that have no RDI/RDA or DRI must also be listed. In the case of herb supplements, the part of the plant used to make the product must also be identified.

But you still have to *read* the label. For example, the term *high potency* may be used for any single-ingredient dietary supplement that contains at least 100 percent of the daily value, which in most cases is regrettably low. In multi-ingredient products, the term *high potency* can be used if two-thirds of the daily value nutrients are present at 100 percent or more of their daily value. In other words, if you want to get the most from your vitamins, read the label not the hype.

240. How Does That Measure Up?

The terminology for measuring vitamin activity is not as confusing as you might think. Fat-soluble vitamins (A, E, D, and K) are usually measured in international units (IU). But a few years ago, an expert committee of the Food and Agriculture Organization/World Health Organization (FAO/WHO) decided to change this order of measurement for vitamin A. Instead of using international units, they proposed that vitamin A be evaluated in terms of retinol equivalents (RE), that is, the equivalent weight of retinol (vitamin A1, alcohol) *actually absorbed and converted.*

Retinol equivalents come out to about five times less than international units (IU). Recommended allowances of 5,000 IU for a male between the ages of twenty-three and fifty would be only 1,000 RE; 4,000 IU for similarly aged females would be only 800 RE.

Most other vitamins and minerals are measured in milligrams (mg.) and micrograms (mcg.). If you know that 1 g. equals .035 ounce, that it takes 28.35 g. to equal 1 ounce (and 1 fluid ounce equals 2 tbsp.), you'll have a better idea of just how much—or rather, how little—it takes for vitamins and minerals to do their job. The following table is a handy guide to refer to:

WHAT'S WHAT IN WEIGHTS AND MEASURES

Metric Measure

1 kilogram equals 1,000 grams
1 gram equals 1,000 milligrams
1 milligram equals 1/1,000th part of a gram
1 microgram equals 1/1,000th part of a milligram
1 gamma equals 1 microgram

Avoirdupois Weight

16 ounces equal 1 pound
7,000 grains equal 1 pound
453.6 grams equal 1 pound
1 ounce av. equals 437.5 grains
1 ounce av. equals 28.35 grams

Conversion Factors

1 gram equals 15.4 grains
1 grain equals 0.085 grams (85 milligrams)
1 ounce apothecary equals 31.1 grams
1 fluid ounce equals 29.8 cc.
1 fluid ounce equals 480 minims

Liquid Measure

1 drop equals 1 minim
1 minim equals 0.06 cc.
15 minims equal 1.0 cc.
4 cc. equal 1 fluid dram
30 cc. equal 1 fluid ounce

Household Measure

1 teaspoon equals 4 cc. equals 1 fluid dram
1 tablespoon equals 15 cc. equals ½ fluid ounce
½ pint equals 240 cc. equals 8 fluid ounces

Abbreviations

AMDR	adult minimum daily requirement
USP Unit	United States Pharmacopeia
IU	international unit
MDR	minimum daily requirement
mg.	milligram
mcg.	microgram
g.	gram
gr.	Grain

241. Breaking the RDA Code

Many people are bewildered by the variances between vitamin standards listed as RDA, US RDA, RDI, DRI, and

DV. It becomes much less confusing when you understand that they are not the same thing.

RDA (recommended dietary allowances) came into being in 1941, when the Food and Nutrition Board of the National Research Council of the Academy of Sciences was established by the government to safeguard public health. The RDA are not formulated to cover the needs of those who are ill—they are not therapeutic and are meant strictly for healthy individuals—nor do they take into account nutrient losses that occur during processing and preparation. Periodically revised, they are *estimates* of nutritional needs necessary to ensure satisfactory growth of children and the prevention of nutrient depletion in adults. *They are not meant to be optimal intakes, nor are they recommendations for an ideal diet.* They are not average requirements but recommendations intended to meet the needs of those *healthy* people with the highest requirements.

US RDA (US recommended daily allowances) were formulated by the Food and Drug Administration (FDA) to be used as the *legal* standards for food labeling in regard to nutrient content. (The RDA were used as the basis for the US RDA.) Serving size, number of servings per container, calories, and ten nutrients—protein, carbohydrate, fat, vitamin A, vitamin C, thiamin, riboflavin, niacin, calcium, and iron—had to be listed on food labels. (Today, unless a food is fortified or a manufacturer claims that it is a good source of vitamin B, levels of B vitamins are excluded.) Information about sodium, cholesterol, and saturated and unsaturated fat, formerly optional, is now mandatory. (US RDA percentages for vitamins D, E, B6, phosphorus, iodine, magnesium, zinc, copper, biotin, and pantothenic acid remain optional.)

RDI (reference daily intakes) and DV (daily values) were established by the FDA for use in nutrition labeling, replacing both the RDA and the US RDA. The RDI are subdivided into the Daily Value (DV), based on both the RDI for vitamins and minerals and the Daily Reference Values (DRV) for protein, fat, and carbohydrates.

DRI (dietary reference intake) is the term that now replaces RDA/RDI. The DRIs are the most recent set of dietary recommendations established by the Food and Nutrition Board of the Institute of Medicine. They replace previous RDAs, and may be the basis for eventually updating the RDIs.

AI (adequate intake) is established only when an RDA cannot be determined. A nutrient, therefore, has either an RDA or an AI. (The AI is based on observed intakes of the nutrient.)

UL (tolerable upper intake level) is the highest daily intake of a nutrient that is likely to pose no risks of toxicity for almost all individuals.

EAR (estimated average requirement) is the amount of a nutrient estimated to meet the requirement of half of all healthy individuals in the population; used by dietitians and others planning diets, developing new foods, and setting food policies.

NOTE: *RDAs, AIs, and ULs are guidelines for individuals. EARs provide guidelines for groups and populations.*

Stress and illness, past or present, affect everyone's nutritional requirements differently. Just because a product claims to provide 100 percent of the US RDA or DV for a nutrient, doesn't necessarily mean that *you* are getting it, or that it's a sufficient amount for *your* individual needs. As far as I and many other leading nutritionists are concerned, the proposed DRIs as well as the RDA/RDIs are still woefully inadequate. Nonetheless, you will find them listed in sections 30 through 73 in the Facts section for each vitamin and mineral.

242. What to Look For—and Look Out for—On Supplement Labels

When buying mineral supplements, look for *amino acid–chelated* on the label. Only 10 percent of ordinary minerals will be assimilated by the body, but when combined with amino acids in chelation, the assimilation is three to five times more efficient.

Hydrolyzed means water dispersible. *Hydrolyzed protein-chelate* means the supplement is in its most easily assimilated form.

Predigested protein is protein that has already been broken down and can go straight to the bloodstream.

Cold pressed is important to look for when buying oil or oil capsules. It means vitamins haven't been destroyed by heat and that the oil, extracted by cold-pressed methods, remains polyunsaturated.

Look out for *serving size*! Most people buying supplements scan the milligrams and the DV percentages without realizing that they might have to take more than one pill or capsule to get that amount. For instance, seeing a supplement that supplies 1,000 mg. of calcium, making it 100 percent of the DV, might look good—until you discover that you'll have to take 6 capsules a day to get it!

243. Labeling on Processed Foods

All processed food must have a Nutrition Facts panel on the label. Once again, unless you don't care if you're nutritionally sandbagged, check the serving size on which all the information is based. This is especially important for dieters who might think they're eating a low-calorie food. For example, 1 cup of popcorn popped might be only 15 calories. But fill a 1 cup measuring cup with that popped popcorn and see if that's really all you eat. I doubt it.

As a rule of thumb, the nutrients toward the top of the label (fat, saturated fat, trans fat, cholesterol, and sodium) are those you want to limit in a healthy diet. The ones below it (fiber, vitamins A and C, calcium and iron) are the ones you want more of.

Ingredients are listed in descending order by weight, so you want to avoid products that show high fructose corn syrup or water as the first ones.

Keep in mind that a manufacturer is allowed to claim 0 grams trans fat if the product has less than 0.5 gram per serving. Again, check the ingredients list. If you see "hydrogenated" or "partially hydrogenated" oils, you're getting trans fats.

The ingredient list can also show if you are getting beneficial fats, such as mono and polyunsaturated fats and omega-3 fats. Although not specified under total fat, if the product contains healthy oils, nuts, and seeds, you're getting the good fats, ones that can help lower bad (LDL) cholesterol. Just remember that—despite their nutritional merits—they should be consumed in limited quantities.

Label Lies: "Wholesome!" "Pure!" "Natural!" These words on labels mean nothing. Wholesome simply means fit for human consumption (i.e., no insect parts). Pure and natural have no official definition, and some products with highly processed high fructose corn syrup can still be labeled "natural."

244. What's Not on the Label May Be Making You Sick

Every day you might be ingesting an endocrine-disrupting chemical that has been linked to breast cancer, cardiovascular disease, obesity, diabetes, ADD, miscarriages, and genital abnormalities in children—and not even know it! It's BPA (bisphenol A), a synthetic estrogen that factories use in plastics and epoxies that's now in our food and turning up in the urine of more than 92 percent of the American public.

Used as an interior coating on cans, BPA was found in almost all brand-name canned foods recently tested by *Consumer Reports*. Although the American Chemical Council has said it's absorbed at safe levels, and the FDA claims that it is not an immediate health risk, bills are already pending to ban BPA from food and beverage containers.

Until that happens:

- Use glass, porcelain, or stainless-steel containers for hot foods and liquids.
- Use glass containers designed for microwaving instead of using polycarbonate plastic containers.
- Use glass or BPA-free baby bottles.
- Cut back on your use of canned foods.
- Make sure you keep your immune system strong (see section 459).

DID YOU KNOW?

- The words *wholesome*, *pure*, and *natural* on labels mean nothing!
- Four out of five supermarket items, 16,000 out of 20,000 products, use clever outright lies in their claims.
- A wide variety of breakfast cereals, baby food, bread, and crackers contain a potential human carcinogen.
- There is no such thing as "hormone-free" milk. All milk produced by cows contains hormones as part of the natural biology of lactation.
- Forty percent of the calories we consume contain a probable carcinogen.

---

245. Any Questions About Chapter X?

Why are Smart Choice labels allowed on foods that even I know are not smart choices—sugary cereals like Fruit Loops, for instance?

Because whatever committee developed the government's guidelines for healthy choices in packaged food was dumb about setting them. All a product has to do to boast a Smart Choice green checkmark on its label is to meet the standards set for levels of vitamins A and C and fiber, while not exceeding the limits for fat. Not only is nothing mentioned about sugar content (Fruit Loops cereal has 12 g. of sugar per serving), but the label can be based on *added nutrients* that can hide the lack of nutrition that's actually in the product—making processed foods appear as healthy as unprocessed ones. At the time of this writing, those standards are still in effect, but the Food and Drug

Administration is planning to propose new ones that will better regulate front-of-container nutrition information. In fact, it's expected that food manufacturers will have to list both positive and negative nutritional information on the front of packages—including information about vitamins, fiber, fats, *and* sugar. Until then, checking the ingredients list is your best bet for making really smart choices.

When buying poultry, which is better, "organic" or "free-range"?

Go for "organic," which means (though there is no guarantee) that the chicken or turkey has not been given antibiotics or hormones, and its feed was herbicide- and pesticide-free. As for "free range," the definition is used pretty...well, freely. Any chicken who has acess to the outside—even just a tiny run—can be called "free range." Not worth paying extra for.

What are emulsifiers?

Emulsifiers are used to homogenize ingredients that do not normally mix well. Lecithin and pectin, which are natural and safe, are commonly used, but unfortunately they're not used exclusively. Polysorbate 60 (which the FDA still has under investigation), locust bean (on the FDA list of additives requiring further study for muta-genic, reproductive, and teratogenic effects), and carra-geenan (another ingredient being studied all too slowly by the FDA), among others, are still being used. Though these are at present generally recognized as safe (GRAS), I personally prefer and recommend products without them.

Are calories counted differently in foreign countries?

Most foreign countries use the metric system, and the

energy value of food is measured in units called joules, our kilocalories, better known as calories. Four of our calories are the equivalent of 17 joules. In other words, a joule is slightly less than one-quarter calorie.

When dealing with vitamin A, how do you convert IUs into mg. or mcg.?

There are no rigid conversions, but 1 IU vitamin A = 0.3 mcg. retinol, and 1 IU beta-carotene = 0.1 mcg. retinol.

I've heard that something called acrylamide is in 40 percent of the foods we eat—and it's a probable carcinogen. Why aren't there warning labels on products that contain it?

Good question. The FDA has not at the time of this writing issued guidelines for manufacturers on reducing acrylamide in food because its presence in products has not been *definitively determined* to present a health risk to humans (tests have only been done on laboratory animals)—but studies are being done.

Acrylamide is a chemical used primarily for industrial purposes, including the treatment of drinking water and sewage, but it is a natural by-product of cooking high-carbohydrate foods at high temperatures. Among the foods that develop acrylamide during cooking are coffee, chocolate, almonds, french fries, potato chips, cereals, crackers, bread, and even some fruits and vegetables when heated to temperatures above 248 degrees Fahrenheit (120 Celsius). Levels of acrylamide in food vary widely depending on the manufacturer, the cooking time, and the method and temperature of the cooking process.

To lower your acrylamide intake, limit your intake of junk-food snacks as well as foods high in saturated fats, *trans* fats, cholesterol, salt, and added sugars. (Cigarette smoke is also a major source of exposure to acrylamide.)

To reduce the formation of acrylamide in your foods:

- Toast bread to a light brown color, rather than a dark brown. (Brown areas contain the most acrylamide.)
- Soaking raw potatoes in water for fifteen to thirty minutes before frying or roasting also helps reduce acrylamide formation.
- Boiling potatoes and microwaving whole potatoes with skin on to make microwaved "baked" potatoes does not produce acrylamide.

XI

YOUR SPECIAL VITAMIN NEEDS

246. Selecting Your Regimen

We all know that not everyone has the same metabolism, but we often forget that this also means that not everyone requires the same vitamins. In the following sections I have outlined a number of personalized regimens for a variety of specialized needs. Look them all over and see which ones best fit your own special situation. If you fall under more than one category, adjust the combined regimens so that you are not double-dosing yourself, only adding the additional supplements.

You will notice that in most cases I advise what I call an MVP, a Mindell Vitamin Program (which can make you an MVP—a Most Valuable Player in the nutrition game). This simple, potent pair—taken with meals—is my foundation for general good health.

MVP MINDELL VITAMIN PROGRAM

- An all-natural, high-potency multiple vitamin/mineral complex (with digestive enzymes for better absorption), plus
- A broad-spectrum antioxidant formula containing natural mixed carotenoids (alpha- and beta-carotene, cryptothaxin, lutein, and zeaxanthin), lycopene, alpha-lipoic acid, L-Carnosine, grape-seed OPCs, white and green tea extract, citrus bioflavonoids, N-Acetyl cysteine, grape skin extract, quercetin from rutin, turmeric, bilberry, vitamin C, vitamin E complex (mixed tocopherols—alpha, gamma, and delta), plus tocotrienols, selenium, ginkgo biloba, coenzyme-Q10, L-gluta-thione, soy isoflavones (genistein and daidzein).

Take twice daily with food. (Dosage is suitable for individuals over twelve years of age.)

WHAT TO LOOK FOR IN RECOMMENDED COMBINATION SUPPLEMENTS

Coenzyme-Q10 complex (look for vitamin E, garlic, cayenne, and hawthorn extract)

Calcium and magnesium (look for amino acid chelation—even better, glycinated amino acid chelation—and a balance of twice as much calcium as magnesium; in a complex, look for vitamin D, boron, and soy isoflavonoids)

Ginkgo biloba complex (look for dimethylamino-ethanol [DMAE], club moss, phosphatidylcholine [PC], phosphatidylserine [PS], and phosphatidylisoleucine [PI])

MSM (methylsulfonylmethane) CAPSULE (look for pharmaceutical grade with vitamin C and bioflavonoids)

I recommend that all powder supplements be mixed

with filtered water or fruit juice—fresh or frozen (not from concentrate). SUPPLEMENTS SHOULD BE TAKEN WITH FOOD UNLESS OTHERWISE NOTED.

247. Women—Teens to Adults

12–18	MVP (see section 246) Calcium (as hydroxyapatite, calcium citrate, and calcium citrate-maleate glycinate) 250 mg. and magnesium, 125 mg. twice daily
19–50	MVP (see section 246) Calcium (as hydroxyapatite, calcium citrate, and calcium citrate-maleate glycinate) 500 mg. and magnesium 250 mg. twice daily *Also:* Organic iron, 15–50 mg. daily, if needed CBD 25 MG DAILY
50+	MVP (see section 246) Vitamin E, 400 IU (dry form) Calcium 500 mg. and magnesium 250 mg., 2 tablets A.M. and at bedtime

For pregnancy, see section 280. For nursing mothers, see section 283. For menstrual irregularities and PMS regimens, see sections 313 and 358. For menopause, see section 312.

248. Men—Teens to Adults

12–18	MVP (see section 246)
19–30	MVP (see section 246) Zinc, 15 mg. daily

30–50	MVP (see section 246)
	Zinc, 15–50 mg. daily
	Arginine time release, 2 tablets A.M. and 2 P.M.
	Prostate formula, 1 twice daily
	Memory formula, A.M. and P.M.
	Cardio support formula, 1 daily
50+	MVP (see section 246)
	Glycinated calcium complex, 500 mg. and 250 mg. magnesium daily
	Prostate formula, 2 tablets A.M. and P.M.
	Memory formula, A.M. and P.M.
	Cardio support formula, A.M. and P.M.
	Arginine (time release) 2 tablets A.M. and P.M.

249. Infants and Toddlers

1–4   One good-tasting chewable multivitamin daily (check label to see that all the primary vitamins are included); there should be no artificial color, flavors, or sugar (sucrose) added. (Liquid vitamins are available for very young children. Remember to check with your pediatrician before making any supplement choice.)

250. Children

4–12   Growing children need a stronger multi-vitamin containing minerals, especially calcium and iron, for normal growth. The tablet should also be high in B complex and vitamin C (50 percent of American children do not even get the RDA for vitamin C). One daily is sufficient (check label to be sure there is no artificial color, flavor, or sugar—sucrose—added).

NOTE: *See sections 247 and 248 for Teens.*

251. Runners and Joggers

During the first fifteen to twenty minutes of running, you burn up almost only glucose. The body then comes in with fats (lipids) for energy (in utilizing lipids for energy, a compound called acegyl-coenzyme-A is formed). If there are only animal fats present, the compound forms slowly and energy is insufficient. If polyunsaturates are present, on the other hand, the compound forms quickly. Increase your intake of polyunsaturates—seeds, peanuts—and anti-oxidants, such as vitamins C, E, and selenium, to avoid free radical reactions.

A good supplement program for both runners and joggers would be:

MVP (See section 246)
Arginine (time release), 2 tablets A.M. and P.M.
B complex, 50 mg. A.M. and P.M.
Soy shake: 1 scoop soy food protein blended in 1–1½ cups soy milk with ice cubes, and fruit if desired, for breakfast (meal replacement)
Two tbsp. MSM powder mixed with filtered water or juice. Drink one glass before, during, or after workout to decrease lactic acid buildup.

252. Executives

With tension and stress an accepted part of your daily life, and energy a necessity, you need a vitamin regimen that won't let you down. Many high-level executives I know use this one:

MVP (see section 246)

B complex, 50 mg. A.M. and P.M.

Standardized ginkgo biloba, 60 mg. complex with DMAE and club moss, 1 tablet twice daily

Chelated calcium 500 mg. and magnesium 250 mg. one to two times daily

If you're in a hurry in the morning, you might want to try my high-energy breakfast drink:

RECIPE:

2 tbsp. whey protein powder	3–4 ice cubes
1 tbsp. whey	2 tbsp. fresh or frozen fruit, or 1 banana
2 tbsp. lecithin granules	1½ cups almond milk

Mix in blender at high speed for one minute.

253. Students

Eating on the run, skipping breakfast, and not getting enough rest is a way of life for most students. And as if this isn't bad enough for good health, student diets usually consist of mostly starches and carbohydrates. If you're in this category, be aware that these factors, as well as your constant stress situations at school, are taking their toll. A good daily supplement program would be:

MVP (see section 246)

Standardized ginkgo biloba, 60 mg. complex, two to three times daily

254. Computer Addicts

If you're spending most of your days—and nights—in front of a computer screen, click on this: The eye lens is dependent on adequate levels of antioxidants to prevent damage by free radicals. My advice is to get online nutritionally with supplements that alleviate eyestrain and protect against oxidative damage. And if you're stressed out from surfing the Web, you'll need something for your strained nerves, too.

MVP (see section 246)

B complex, 50 mg. A.M. and P.M.

Calcium 500 mg. and magnesium 250 mg. twice daily (and 1 at bedtime if needed)

Standardized ginkgo biloba, 60 mg. twice daily

Coenzyme-Q10 and vitamin E complex, 1 capsule daily

CBD, 25 mg. twice daily

255. Seniors

The nutritional needs of seniors may vary widely, depending on the individual. As a general rule, however, if you're over sixty-five, you need extra minerals and vitamins, especially calcium, magnesium, and vitamin D (see section 47), as well as B complex and C. Vitamin E can help alleviate poor circulation, which is often responsible for leg cramps. And don't forget about fiber. If chewing is a problem, high-fiber foods can be ground to convenient sizes and textures and are just as effective. Also, sweets should be discouraged; there is a high incidence of diabetes mellitus among older people.

A good supplement regimen would be:

MVP (see section 246)

Vitamin E 200–400 IU

Calcium 500 mg. and magnesium 250 mg. twice daily

Standardized ginkgo biloba, 60 mg., complex with DMAE two to three times daily

Coenzyme-Q10 200 mg. complex; 1 capsule daily

256. Athletes

Athletes have very demanding nutritional needs. The prime nutritional requirement for performance is energy, and high-energy foods—as opposed to quick-energy foods— are what should be eaten. If you're involved in action sports, you need a diet with more complex carbohydrates and protein than someone involved in a low-energy sport. Then again, even golf can become a high-energy game when carried on intensively for a long time. Keep in mind that excess amounts of glucose, sugar, honey, or hard candy tend to draw fluid into the gastrointestinal tract. This can add to dehydration problems in endurance performance. A thirst-quenching tart drink of frozen or fresh fruit juice is a great quick-energy beverage.

For supplements, I recommend:

MVP (see section 246)

B complex, 50 mg., twice daily

Coenzyme-Q10, 200 mg. daily

Octacosanol, 1,000 mcg. three times daily

Creatine monohydrate, 1 tbsp. (5,000 mg.) in juice (not from concentrate) or water daily

OPTIONAL: Branched chain amino acids (see Body-builders)

MSM powder, 1–2 spoonfuls dissolved in 8 oz. water; drink before, during, or after workout.

257. Bodybuilders

If you work out with weights, being on the right diet is as important as your warm-ups and cooldowns. In fact, without combining them, you may wind up with bulging muscles that will be layered with fat and won't do much for your overall shape.

While it's true that protein builds and repairs muscles, it is complex carbohydrates that supply energy for the continuous and repeated muscular contractions that occur during prolonged exercise. For best results, I'd advise getting 80–90 percent of your calories from complex carbohydrates and no more than 10 percent from meat protein. You might also want to try branched chain amino acids (see section 90), which are natural anabolic muscle builders.

My supplement suggestion:

MVP (see section 246)

B complex, 50 mg. twice daily

Octacosanol, 1,000 mcg. one to three times daily

Creatine monohydrate, 1 tbsp. (5,000 mg.) in juice (not from concentrate) or water daily

Arginine, 1–3 g. with lysine (on empty stomach one hour before bedtime)

Whey shake (see section 252 recipe) for breakfast and between meals if desired

MSM powder, 1–2 spoonsful dissolved in 8 oz. water after workout to decrease lactic-acid buildup

OPTIONAL: Branched chain amino acids (BCAA) 600 mg.

For heavy workout 4–6, taken a half hour
    before workout

For moderate workout 3–4, taken a half
    hour before workout

For light workout, 1–2, taken a half hour
   before workout

258. Night Workers

The Center for Research on Stress and Health at the Stanford Research Institute has found that "the rotating shift exacts a heavy physical and emotional toll from workers." When eating and sleeping patterns are disrupted, so are the body's biological rhythms, and it takes "three to four weeks for the circadian rhythms to become synchronized." If you change from day to night shifts, often your body is under much stress, your chances of illness are greater, and your risk of ulcers is high. I feel that supplements are essential:

   MVP (see section 246)
   1 vitamin D, 4000 IU with largest meal

If you switch to regular hours on the weekend, take calcium 500 mg. And magnesium 250 mg. 1–2 tablets half an hour before bedtime. Or take 5 mg. melatonin, sublingually (allow to dissolve under the tongue) fifteen minutes before bedtime.

259. Truck Drivers

Tension, stress, and a diet that is all too often high in greasy foods are important reasons for considering the following supplements:

   MVP (see section 246)
   B complex, 50 mg. A.M. and P.M.
   CBD, 50 mg. daily

260. Dancers

Dancers have energy requirements that rank with those of athletes, but because of weight restrictions they cannot consume the same amount of carbohydrates. Good supplements are indispensable, as most dancers will tell you. I suggest:

MVP (see section 246)

Calcium-magnesium complex (with soy isoflavones), 2 tabs A.M. and P.M.

B complex, 50 mg. A.M. and P.M.

Coenzyme-Q10, 200 mg. daily

Octocosanol, 1,000 mcg. daily

261. Construction Workers

One out of every four workers is exposed to substances considered hazardous, according to the National Institute for Occupational Safety and Health (NIOSH). Construction workers are particularly vulnerable. Depending upon the sort of construction you're doing and where you're doing it, you're exposed to a variety of harmful conditions from general pollution to inhaling lead oxide, which can happen if you're soldering scrap metal or plastics. In any event, a diet rich in antioxidants such as vitamins A, C, and E will help detoxify your body. The following supplements are recommended:

MVP (see section 246)

B complex, 50 mg. twice daily

Coenzyme-Q10, 200 mg. daily

Octocosanol, 1,000 mcg. daily

262. Poker Players

If you're a poker player, I don't have to tell you about stress, lack of sleep, and less than optimal nutrition. It's a safe bet that you're aware all three have become part of your life. What you might not realize, though, is that they could be undermining your game mentally and physically. Because of lack of sunlight, there's a good chance that you're in need of vitamin D supplementation (see section 47). For putting yourself on a nutritional winning streak, I suggest the following supplements:

MVP (see section 246)

Coenzyme-Q10 complex, 200 mg. daily

Calcium-magnesium complex, A.M. and P.M.

263. Salespersons

The daily grind of having to deal with the public cannot be underestimated. Whether you're selling automobiles, books, electronics, or furniture, doing it on the road or from behind a counter, the emotional and physical stress on your body is significant. And because appearances are often as important as products in your line of work, you'd be wise to keep the right supplements within easy reach. You'll be happily surprised with the results.

MVP (see section 246)

B complex, 50 mg. A.M. and P.M.

Calcium, 500 mg. and magnesium, 250 mg., A.M. and P.M.

Coenzyme-Q10 complex, 200 mg. daily

Ginkgo biloba, 60 mg. A.M. and P.M.

CBD, 25–50 mg. daily

264. Actors—Stage, Screen, Radio, and TV Performers

There's not an actor I know who doesn't need a B-vitamin supplement. The stress and tension of performing is an occupational given. And if you're like most theatrical performers, dieting is the only form of eating you know, too often denying yourself necessary vitamins. A helpful supplement scenario would be:

MVP (see section 246)

B complex, 50 mg. A.M. and P.M.

Coenzyme-Q10, 200 mg., and vitamin E complex, 1 daily

Calcium 500 mg. and magnesium, 250 mg., A.M. and P.M.

CBD, 50 mg. daily

265. Singers

Like actors, singers are also under high levels of stress, whether performing or rehearsing If you worry about laryngitis or other throat infections, it's advisable to keep your vitamin C levels high at all times.

MVP (see section 246)

Additional vitamin C, 1,000 mg. A.M. and P.M. when necessary

266. Doctors and Nurses

If you work with illness, you need all the protection you can get. Long hours, stress, and germs themselves all contribute to your need for vitamin and mineral supplementation.

MVP (see section 246)

B complex, 50 mg. A.M. and P.M.

Extra vitamin C, 500 mg., to ward off infections

Calcium, 500 mg. and magnesium, 250 mg. complex A.M. and P.M.

267. Manicurists and Hair Colorists

You may be in the beauty business, but your daily exposure to chemical fumes creates destructive free radicals, and healthwise that's not a pretty picture. As free radical levels rise, so does your body's need for additional antioxidants to disable them.

MVP (see section 246)

B complex, 50 mg. A.M. and P.M.

Extra vitamin C, 500 mg. one to two times daily

Ginkgo biloba complex, 60 mg. A.M. and P.M.

Coenzyme-Q10, 200 mg., and vitamin E complex, 1 daily

268. Bicyclists

Cycling is great aerobic conditioning. But if you're on the road taking in the scenery, you're also taking in pollution and ultraviolet radiation from the sun. And since the intensity of your exercise is already generating unwanted free radicals, your natural antioxidants need nutritional backup.

MVP (see section 246)

Coenzyme-Q10, 200 mg. and vitamin E complex, 1 daily

Calcium 500 mg., and magnesium 250 mg. complex, twice daily

Octocosanol, 1,000 mcg. one to three times daily

MSM powder, 1–2 tbsp. in 8 oz. water or juice before, during, or after cycling

269. Swimmers

If you take the plunge regularly, you're giving your entire body a fine all-over workout. But you are also subjecting it to stress and generating extra free radicals. A high-antioxidant diet along with supplements will keep you in the swim.

MVP (see section 246)

B complex, 50 mg. A.M. and P.M.

Coenzyme-Q10, 200 mg. daily

MSM powder, 1–2 tbsp. dissolved in 8 oz. water or juice, before or after swimming

270. Persons with Disabilities

If you have a disability, your needs for vitamins are usually increased. More often than not, if one part of your body is not functioning properly, another part is working twice as hard—and needs nourishment. Helpful basic supplements would be:

MVP (see section 246)

B complex, 50 mg. A.M. and P.M.

Calcium (500 mg.) and magnesium (250 mg.) complex A.M. and P.M.

CBD, 50 mg. daily

271. Golfers

As much as you enjoy it, golfing takes a lot out of you. The stress and tension of the game can use up B vitamins at a rapid clip. The right supplements might not get you down into the seventies, but they can help you stay energetic throughout the game.

MVP (see section 246)

B complex, 50 mg. A.M. and P.M.

Zinc, 15–50 mg. daily

Calcium (500 mg.) and magnesium (250 mg.) complex A.M. and P.M.

Coenzyme-Q10, 200 mg. daily

CBD, 50 mg. daily

272. Tennis Players

If you play tennis often, you might look good on the outside but be a nutritional mess inside. I've found that far too many tennis buffs skip meals, or eat only protein—both bad habits. A demanding game like tennis requires that you serve yourself all the vitamins you need.

MVP (see section 246)

B complex, 50 mg. A.M. and P.M.

Calcium (500 mg.) and magnesium (250 mg.) complex A.M. and P.M.

MSM powder, 1–2 tbsp. dissolved in 8 oz. water or juice; drink after match to decrease lactic-acid buildup

Coenzyme-Q10, 200 mg., and vitamin E complex, 1 daily

Octocosanol, 1,000 mcg. one to three times daily

273. Racquetball Players

Few sports require as intense physical stamina as racquetball, so if you intend to play it on a regular basis (or even on an occasional lunch hour), you'd better be prepared to meet not only your opponent, but the nutritional challenge as well.

MVP (see section 246)

Octocosanol, 1,000 mcg. one to three times daily

Coenzyme-Q10, 200 mg., and vitamin E complex, 1 daily

B complex, 50 mg. A.M. and P.M.

MSM powder, 1–2 tbsp. dissolved in 8 oz. water or juice; drink before, during, or after game

274. Teachers

School days are as stressful for teachers as they are for students, if not more so. To keep your immune system, energy and spirits up, a good vitamin program is important.

MVP (see section 246)

B complex, 50 mg. A.M. and P.M.

Calcium (500 mg.) and magnesium (250 mg.) A.M. and P.M.

Coenzyme-Q10, 200 mg., and vitamin E complex, 1 daily

CBD, 50 mg. daily

275. Smokers

Every cigarette you smoke destroys about 25–100 mg. of vitamin C. Also, lung cancer risks aside, you're more prone to cardiovascular and pulmonary disorders than nonsmokers. Without going into the long list of deleterious effects cigarettes can have, I feel confident in telling smokers that they need all the nutritional help they can get, especially from antioxidants such as vitamins A, C, E, and selenium. Your life expectancy can be up to fifteen years less than nonsmokers'.

MVP (see section 246)

Vitamin C, 500 mg. A.M. and P.M.

Ginkgo biloba complex, 60 mg. A.M. and P.M.

Selenium, 200 mcg. daily

276. Drinkers

Alcoholism is the chief cause of vitamin deficiency among civilized people with ample food supplies. If you're a heavy drinker, the alcohol you consume usually takes the place of needed protein, or, in some cases, prevents absorption or proper storage of ingested vitamins.

MVP (see section 246)

B complex, 100 mg. twice daily (especially needed are B1, B6, and folic acid)

Calcium (500 mg.) and magnesium (250 mg.) two to three times daily

Silymarin (milk thistle), 1 capsule three times daily for liver rejuvenation

Kudzu, 500 mg., 1–3 capsules before or after drinking alcohol

277. TV Couch Potatoes

Just because you spend a lot of time relaxing in front of your set doesn't mean you're not in need of extra vitamins. For the eyestrain it's more than likely that you need additional vitamin A. And if you rarely get to see the light of day, you might need vitamin D also.

MVP (see section 246)

Beta-carotene, 10,000 IU with breakfast (take for five days, stop for two)

Vitamin D, 2000 IU daily

278. Frequent Fliers

Whether you travel for business or pleasure, stress may go unnoticed, but it can be significant. Varying time zones and temperatures (to say nothing of recycled air in the airplane cabin) take their toll, which is why you should take supplements wherever you go.

If you're heading to warm or tropical places, be sure that the vitamins you take are in opaque containers and that you keep them in a cool place, not out in the sun. If you're headed for chillier environs, be sure to bring along plenty of vitamin C and take it with all your meals, not just breakfast and dinner. And if you're traveling to foreign ports, keep in mind that *acidophilus* (3 capsules or 2 tbsp. liquid) three times a day is a good diarrhea preventive.

MVP (see section 246)

Coenzyme-Q10, 200 mg., and vitamin E complex, 200 IU daily

B complex, 50 mg. A.M. and P.M.

If you're having trouble sleeping in a new time zone, take:

- Calcium (500 mg.) and magnesium (250 mg.), 2 tablets before bedtime; or 5 mg.
- Melatonin sublingually (let dissolve under your tongue) fifteen minutes before bedtime.

DID YOU KNOW?

- There is a one in five chance of developing colds, flu, and respiratory infection among all passengers who fly.
- A high-carbohydrate diet is recommended for anyone involved in an endurance sport.
- Daily vitamin C supplements can reduce the risk of developing cataracts.
- Life expectancies between smokers and non-smokers differ by eighteen years.

---

279. Any Questions About Chapter XI?

Are foreign vitamins different?

Vitamins the world over are the same, only dosages vary. The metric system is used internationally for measurement, and nutrients are measured by weight. (See section 240 for a better understanding of what equals what.)

I'm a twenty-two-year-old ballet dancer. Although I've been told it is not unusual for ballet dancers to stop menstruating for several months at a time, are there special supplements I should be taking because of this—particularly when I'm performing?

You definitely need to up your calcium intake. A dancer who doesn't get her period is more like a postmenopausal woman. I'd suggest that, along with the supplement regimen I've outlined in section 260, you take an additional 1,500 mg. of calcium citrate daily. If you are currently taking an iron supplement, be sure to take the calcium at a different time of day. Taken together, these supplements can cancel each other out, undermining the benefits of both.

Are older people subject to any specific nutrient deficiencies?

As a general rule, they are. Aside from the fact that they consume more drugs than any other age group, they usually suffer from subclinical nutritional deficiencies because of their lifestyle and marginal intakes of key nutrients owing to malabsorption, poor teeth, loneliness, and other social problems.

Their most common nutrient deficiencies are folic acid, calcium, vitamin B12, vitamin D, and vitamin C. Also, because older people have a tendency to take stimulant laxatives on a regular basis, they lose large amounts of vitamins A, D, E, and K as well as calcium and potassium. (See section 381 for other drug-related vitamin deficiencies.)

I'm a thirty-five-year-old woman and I work out daily. And I mean WORK OUT—weights, Nautilus, the whole nine yards. I know I must need more of certain nutrients than ordinary people do. But what are they?

They are vitamins A, B6, and C; calcium (for optimal protein utilization); magnesium (lost through workout sweating and essential for muscle relaxation); and branched chain amino acids (for repair and reconstruction). For extended energy to keep you going through workouts, some nutrients and foods are better than others. For instance: soybeans would be better for you than peas; whole wheat spaghetti better than white; beets preferable to carrots; grapefruit better than oranges, apples, or bananas.

I work at a loom all day, and I think I'm developing carpal tunnel syndrome. Are there any supplements you could recommend?

Well, your occupation does put you at risk for developing it. Repetitive stress injury, which is another name for carpal tunnel syndrome, is brought on by overuse of the muscles and tendons of the fingers, hands, arms, and shoulders. I'd suggest a vitamin B complex with B6, 50 mg. three times daily; MSM, 1,000 mg. with a vitamin C complex A.M. and P.M.

Did You Know

- Vitamin D deficiency weakens your immune system and could lead to an increased risk of complications from infections.
- More than 23 million Americans, including millions of children, live in a food deserts—areas that are more than one mile (1.6 kilometers) from a supermarket at which they can find and buy fresh fruits and vegetables.

- 95 percent of adults and 90 percent of teens do not have adequate vitamin D intake.
- 31 percent of the US population is at risk for at least one vitamin deficiency or anemia. Twenty-three percent are at risk of deficiency of one, two, or three to five vitamins.
- 32 percent of Americans have insufficient vitamin B6 intake.
- 1 percent are not getting enough B12.
- 3 percent are not getting enough folate.
- 46 percent are not getting enough vitamin C.
- 84 percent are not getting enough vitamin E.
- 3 percent have an inadequate iron intake.
- 15 percent of adults have inadequate intake of zinc.[1]

---

[1] Source: National Health Nutrition Examination Survey (NHAMES) a bi-yearly study of the US population, conducted by the US Centers for Disease Control (CDC). The CDC surveyed 2,862 adults between the ages of 19 and 99. This data was sourced from NHAMES, spanning 2005 to 2016.

XII

HAVING BABIES 101

280. So You Want to Have a Baby

If you're thinking of becoming pregnant, now is the time for you and your partner to make sure that you're getting the nutrients most beneficial for fertility and conception.

FERTILITY-ENHANCING SUPPLEMENTS FOR
WOMEN AND MEN

Folate, 800 mcg. daily (See section 43 for best natural sources.)

Vitamin B6, 50 mg. daily (See section 36 for best natural sources.)

Vitamin B12, 50 mcg. daily (See section 37 for best natural sources.)

Vitamin C, 1,000 mg. daily (See section 46 for best natural sources.)

Vitamin D, 800–1,000 IU daily (See section 47 for best natural sources.)

Vitamin E, 50–100 IU daily (See section 48 for best natural sources.)

Selenium, 50–100 mcg. daily (See section 68 for best natural sources.)

Zinc, 15–50 mg. daily (See section 72 for best natural sources.)

Omega-3, 1,000 mg. capsules three times daily

CBD, 25–50 mg. daily for anti-stress

CAUTION: *Do not take a prenatal formula in addition to a multivitamin or a prescription prenatal version. Also, check labels to be sure you're not double-dosing on any of the above supplements. When it comes to prenatal supplementation, too much of a good thing can be bad for you.*

PERSONAL ADVICE: *Drinking more than one cup of coffee—or the equivalent in other caffeinated beverages—can reduce your chances of conceiving. Also, avoid relaxation drinks that contain melatonin; it can alter sperm count and adversely affect other hormones. STAY CLEAR OF ARTIFICIAL SWEETENING AGENTS (THE NO-CALORIE SWEETENERS). STEVIA, A NATURAL SWEETENER WITH NO CALORIES, IS AVAILABLE.*

281. When Baby's on Board

Now that you're pregnant, you're in charge of precious cargo for the next nine months, so you want to do everything you can to make sure it arrives in the best posssible nutritional condition.

THINGS TO THINK ABOUT

Low vitamin D levels during pregnancy may mean cavities for your baby. (Baby teeth begin developing as early as six weeks in utero, and vitamin D is known to be involved in the formation of protective tooth enamel.)

Recommended Prevention: Take your prenatal vitamins, drink milk fortified with vitamin D, and get a *small* amount of sunlight when possible. Before taking any supplements, it's important to check with your doctor. But the right vitamins *are* essential at this time:

MVP (see section 246) twice daily

Folate, 800 mcg., (at bedtime)

Glycinated calcium (500 mg.) and magnesium (250 mg.) A.M. and P.M.

MSM, 1,000 mg., with vitamin C complex, 1 tablet with each meal

Ginger extract, 1 capsule one to three times daily if needed for morning sickness

Acidophilus, 1 capsule daily

282. Be Careful When Eating for Two

You may be eating for two, but only one of you is making the decisions about what foods to pick. And when you're pregnant it's more important than ever not to pick the wrong ones.

FOODS TO STAY AWAY FROM

Fish is an important source of omega-3 fatty acids, but those with high levels of mercury can damage the development of your baby's brain. Avoid large fish like swordfish and tilefish, and limit tuna and snapper to no more than one serving a week. Sushi and sashimi are definite no-nos. See section 102 for more warnings and recommendations.

Ready-to-eat deli meats (ham, turkey, salami, and bologna), as well as hot dogs, which can contain listeria, unless thoroughly heated and steaming hot.

Cured meats such as prosciutto.

Uncooked or runny eggs (as well as sauces made with raw eggs, like some remoulades and hollandaises).

Unpasteurized milk.

Paté.

Soft cheeses made with unpasteurized milk.

Caffeinated beverages, especially during the first trimester; try to limit yourself to no more than 200–300 mg. a day.

MY ADVICE: When in doubt—don't. Or at least consult with your healthcare provider before you do.

283. Making Breast-Feeding the Best

Your body and your baby need the best nourishment you can give them. Diet at this time is particularly important. Nursing mothers' supplement needs are essentially the same as those recommended for pregnant women—although nursing mothers do need a little more biotin because it is passed through breast milk. The Institute of Medicine recommends that breast-feeding women get a daily biotin adequate intake (AI) of 35 mcg. (as opposed to 30 mcg.), preferably through food (see section 41). Additional vitamins B6, B12, C, and D may also be called for.

Lactating mothers with preterm infants might want to check with their doctor about taking DHA (1,000 mg.) supplements. According to results of a six-year study published in the *Journal of the American Medical Association*, the omega-3 fatty acid DHA (docosahexaenoic acid), a major lipid in the brain, is not developed sufficiently in premature babies, leading to possible impaired mental development. Supplemental DHA supplied via the mother's breast milk (or infant formula) was found to significantly reduce this incidence of mental delay.

Vitamin D is deficient in breast milk; therefore, breast-fed infants may require supplementation. On the other hand, use of excessive amounts of vitamin D in nursing mothers may result in hypercalcemia in infants. I'd suggest checking with your healthcare provider before taking any supplements.

CAUTION: *Many herbals contain ingredients that pass through breast milk and could be potentially dangerous to a nursing mother and her baby. For example, coumarin and nicotinic acid found in fenugreek can have very potent effects on heart rate, blood pressure, blood sugar, and other bodily functions, which your baby can experience as well. For other herbs to definitely stay away from during pregnancy and lactation, see section 229. Again, I strongly advise consulting a healthcare professional before taking* any *dietary supplement.*

284. Postpartum Depression

About 80 percent of new mothers experience some form of postpartum depression (PPD). "Baby Blues," with symptoms such as crying for no apparent reason, irritability, and restlessness, are a mild, short-lived form of PPD, an understandable letdown after the emotionally charged experience of birth. PPD, on the other hand, is more severe and can last longer.

You can reduce your chances of PPD by proactively taking omega-3 supplements during pregnancy. A deficiency of omega-3s not only depletes the neuroprotective, depression-combating emotional stamina you need to get through the early postpartum days but can hinder your baby's brain development as well.

Supplementing may be even more necessary after giving birth. While breast-feeding offers some protection against PPD, it could deplete your reserves of omega-3s and worsen postpartum depression.

DID YOU KNOW?

- Pregnant women need only 300 extra calories a day.
- Most of the iron in spinach cannot be absorbed through your intestines.
- Nonfat foods can cause you to gain weight.
- Eighty percent of American women are deficient in calcium.

---

285. Any Questions About Chapter XII?

What herbs are okay under ordinary circumstances but contraindicated during pregnancy and breast-feeding?

There are lots of them. For example, goldenseal should definitely be avoided during pregnancy and lactation. (Berberine, the alkaloid in goldenseal, is quite similar to morphine.) Also, steer clear of caffeine-containing herbs, such as guarana and kola nuts.

Laxatives, be they natural or manufactured, should not be taken during the first few months of pregnancy, as they could cause miscarriage. (Buckthorn, rhubarb, and senna are natural laxatives.) Strong sedative herbs like skullcap and valerian are not advisable, nor are strong spices such as capsicum and horseradish. Emetics, such as lobelia, can be dangerous early in pregnancy and in the last trimester.

Though garlic and onions are great for many things, it might be wise to avoid them, especially if you're nursing, as they have been known to pass through the breast milk and produce colic in infants. I'd suggest that if you are pregnant or breast-feeding, play it safe and consult a healthcare professional before taking any supplemental herbs.

My obstetrician doesn't say too much to me except "Take your vitamins." Since you're a pharmacist as well as a nutritionist, could you tell me what drugs or medicines could be dangerous to me and my baby?

I'd feel safest in saying all of them—unless specifically prescribed by your doctor. No drug—whether it's OTC (over-the-counter) or prescription, alcohol, nicotine, or caffeine—should be considered safe during pregnancy. Most drugs can cross the placenta and thus affect fetus as well as mother. Especially avoid any products containing aspirin during the last three months of pregnancy and while breast-feeding. Also, considering that the major stages in an embryo's development occur during life's first few weeks, if you're even *thinking* about being a mother, check with your doctor before taking *any* medication.

My husband and I have been trying to have a child for over a year. Recently we learned that he has a low sperm count, which is most likely why we haven't been successful. Before we invest in conventional medical treatments, are there any natural supplements you can recommend?

There are and they're definitely worth a try. Free radicals, which cause oxidative damage (see section 104), can adversely impact male fertility. The antioxidant effect of L-carnitine, which provides cells with energy, has been found to play an important role in improving sperm development and motility. My recommendation is that your husband take two 500 mg. L-carnitine capsules daily along with 50 mg. of grape-seed extract, which is also a potent antioxidant. I'd also suggest that he steer clear of products containing cyclamate (the no-calorie sweetener in diet beverages and other low-calorie foods) and relaxation drinks that contain melatonin, which may decrease fertility in men.

XIII

THE RIGHT VITAMIN AT THE RIGHT TIME

286. Special Situation Supplements

Your body's vitamin needs are not always the same, and special situations require special food regimens and supplements. What follows is a list of such situations, most of them temporary, with supplement suggestions. (For foods that offer specific vitamins and minerals, see sections 30 through 73.) Once again, this information is not prescriptive. (See section 246 for MVP.)

287. Acne

This scourge of teenage years has been treated in a variety of ways, from X-rays to tetracycline, with only varying degrees of success. I encourage more natural treatment of the condition and have been delighted by the results.

MVP (See section 246)

Vitamin E (dry form), 400 IU daily

Beta-carotene, 10,000 IU daily

Zinc, 15–50 mg. chelated, 1 tablet daily with a meal

Acidophilus liquid, 1–2 tbsp. three times daily, or 3–6 capsules three times daily

Cysteine, 1 g. daily half an hour before meals with vitamin C, 1,000 mg., three times daily

MSM, 1,000 mg., 1 CAPSULE daily

MSM lotion, apply three times daily

Eliminate all processed foods. They are usually high in salt that has been iodized.

CAUTION: *If you are taking a prescription medication for acne, do NOT take extra vitamin A unless advised by your doctor.*

288. Athlete's Foot

Vitamin C powder or crystals applied directly to the affected areas seem to help this fungus infection. Keep your feet dry and out of shoes as much as possible until the infection clears. Tea tree oil applied to the affected area can help as well.

289. Bad Breath

Along with proper brushing and flossing, you might try:

MVP (see section 246)

1 chlorophyll tablet or capsule one to three times daily

3 *acidophilus* capsules three times daily, or 1–2 tbsp. flavored *acidophilus*

1–3 multiple digestive enzyme capsules with each meal

Zinc, 50 mg. daily

290. Baldness or Falling Hair

There are no guarantees, but many people report a definite diminution of hair loss with this regimen:

B complex, 50 mg. twice daily

Choline and inositol, 1,000 mg. of each daily

Daily jojoba oil scalp massage and shampoo

Calcium (500 mg.) and magnesium (250 mg.) complex, 1 daily

Cysteine, 1,000 mg. daily

Vitamin C, 500 mg. A.M. and P.M.

Saw palmetto standardized extract, 160 mg. twice daily

291. Bee Stings

The best thing to do about bee stings is try to avoid them. Vitamin B1 (thiamin) has been shown to be a fairly good insect repellent. Taken three times daily, 100 mg. B1 creates a smell at the level of your skin that insects do not like. If you're too late with the B1 and do get stung, 1,000 mg. vitamin C could help ease allergic reactions. Also, 1 MSM capsule 1,000 mg., taken three times daily for a week is a good idea.

292. Bleeding Gums

The most effective supplement therapy for bleeding gums, usually caused by a buildup of plaque along the gum line and known as gingivitis, is:

1,000 mg. vitamin C complex, with bioflavonoids, rutin, and hesperidin, taken three times daily. Zinc, 15 mg., once or twice daily. Vitamin E, 400–500 IU daily. Coenzyme-Q10, 200 mg. one to three times daily.

Quercetin, 400 mg. before eating, one to three times daily. I'd also suggest brushing regularly with tea tree oil toothpaste.

293. Broken Bones

If you've ever broken a bone, you know how frustrating it is waiting for it to mend. That feeling can be alleviated, and bone-healing accelerated, by increasing your calcium and vitamin D intakes. Doses of 1,000 mg. calcium and 500 mg. magnesium in a complex with vitamin D are recommended two to three times daily, along with 80 mcg. of vitamin K once a day.

294. Bruises

Vitamin C complex, 1,000 mg., with bioflavonoids, rutin, and hesperidin, taken three times daily will help prevent capillary fragility, those black-and-blue marks that occur when the tiny blood vessels beneath the skin rupture. For healing I recommend coenzyme-Q10, 60 mg. one to three times daily. Vitamin A, 5,000–10,000 IU daily. Vitamin E, 400–500 IU daily. Herbs such as aloe vera gel, calendula ointment or gel, comfrey, and witch hazel applied topically as directed on the label can speed recovery time and help bruises fade quickly.

295. Burns

The most important thing to do with a burn is to put cold water on it immediately. To effectively stimulate wound healing, 50 mg. zinc daily has been found useful and is worth trying. Vitamin C complex, 1,000 mg. with bioflavonoids, taken in the morning and evening is recommended to prevent infections. Vitamin E, 1,000 IU used orally and topically, can help prevent scarring. MSM lotion applied three times daily and 1 MSM tablet, 1,000 mg., taken three times daily, are advised for a month.

296. Chemotherapy

A complete antioxidant formula can enhance the effectiveness of chemo in reducing cancerous tumors while at the same time protecting healthy tissue and fortifying your immune system. Ginger aids in alleviating some of the unwanted side effects such as nausea and vomiting. I'd suggest taking 50 mg. of CBD daily as well.

CAUTION: *If you are undergoing chemotherapy, be sure to check with your doctor before adding any new supplements.*

297. Cold Feet

If you're embarrassed by wearing socks to bed all the time, you could try a good multimineral supplement with iodine twice a day, along with kelp tablets. The cold feet could be due to the fact that your thyroid glands are not producing enough thyroxin. Niacin and vitamin E can also help circulation. I also suggest ginkgo biloba, 60 mg. one to three times daily and 2 arginine tablets, 1,500 mg., twice daily.

298. Cold Sores and Herpes Simplex

Few things are more annoying than cold sores. The best supplement remedy I've discovered is:

Lactobacillus acidophilus, 3 capsules three times a day

Vitamin E oil, 28,000 IU, applied directly to affected area

Lysine, 3 g. (3,000 mg.) daily (in divided doses) between meals (with water or juice—no protein)

As a preventive: Lysine, 500 mg. daily (with water or juice—no protein)

Vitamin C, 1,000 mg. A.M. and P.M.

299. Constipation

Everyone is bothered by constipation at some time or other. Usually this is due to a lack of bulk in the diet or because of certain medications, such as codeine. Harsh laxatives can rob the body of nutrients, as well as cause rebound constipation and laxative dependency, so natural remedies should be your first choice.

Dietary fiber, 2 g. in tablet form, twice daily, or 1 rounded tsp. psyllium fiber (if not allergic to it) in juice or nonfat milk

1 tbsp. *acidophilus* liquid three times daily or one 25-billion-organisms capsule twice daily

A vegetable laxative and sugar-free stool softener for a short time if necessary

8–10 glasses of water daily (and a little exercise wouldn't hurt)

300. Cuts

Vitamin C complex, 1,000 mg. with bioflavonoids, twice daily, along with 50 mg. zinc and 400 IU vitamin E.

301. Dry Skin

Vitamin E (dry form) oil seems to work wonders when applied to dry skin, as do oils rich in vitamins A and D. As a dietary supplement, I recommend 200–400 IU vitamin

E daily and 10,000 IU vitamin A (take for five days and stop for two). I also recommend an MVP (see section 246) and omega-3 fatty acids, 1–3 capsules three times a day. (See section 100 for the complete lowdown on omega-3 fatty acids.)

If you don't want to take fish oils (omega-3 fatty acids are marketed primarily as EPA [eicosapentaenoic and docosahexaenoic acid]), other natural sources of omega-3 fatty acids are flaxseed oil, pumpkin oil, canola oil, and soy oil (1–2 tsp. added to a salad dressing should help). Significant amounts are also found in walnuts, navy beans, kidney beans, soybeans, and great northern beans.

302. Hangovers

To prevent them, take 1 B complex, 100 mg., before going out, 1 again while you're drinking, and another right before going to bed. (Alcohol destroys B complex.) Cysteine, 500 mg., with vitamin C, 1,500 mg., can help, too. (See section 276.)

303. Hay Fever

Stress can cause hay fever attacks to worsen. If you're one of the many who suffer, you might find relief with 1 B complex twice daily; pantothenic acid, 1,000 mg. three times daily; and the same dose of vitamin C, which has evidenced effective antihistamine properties. Also, standardized extract of sting nettles, Chinese skullcap, feverfew leaf, horseradish root, and yerba santa, taken with an MSM capsule 1,000 mg., twice daily may help you through the sneeze season.

304. Headaches

A surprisingly effective vitamin-mineral regimen for head-aches is:

100 mg. niacin (inositol hexanicotinate) three times daily

100 mg. B complex (time release) twice daily

CBD, 25 mg. twice daily

Calcium and magnesium (twice as much calcium as magnesium is the proper ratio), which are nature's tranquilizers

For migraines, see section 314.

305. Heartburn

Over-the-counter antacids, such as Gelusil, Kolantyl, Maalox, Di-Gel, and Rolaids, contain aluminum, which disturbs calcium and phosphorus metabolism. You'll probably be better off taking one MSM 1,000 mg. capsule three times daily to decrease the acid (or 2 calcium [250 mg.] and magnesium [125 mg.] tablets three times daily); multiple digestive enzymes one to three times daily; chewable papaya; drinking fluids before or after meals, *not* during; and eating more slowly.

306. Hemorrhoids

Just about half the people over fifty are afflicted by hemorrhoids. Improper diet, lack of exercise, and straining at stool are all contributing factors. And coffee, chocolate, cola, and cocoa are accessories to the discomfort by promoting anal itching. If you're bothered by hemorrhoids, 1 tbsp. of unprocessed bran three times a day or 2 g. of dietary fiber twice daily is helpful, along with 1,000 mg.

vitamin C complex twice a day for healing membranes, and 3 *acidophilus* capsules three times a day (or 1–2 tbsp. of *acidophilus* liquid one to three times a day). Vitamin E oil, 28,000 IU per ounce, can be applied to the affected area with a cotton swab.

307. Impotence/Erectile Dysfunction (ED)

If you have trouble maintaining an erection adequate for satisfactory sexual performance, you might want to try some natural remedies before you go for a Viagra or Cialis prescription. I suggest ginkgo biloba, 60 mg. three times daily; 2–4 saw palmetto, zinc, and pumpkin seed oil combination capsules daily; and arginine (time release), 1,500 mg. taken twice daily. If you are over fifty years of age, I also recommend one 25–50 mg. DHEA tablet daily. (DHEA should *not* be taken by anyone under forty unless blood level of that hormone is low. Men over fifty can take 50 mg. daily, women, 25 mg. daily.)

308. Insomnia

Can't sleep? Maybe you need a more naturally effective anti-insomnia program:

1 chelated calcium (250 mg.) and magnesium (125 mg.) tablet three times daily—and 3 tablets a half hour before bedtime.

Vitamin B6, 100 mg., and niacinamide, 100 mg., work together to produce the brain chemical serotonin, which is essential for restful REM sleep.

Turkey is a good source of tryptophan. Therefore, an open-faced turkey sandwich and a cup of herbal tea (chamomile, valerian, skullcap) before bedtime could be the sleep remedy of your life.

For more difficult insomnia, try 5 mg. of melatonin thirty minutes before bedtime.

309. Itching

As an antihistamine, one 1,000 mg. vitamin C tablet, plus a 1,000 mg. MSM capsule, in the morning and in the evening, with food, might be helpful. I would also recommend 1,000 mg. pantothenic acid one to three times daily, and vitamin E cream (20,000 IU per ounce) applied to afflicted area three times daily.

310. Jet Lag

So your plane from London lands at 9 A.M. and you're supposed to be at a meeting at 10 A.M. No problem, except for the fact that as far as your body is concerned, it's still only 4 A.M. and you should be asleep. Your best bet is to help your system catch up with your schedule by giving it the vitamins it needs.

B complex, 50 mg. A.M. and P.M. (start while still on the plane).

MVP with food, twice during flights of five or more hours (see section 246).

Melatonin, 1 mg., can also be taken.

If you're feeling run-down as well as tired, be sure to take additional vitamin C.

NOTE: *Intestinal gas expands at high altitudes, so pass on the beans and other gas-inducing foods right before and during the flight if you want to feel fit on arrival. Also, keep in mind that alcohol destroys vitamin B complex, which is one of the best jet-lag fighters around. And be sure to drink water every hour on the plane; the pressurized cabin causes your body to dehydrate faster.*

311. Leg Pains

Increase your calcium. Try 1 chelated calcium and magnesium tablet with breakfast and dinner. Vitamin E has been reported to be quite helpful in cases of charley horse. The most common doses for it are 400–1,000 IU vitamin E one to three times daily. And ginkgo biloba, 60 mg. one to three times daily can also help the circulation to your legs. The herb horse chestnut can be taken, 50 mg. twice daily.

312. Menopause

Because of health concerns that have been brought to light about estrogens and hormone replacement therapy (HRT)—including increased risk of breast and ovarian cancer, strokes, adult-onset asthma, cardiac events, serious blood clots, dementia, and loss of libido—many women have been seeking other ways to relieve the discomforts of menopause. A good number of menopausal women have found that 200–400 IU vitamin E (mixed tocopherols) with selenium one to three times a day does indeed alleviate hot flashes. If you're at that time of life, MVP and a 50 mg. B complex twice a day also seem to help. Chelated calcium (250 mg.) and magnesium (125 mg.) can be taken with a soy isoflavonoid complex (containing daidzein, genistein, vitamin D, and boron) twice daily. And for a soothing, mood-elevating, and muscle-relaxing aid, try a St. John's wort complex and black cohosh extract combination tablet once or twice daily. There are many other herbs with estrogenic plant components that can add to estrogen levels in the body and help stem hot flashes, vaginal dryness, fatigue, depression, and other symptoms of menopause. (See section 461 for natural Alternatives to HRT.)

313. Menstruation

Between the cramps and the bloating, menstruation is for most women a monthly annoyance. But this annoyance can dwindle down to a mere distraction once the discomfort is alleviated.

MVP (see section 246)

Vitamin B6, 50 mg. three times daily (most effective as a natural diuretic)

B complex, 50 mg. A.M. and P.M.

Evening primrose oil, 500 mg. three times daily

314. Migraines

Migraines are headaches on steroids. If you've ever had one you don't want another. New research has shown that B vitamins can help reduce the severity and incidences of migraine attacks.

Folic acid, 800 mcg. daily

Vitamin B6, 50 mg. daily

Vitamin B12, 400 mcg. daily

Vitamin B2, 200 mg. daily

Feverfew, 500 mg. daily (see section 192)

NOTE: *This regimen can be divided in half and taken with food* A.M. *and* P.M.

315. Motion Sickness

This is one condition where remedies are most effective if taken beforehand. Vitamins B1 and B6 are the nutrients of choice (in fact, many prenatal antinausea preparations contain vitamin B6). Taking 50 mg. B complex the night before you leave and the morning of your trip has been found to be effective by many queasy travelers.

Ginger extract capsules taken three times daily work also!

316. Muscle Soreness

For that achy-all-over feeling after a workout, or just general muscle soreness, I've seen many people find relief with vitamin E, 400–800 IU, taken one to three times daily. A chelated calcium and magnesium tablet in the morning and at night also has helped.

317. The Pill

If you take oral contraceptives, not only are you more vulnerable than other women to blood clots, strokes, and heart attacks, but you're also more likely to be deficient in zinc, folic acid, vitamins C, B6, and B12 (which accounts for much nervousness and depression among pill-takers).

Supplements are important:
MVP (see section 246)
Zinc, 15 mg. chelated, 1 tablet daily
Folic acid, 800 mcg. daily
B6, 50–100 mg. daily

318. Poison Ivy/Poison Oak

MSM lotion, vitamin E oil, or aloe vera gel applied externally three times daily can help healing. A 1,000 mg. vitamin C tablet taken A.M. and P.M. should alleviate the itching.

319. Polyps

These small annoying growths should definitely be seen by a doctor, and in most instances surgical removal is necessary. But as far as supplements go, Dr. Jerome J. DeCosse, professor and chairman of surgery at the Medical College of Wisconsin, used 3,000 mg. vitamin C daily on patients with polyps, and had noteworthy success with the treatment.

320. Postoperative Healing

After surgery, your body needs all the nutritional support it can get.

MVP (see section 246) three times daily, with meals

2 vitamin C complex, 1,000 mg., with bioflavonoids, hesperidin, and rutin, A.M. and P.M.

This regimen can be used for two weeks before and two to four weeks after surgery.

For post–plastic surgery add:

Arnica, 4 pellets sublingually (under tongue) on an empty stomach, before meals, three to four times daily (for bruising)

Bromelain, 500 mg., 1–2 tablets daily (to reduce swelling)

CAUTION: *Do not take large doses of vitamin E for two weeks before or after surgery.*

321. Prickly Heat

Much like itching, prickly heat seems to respond to the antihistamine properties of vitamin C. (See section 309 for regimen.)

322. Prostate Problems

Chronic prostatitis, where inflammation of the gland is often combined with infection, has been found to respond to treatment with zinc. (The prostate gland normally contains about ten times more zinc than any other organ in the body.) In many cases, symptoms have completely disappeared, especially with supplements that also contain pygeum and saw palmetto.

MVP (see section 246)

Combination saw palmetto, pygeum, selenium, stinging nettle, beta-sitosterol, zinc, and lycopene tablet twice daily.

NOTE: *See section 359 for a dietary and supplement regimen designed to protect the prostate from BPH (benign prostatic hyperplasia).*

323. Psoriasis

Though many jokes have been made about this disease, it is no laughing matter to the millions who suffer from it. No one treatment has been found to be totally effective, but the following has met with much success:

MVP (see section 246)

Beta-carotene, 10,000 IU daily

B complex, 50 mg. A.M. and P.M.

Rose hips vitamin C, 500 mg. A.M. and P.M.

Vitamin E (dry form), 200–400 IU twice daily

Evening primrose, borage, or flaxseed oil capsules, 500 mg. three times daily

Selenium, 100–200 mcg. daily

324. Stopping Smoking

It's no mean feat to stop smoking, and your body knows it. Those withdrawal symptoms are real. For the irritability that occurs, take one CBD (50 mg.); a chelated calcium (250 mg.) and magnesium (125 mg.) tablet; and a B complex, 50 mg. in the morning or afternoon with food. Between meals take 1,000 mg. cysteine. With the evening meal, take another calcium and magnesium tablet and a 50 mg. B complex. And don't forget your MVP (see section 246).

CAUTION: *If you are using a nicotine gum to help you quit smoking, be aware that consuming coffee, cola, or acidic drinks before chewing nicotine gum* significantly inhibits its absorption.

325. Stress

Stress can be physical or psychological, result from injury, disease, infection, overwork, financial worries, relationship conflicts, or even too much of a good thing. We all know what it feels like, but we don't always know how to deal with it nutritionally. Before racing off for prescription drugs, be aware that natural remedies can help a lot.

MVP (see section 246)

Calcium, 500–1,000 mg. daily (1,500–2,000 mg. for women over forty)

DHEA, 25 mg. daily for women over forty and 50 mg. daily for men over forty

Magnesium, 250–500 mg. daily

Melatonin, one to three 1 mg. time-release tablets before bedtime

Vitamin B complex, 25–50 mg. daily

Chamomile, as directed on label

CBD, 50 mg. daily

326. Sunburn

A good sunscreen preparation should always be used before exposing yourself to the sun's ultraviolet rays for any length of time. What most people don't realize is that the sun actually burns the skin, and bad burns can break the skin and leave it vulnerable to infection.

If it's too late for preventives, try this:

Aloe vera gel, applied three to four times daily

An MSM lotion or vitamin E cream (20,000 IU), also applied three to four times daily

MVP (see section 246)

Additional vitamin C, 500 mg. A.M. and P.M. until burn heals

327. Teeth Grinding

People are usually unaware of grinding their teeth. It occurs more often in children than adults, and most often during sleep. To get out of the "grind," try MVP (see section 246); B complex, 50 mg. A.M. and P.M.; 1 dual-action St. John's wort complex once or twice daily; and chelated calcium (250 mg.) and magnesium (125 mg.) taken at bedtime.

328. Varicose Veins

Age, lack of exercise, and chronic constipation are contributing factors to varicose veins. Watching your diet and exercising regularly can do a lot toward preventing them. MVP with an extra 500 mg. vitamin C complex (especially combined with butcher's broom extract) twice daily has been found to help, along with 400–800 IU of vitamin E. I'd also suggest a horse chestnut extract supplement twice daily, and ginkgo biloba, 60 mg., two to three times daily for improved circulation.

Suggestion: Topical application of a witch hazel ointment three or more times daily may be useful. Allow two or more weeks before expecting results.

329. Vasectomy

Men with vasectomies are more susceptible to infections and would be wise to take an additional 1,000 mg. vitamin C complex daily, along with regular MVP diet supplementation. Extra zinc, 15–50 mg. every day, is also a good idea.

330. Warts

They don't come from handling frogs, but they do seem to effectively disappear when treated with vitamin E oil. The most successful regimen appears to be 28,000 IU vitamin E applied externally one to two times daily and 400 IU vitamin E (dry form) taken internally three times a day. Vitamin C complex, 1,000–2,000 mg. daily, can help build up the body's immunity and possibly prevent warts from occurring at all.

DID YOU KNOW?

- Coffee can inhibit the absorption of nicotine chewing gum.
- Men with vasectomies are more susceptible to infections.
- Vitamin B1 can fight air- and seasickness.

331. Any Questions About Chapter XIII?

You talk about digestive enzymes being helpful for heart-burn. What are they and what do they do?

Enzymes, which can be purchased as supplements, can help your own digestive system assimilate the foods you eat. *Bromelain,* for instance, is a digestive enzyme from pineapple. *Cellulose* is an aid to digesting vegetable matter and breaking down food fiber. *Hydrochloric acid (HCl)* works in the stomach on tough foods, such as fibrous meats, vegetables, and poultry (betaine HCl is the best form available). *Lipase* assists in fat digestion, and *mylase* dissolves thousands of times its own weight in starches so you can more easily assimilate them. *Papain* is a protein-digesting enzyme (from papaya), and *prolase* is a concentrated protein-digesting enzyme derived from papain.

Both of my parents developed cataracts in their sixties. I'm forty years old and would like to know if there are any nutritional preventive measures I could be taking now that might lessen my risk.

Cataracts in older people involve progressive oxidative changes in the lens of the eye. Starting an antioxidant regimen now would be your best defense. Glutathione, which is synthesized from three amino acids (cysteine, glutamic acid, and glycine), has been found to deactivate free radicals that speed the aging process and appears to be a key factor in preventing lens oxidation. I'd suggest taking a 50 mg. capsule twice daily, as well as one 125 mcg. capsule of superoxide dismutase (SOD) and a high-potency multivitamin-mineral complex.

Is there a specific reason for your recommending a soy isoflavonoid complex in the treatment of menopause?

Definitely. Since estrogen replacement began in the 1950s, it has been linked to a 35 percent increase in uterine cancer. Soy isoflavones, particularly genistein and daidzein, are estrogenlike compounds that can not only help relieve the symptoms of menopause, such as hot flashes, irritability, and vaginal dryness; they can help protect against cancer as well. In fact, the combination of soy isoflavones and calcium, magnesium, vitamin D, and boron has also been found helpful in preventing osteoporosis (see section 357)!

I've been told that I'm prone to gallstones. Can you recommend a supplement or regimen to reduce my risk of developing them?

Gallstones are crystallized masses of mostly cholesterol, so I would suggest taking 1 tablespoon of lecithin granules one to three times daily, and 500–1,500 mg. of taurine daily. I'd also recommend that you avoid refined carbohydrates and saturated fats and eat more oat bran.

XIV

GETTING WELL AND STAYING THAT WAY

332. Why and When You Don't Need Antibiotics

Listen to me: You don't need to take an antibiotic for a cold, flu, sore throat, or even a sinus, bronchial, or urinary tract infection, unless that infection has been diagnosed as bacterial or symptoms have lasted more than a week and your temperature has been higher than 100.4.

Antibiotics are ineffective against viral illnesses, not even limiting their duration or severity. Taking them for viral infections simply kills off weak bacteria and allows the strongest to survive—creating dangerous antibiotic resistance. In other words, lifesaving antibiotics may become ineffective just when you need them the most.

Try a natural remedy first.

Sore throat: Dissolve 1 drop bitter orange essential oil (a natural antibacterial/anti-inflammatory) and ¼ teaspoon salt in ½ cup warm water and gargle twice daily. Don't swallow. Tea that contains licorice root as well as echinacea and goldenseal (see section 185) can alleviate symptoms and speed recovery.

Sinus infection (sinusitis): Mix 20 drops of grape-seed liquid extract in water, juice, or tea daily. Also, a beta-carotene supplement can help heal mucous membranes.

Urinary tract infection: Drink four 8-ounce glasses of unsweeted cranberry or blueberry juice daily. Also effective is the herb uva ursi. Suggested dose is 2 capsules twice daily.

Bronchitis: Black elder tea has been found to be antiviral. Steep 1 tsp. elder flowers and ½ tsp. elderberries for ten minutes in 1 cup of boiled water; add ½ tsp. honey. Drink 2–3 cups daily.

If your symptoms don't start improving within 24 hours of taking natural supplements (or if fever is above 100.4) see your doctor or healthcare provider for a bacterial culture to determine if you need an antibiotic.

If antibiotics are prescribed:

- Maximize their effectiveness by taking them with green tea.
- Avoid antacids, which can decrease antibiotic effectiveness by 90 percent.
- Take probiotics (see section 131) two hours before or after taking medication to prevent diarrhea and yeast infections.

333. Why You Definitely Need Supplements During Illness

During illness the body is under stress. Cells are destroyed, exhausted adrenal glands deprived of nutrients are unable to function properly, and the body's stress-fighting team of vitamin C, B6, folic acid, and pantothenic acid is severely depleted. Zinc and vitamin C are also needed in greater amounts.

Because these vitamins are required to utilize other nutrients effectively and to keep your metabolism functioning, the need for them is obviously increased when you are ill. And since we know that fever and stress rob the body of its most essential nutrients, the importance of supplements is self-evident. Keep in mind that all supplements should be taken with food, unless otherwise indicated.

Again, the following regimens are not intended as medical advice, only as a guide in working with your doctor.

334. ADD/ADHD

Attention deficit disorder (ADD) is a condition characterized by a short or poor attention span and inappropriate, impulsive behavior. Attention-deficit/hyperactivity disorder (ADHD) is ADD with hyperactivity. These disorders usually affect school-age children, but may continue into adulthood and not be recognized until then. Symptoms include fidgeting, excessive talking, disregard of consequences, and an inability to concentrate. Psychostimulant drugs such as Ritalin (methylphenidate) and Adderall (an amphetamine) are often (too often, as far as I'm concerned) prescribed to control ADD/ADHD, but nutritional supplements have in many cases worked as nonprescription alternatives.

MVP (see section 246) A.M. and P.M.

Calcium, 500–1,000 mg. daily

Magnesium, 250–500 mg. daily

MSM, 1,000 mg. one to three times daily

Bacopa extract, 100 mg. daily

Huperzine A (extract from club moss), 50 mcg. one to three times daily

Ginkgo biloba, 60 mg., one to three times daily

Grape-seed/green tea complex, 100 mg. of each twice daily

Phosphatidylserine (PS), 300–600 mg. daily

St. John's wort complex, 300 mg. one to two times daily

NOTE: *Recent findings have shown that when children with ADD received a formula that provided EPA, DHA, and GLA, significant improvements were noted. In light of this, a daily intake of EPA (300 mg.), DHA (150 mg.), and borage oil (150 mg.), which will provide 80 mg. of GLA, might be advisable—especially since formulas with these fatty acids are currently available in kid-friendly chewable gelatin capsules as well as liquids.*

335. Allergies

Allergies come in all shapes and sizes, with all sorts of symptoms, and you can contract them from just about anything. Nonetheless, they take their nutritional toll, and supplements can help.

MVP (see section 246) A.M. and P.M.

Vitamin B complex, 50 mg. two times daily

Pantothenic acid, 500 mg. A.M. and P.M.

MSM, 1,000 mg., with vitamin C complex, one to three times daily

Herbal extract of stinging nettle, skullcap, feverfew leaf, horseradish root, and yerba santa tablet twice daily

If you have an allergy, it would be a good idea to take a hard look at your present diet. Many allergies are caused by MSG, food coloring, additives, and preservatives.

336. Arthritis

Thousands of people suffer from this painful chronic condition. Because it puts so much stress on the body, vitamin-mineral supplementation is really essential.

MVP (see section 246)

Extra vitamin C, 500 mg. one to two times a day (if you're taking lots of aspirin, you're losing vitamin C)

Pantothenic acid, 100 mg. three times daily

1 omega-3 capsule, two to three times daily

Copper, 2 mg. daily

MSM, 1000 mg. two to three times daily

Curcumin, 50 mg. twice daily

CBD, 50 mg. daily

Increase your consumption of fatty fish, such as cod, salmon, and halibut. They are a great source of omega-3 fatty acids, which have anti-inflammatory properties. I'd also suggest you eliminate the nightshades, such as potatoes, tomatoes, and eggplant, from your diet, as they may aggravate your condition.

337. Asthma

Asthma is a chronic allergic condition that affects the bronchial tubes. When an attack occurs, the muscle tissue of the tubes constricts spasmodically, squeezing the air passages and causing labored breathing and a feeling of suffocation. Allergies, heredity, and emotional stress have all been implicated as contributing factors to asthmatic conditions, but many nutrients have been found to provide remarkable natural relief.

MVP (see section 246) A.M. and P.M.

Extra vitamin C, 500 mg. A.M. and P.M.

2 evening primrose oil capsules, 500 mg. three times

daily for three to four months; then 1 capsule three times daily. (If you are taking steroids, you won't benefit from EPO, because steroids interfere with EPO's action.)

CBD, 50 mg. daily
Curcumin, 50 mg. twice daily
Omega-3, 1,000 mg. three times daily
MSM, 1,000 mg., two to three times daily
Vitamin B complex, 50 mg. twice daily
Ginkgo biloba, 60 mg., two to three times daily

338. Blood Pressure—High and Low and In Between

According to revised new guidelines, only blood pressure of *less than* 120 over 80 is considered normal for adults. A blood pressure reading equal to or greater than 140 over 90 is considered high.

HIGH

More than eighty million Americans have high blood pressure (hypertension), which has been intimately linked to heart attacks and strokes. Additionally, evidence also suggests that it can contribute to kidney failure, the progression of mental deficits, and dementia. The importance of keeping your blood pressure down cannot be overestimated, and there are a number of natural ways that can help.

- Talk slower (fast talkers often don't breathe properly, and this can result in elevated blood pressure).
- Reduce if you are overweight (controlled, sensible dieting can significantly lower blood pressure in overweight individuals).
- Decrease sodium and increase potassium in your diet (see section 427 on hidden salt in foods).

- Decrease your sugar intake (see section 425).
- Eliminate or moderate alcohol intake—no more than 1 drink a day for women and 2 for men.
- Eliminate caffeine (see section 371).
- Eat more onions and garlic.
- Stop smoking.
- Avoid stress or anxiety-provoking situations (jangling everyday noises, even loud televisions, can cause stress and elevate blood pressure).
- Exercise regularly (brisk walking) and get adequate rest.
- Eat 3–4 celery stalks daily (celery contains natural blood pressure–lowering properties).

Regimen

Potassium may be necessary if you are taking an antihypertensive, but check with your doctor to be sure it's not contraindicated for your particular medication.

MVP (see section 246)

Calcium, 1,000 mg. daily

Magnesium, 500 mg. daily

Coenzyme-Q10, 200 mg. with vitamin E, daily

IN BETWEEN (PREHYPERTENSION)

Recent revamping of guidelines for "normal" blood pressure has led to the establishment of a condition called "prehypertension" to describe people with blood pressure readings from 120 to 139 (the upper number, or systolic pressure) over 80 to 90 (the lower, or diastolic pressure). If your blood pressure falls in this range, you are at high risk of developing dangerous hypertension and should start following the advice I've given above to lower that risk as soon as possible. Be aware that as you age your blood pressure tends to rise.

(According to the Framingham Heart Study, 90 percent of all people who may have normal readings when they are fifty-five eventually develop high blood pressure.)

LOW

Low blood pressure, unless extreme, is a far better condition to have than its alternative. Nonetheless, hypotensives often suffer from dizziness and occasional fainting spells and blackouts.

Regimen

1–3 kelp tablets daily (If you're taking thyroid medication, check with your doctor, as kelp might decrease the need for the amount you're currently taking.)

MVP (see section 246)

339. Bronchitis

This inflammation of the bronchial tube lining is quite common and extremely enervating. The stress it puts on the body is high, and even antibiotics are the bad guys as far as nutrients are concerned (see section 381).

Beta-carotene, 10,000 IU daily

Rose hips vitamin C, 1,000 mg. A.M. and P.M.

MVP (see section 246)

Vitamin E (dry form), 400 IU one to three times daily

MSM, 1,000 mg., with vitamin C complex two to three times daily with food

Water, 6–8 glasses daily

3 *acidophilus* caps three times daily, or 1–2 tbsp. liquid three times daily

340. *Candida Albicans*

This yeast infection takes advantage of circumstances in the body that are conducive to its growth, and there are many. For example: antibiotics, birth control pills, cortisone, diabetes mellitus, nutritional deficiencies, chronic constipation or diarrhea, and physical or emotional stress.

Symptoms can range from all those associated with vaginitis (discharge, itching, bladder infection, menstrual irregularities and cramps) to severe depression, acne, anxiety, fatigue, nervousness, and mental confusion.

The first step in treating *Candida albicans* is to deprive the body of all yeast-containing foods. For example: cheese, leavened breads, sour cream, buttermilk, beer, wine, cider, mushrooms, soy sauce, tofu, vinegar, dried fruits, melons, and frozen or canned juices.

If your doctor has not yet put you on a yeast fungus–killing drug, such as nystatin, there are many natural and surprisingly effective dietary combatants. Among them are garlic, broccoli, cabbage, onions, plain yogurt, turnips, and other vegetables.

And an effective supplement regimen would be:

MVP (see section 246)

MSM, 1,000 mg. three times daily

Vitamin E (dry form), 200–400 IU daily

Caprylic acid supplement one to three times daily

Acidophilus (yeast-free), 1 capsule three times daily

341. Chicken Pox

This childhood staple is caused by a virus closely related to that of shingles. The fever and itching deplete a good amount of nutrients. Many mothers have found their children up and about faster by adding the following supplements to their diets:

Rose hips vitamin C, 500 mg. three times daily

Vitamin E (dry form), 100–200 IU one to three times daily

Beta-carotene, 10,000 IU daily (check pediatrician for proper dosage according to age and weight)

All-natural chewable vitamin and mineral MVP if child is over twelve years of age

MSM therapeutic lotion applied to affected areas three times daily

342. Chronic Fatigue Syndrome

It's known by different names in different countries, but the common symptoms are: sudden onset, extreme fatigue, chills or low-grade fever, sore throat, tender lymph nodes, muscle pain, headaches, joint pain (without swelling), confusion, memory loss, visual disturbances, and sleep disorders, among others.

Two to five million Americans have been stricken with this illness. The British and Canadians know it as ME (myalgic encephalomyelitis), and the Japanese refer to it as low natural killer cell syndrome. In this country it's referred to as chronic fatigue immune dysfunction syndrome (CFIDS) or chronic fatigue syndrome (CFS).

Originally thought to be caused by the Epstein-Barr virus (the herpes virus that causes infectious mononucleosis), it is now known that CFS victims develop high amounts of antibodies to numerous other bugs.

According to a report in *Newsweek* magazine, Dr. Jay Goldstein, a Southern California physician, has theorized that the illness begins "when an unknown chemical or contagion damages the immune system...enabling viruses ordinarily held in check to start running amok. The immune system's helper T cells then start churning out tougher chemicals called 'cytokines,' which can themselves cause CFS symptoms." And the normal killer T cells that should attack anything foreign become mysteriously underactive (or, in some cases, unhealthily overactive).

There's no "silver bullet" treatment for CFS, but the body's immune system can use all the nutritional help it can get.

MVP (see section 246) A.M. and P.M.

Beta-carotene, 10,000 IU daily, five days a week (stop for two days)

Vitamin C, 1,000 mg. one to three times daily

Vitamin E (dry form), 200–400 IU, one to three times daily

Cysteine, 1 daily, with vitamin C (three times as much vitamin C as cysteine)

Selenium, 200 mcg. daily

Zinc, chelated, 15–50 mg. daily

Evening primrose oil, 500 mg., one to three times daily

MSM, 1,000 mg. three times daily

My Advice:

Because the herpes virus is implicated, I'd suggest avoiding arginine-rich foods (see section 85). I'd also advise steering clear of refined carbohydrates, caffeine, alcohol, highly allergenic foods, and foods containing artificial flavors, colors, and other additives that can stress the immune system.

343. Colds

No one pays too much attention to a cold, except the body—it pays plenty.

MVP (see section 246)

Rose hips vitamin C, 1,000 mg. three to six times daily for two days

Beta-carotene, 10,000 IU one to three times daily (take for five days and stop for two)

Water, 6–8 glasses daily

3 *acidophilus* capsules three times daily, or 1–2 tbsp. liquid three times daily

Zinc lozenge (let dissolve in mouth) three to four times daily

Echinacea, American feverfew, and elderberry extract, 1 dropper every three to four hours as needed

344. Colitis

As a rule, this illness is more common in women than men and often is triggered by emotional upset. Alternating diarrhea and constipation, as well as abdominal pain, are its distressing hallmarks. Diet is of prime importance and vitamins are recommended.

MVP (see section 246)

Potassium, 99 mg. (elemental) one to three times daily

Raw cabbage juice (vitamin U), 1 glass three times daily

Water, 6–8 glasses daily

Aloe vera juice (for internal use), 1 tbsp. three times daily or 1–3 capsules three times daily

3–6 *acidophilus* caps three times daily, or 2 tbsp. liquid three times daily

1 tbsp. bran flakes 3 times daily, or 2 grams of fiber in tablet form twice daily

MSM, 1,000 mg. three times daily

CAUTION: *Colitis sufferers are fructose intolerant. Because of this, colitis is one of those medical conditions, like Crohn's*

*disease, celiacs, and irritable bowel syndrome, where normally
healthy dietary choices can be harmful. Eating fruits, and
some vegetables like onions, leeks, green beans, artichokes, and
asparagus, which contain fructans, can trigger painful flare-
ups. (High fructose corn syrup, which is in many processed
foods, should also be avoided.)*

345. COPD (Chronic Obstructive Pulmonary Disease)

This chronic disease, which worsens over time, encompasses emphysema and chronic bronchitis. Characterized
by coughing and breathlessness, people with COPD are
more prone to chest infection because the lining in the
lungs loses its normal defense mechanism. Also, because it
is an inflammatory disease, sufferers are subjected to high
levels of oxidated stress. COPD is irreversible, but its progress can be slowed.

Regimen

Vitamin A (from fish oil), 2,500 IU
Vitamin C, 500 mg.
Vitamin E, 200 IU
N-acetylcysteine, 500 mg.
L-Carnitine, 250 mg.
Bromelain, 250 mg.
Omega 3 (EPA/DHA), 1,000 mg.
This regimen can be taken twice daily with food.

Flavonoids from soy food act as anti-inflammatory
agents in the lungs and can help protect against tobacco
carcinogens. Broccoli may also help protect against respiratory inflammation.

346. Diabetes

What happens in diabetes, primarily, is that the pancreas fails to produce adequate insulin and the blood sugar rises uncontrollably. In mild cases diet alone can control the condition. (Beware of hidden sugars. See section 425.) In severe cases, replacement insulin is necessary. In all cases, the care of a physician is essential.

There is an herbal, though, that's been found to help many diabetics—banaba leaf. The banaba is a medicinal plant grown in the Philippines and Asia where its leaves have long been used to brew tea as a folk remedy for treating diabetes and kidney disease. New research has found that it contains a plant chemical called corosolic acid that acts like a natural insulin, helping transport glucose into cells and thereby lowering the unwanted levels of glucose in the blood. Unlike supplemental insulin, banaba is not fat-forming and has been shown to lower glucose in patients with type 2 diabetes without promoting weight gain. Additionally, because fluctuations in blood glucose often lead to sugar cravings, keeping blood sugar levels even could help control weight, too.

Banaba leaf extract is available in supplemental form. The recommended dosage is from 16 to 48 mg. daily. (I'd suggest 16 mg. at the end of each meal.) It is also found in combination products for diabetes and weight loss, supplements formulated with minerals and metabolism-boosting nutrients. If taking a combination supplement, follow directions on the label.

Other supplements that aid diabetics are:

MVP (see section 246)

Chromium picolinate, 200 mcg.

Alpha-lipoic acid, 50 mg. daily

Potassium, 99 mg. three times daily

Chelated zinc, 50 mg. one to three times daily
Water, 6–8 glasses daily

347. Eye Problems

From simple inflammations to refraction difficulties to serious diseases, eye problems should never be ignored, nor should visits to the ophthalmologist be postponed. There are, however, generally beneficial supplements you can take.

MVP (see section 246)
Beta-carotene, 10,000 IU daily
Vitamin C complex, 500 mg. A.M. and P.M.
Vitamin E (dry form), 400 IU daily
Lutein, 20 mg. daily

348. Flu (Influenza/H1N1)

The best way to deal with a flu is to fight it off before it gets to you. And the best way to do that is to be well armed with a strong immune system. Although vaccines are available, influenza viruses mutate from year to year, and no one vaccine can combat all strains without time-consuming tweaking that can cost lives, as attested to by the swine flu (H1N1) epidemic. Having a powerful immune system is your best defense and could mean the difference between life and death.

SUPPLEMENTS TO SIDESTEP SWINE FLU (H1N1)

At the first sign of symptoms take:

MVP (see section 246)
Vitamin C, 500 mg. every hour until symptoms subside (discontinue if diarrhea occurs)
Beta-carotene, 5,000 IU daily

Vitamin A, 3,000 IU daily

Quercetin, 50 mg. twice daily

Zinc gluconate, 15 mg. twice daily

Citrus bioflavonoids, 50 mg. twice daily

Odorless aged garlic, 160 mg. daily

B-complex, 25 mg. twice daily with food

Selenium, 200 mcg. up to three times daily for three days

N-acetyl-cysteine, 500 mg. twice daily for three days

(Drink plenty of fluids and avoid dairy and beverages that can dehydrate the body, such as coffee and caffeinated sodas.)

FIVE FAB FLU-FIGHTING FOODS

- Probiotics
- Green tea
- Cayenne
- Blueberries
- Ginger

349. Gout

Dietary factors, such as high protein consumption, play a role in the development of this painful condition, which occurs when excess uric acid crystallizes in a joint or joints and causes inflammation. Feet, knees, wrists, and elbows are the joints most commonly affected. Because obesity can be linked to high uric acid levels in the blood, people who are overweight should consult their healthcare provider about starting a weight-loss program.

CAUTION: *Fasting or extreme dieting can actually raise uric acid levels and cause gout to worsen, as can the consumption of alcohol.*

FOODS TO AVOID

High purine-rich foods such as: hearts, sweetbreads, sardines, yeast, mussels, smelt, and herring.

Moderately purine-rich foods such as: turkey, scallops, salmon, bacon, liver, anchovies, veal, mutton, trout, and haddock.

The following supplements and herbal remedies are helpful in ridding the body of excess uric acid and reducing inflammation, especially taken in conjunction with drinking 10–12 glasses of nonalcoholic fluids daily.

MVP (see section 246)

MSM, 1,000 mg. one to three times daily

Vitamin B complex, 50 mg. daily

Ginger extract, one to two 170 mg. capsules daily

PCOs (grape-seed extract), 100 mg. one to three times daily

NOTE: *Low-fat dairy products have been found to* decrease *the risk of gout.*

350. Heart Conditions

With any heart condition, you should be under a doctor's care. Though the following supplements have been found to be quite safe and helpful, you should check with your physician to make sure they are not contraindicated in your particular case. (Vitamin E can increase the imbalance between the two sides of the heart for some people with rheumatic hearts.)

MVP (see section 246)

Coenzyme-Q10 complex two to three times daily

Vitamin B, 100 mg. A.M. and P.M.

Soy isoflavonoid complex twice daily

EPA and DHA, 1–3 capsules daily (fish oil or flaxseed oil)

TOP HEART-PROTECTING SUPPLEMENTS

Coenzyme-Q10—Frequently prescribed heart medications such as statins and beta-blockers can lower Co-Q10 levels. Supplements of Co-Q10 can normalize them. (See section 119.)

Niacin—Taken in combination with statins, niacin further lowers LDL levels, improves blood level function, and can help prevent a second heart attack. (See section 33.)

Omega-3 fatty acids—Reduce likelihood of blood clots, clogged arteries, high triglycerides, and irregular heartbeats. (See section 100.)

Red yeast rice—Lowers LDL cholesterol and triglycerides while raising HDL cholesterol. Combined with fish oil supplements, can match the cholesterol and triglyceride lowering achieved with prescription statin drugs.

Phytosterols/sterols—Increasingly added to food and drinks, these related compounds are available as supplements in doses proven to lower LDL cholesterol beyond the effects of diet and drugs.

Vitamin D—Calcitrol, manufactured from 25-hydroxyvitamin D, is now considered essential for proper functioning of heart muscle cells and can reduce risk of attacks, congestive heart failure, hypertension, and diabetes.

HEART ATTACK *PREVENTION* TACTICS

- Decrease sugar and salt consumption.
- Use alcohol in moderation.
- Stop smoking.
- Exercise regularly.
- Watch your weight.
- Practice relaxation techniques such as meditation and biofeedback to reduce stress.

- Decrease intake of saturated fats, hydrogenated oils, and cholesterol.
- Eat more garlic, fresh fruit, and fish.
- Increase your soy protein intake (use in place of animal protein whenever possible).
- Get enough calcium and magnesium in your diet; supplements of 1,000 mg. calcium and 500 mg. magnesium daily are recommended. (See section 63 for more on how magnesium can help.)
- Supplement lecithin in your diet.
- Take supplements of B6, B12, and folic acid, as well as vitamins C and E. (This will help prevent overproduction of the toxic amino acid homocysteine, which is a greater contributor to heart disease than elevated cholesterol!)
- Laughter is great medicine (not only does it release pent-up emotions and stress…it's fun and feels good, too).

NOTE: *Heart disease is the leading killer among women, yet millions of women remain at risk, and increasingly at a younger age. According to the National Heart, Lung and Blood Institute, 60 percent of women ages twenty to thirty-nine have one or more of the top risk factors (high blood pressure, high cholesterol, being overweight, being physically inactive, smoking, and diabetes), but these can be modified to reduce the risk of heart disease (even by women already in their forties and fifties) by following the heart attack prevention tactics I've listed above.*

351. HIV (AIDS)

When human immunodeficiency virus (HIV), the virus that causes AIDS, attacks disease-fighting T cells and multiplies, it brings about the breakdown of the body's immune system. Anyone with HIV or AIDS needs higher amounts of nutrients because malabsorption is a common problem. My best advice is to contact a nutritionally oriented practitioner (see section 462) who can personalize a regimen that will be most effective for you. The internet, also, has some solid HIV and AIDS websites with the latest in alternative as well as traditional treatments that are worth checking out: www.hivinsite.ucsf.edu and www.tpan.com. For a general immune system–boosting regimen, though, I suggest the following:

MVP (see section 246)

Selenium, 200 mcg. daily

Vitamin C (buffered), 500 mg. one to three times daily

Acidophilus caps, 2, taken three times daily a half hour before or after meals

Coenzyme-Q10 complex, 200 mg., once daily

1 standardized maitake mushroom extract tablet daily

Beta-1,3-glucan, 2.5 mg. capsule, 1 daily a half hour before a meal or two hours after eating

Cat's claw (una de gato), 500 mg., 1–3 capsules daily

CAUTION: *If you are currently taking any medication, be sure to check with your physician before adding any supplements to your diet. (See section 459 for more immune system boosters at a glance.)*

352. Hypoglycemia

Though an estimated 20–40 million Americans have it, this disease is one of the most often undiagnosed. It is a condition of low blood sugar and, like diabetes, presents a situation where the body is unable to metabolize carbohydrates normally. Since a hypoglycemic's system overreacts to sugar, producing too much insulin, the key to raising blood sugar levels is not by eating rapidly metabolized refined carbohydrates but by eating more complex carbohydrates and protein.

Recommended supplements:

Beta-carotene and vitamin D capsules (500 and 400 IU), daily

Vitamin C, 500 mg. with or after each meal

B complex, 50 mg. three times daily

Fish oil capsules, 1,000 mg. three times daily

Digestive enzymes if necessary

GTF chromium or chromium dinicotinate glycinate, 200 mcg. two to three times daily

Banaba gymnema sylvestre leaf standardized extract, taken with each meal

St. John's wort, 1 daily

353. Impetigo

Caused by germs similar to those that cause boils—staphylococcus or streptococcus—impetigo occurs more in children than adults, but no one is immune. It often results from scratching and infecting insect bites, allowing the germs to get into broken skin.

Vitamin A and D capsules (10,000 and 400 IU) daily (reduce dose for child) for five days, then stop for two

Vitamin E (dry form), 100–400 IU once a day

Rose hips vitamin C, 500 mg. A.M. and P.M.

MSM, 1,000 mg. A.M. and P.M.

MSM lotion applied three times daily

354. Measles

You can get measles at any age, though it's more common among children. It is the most contagious of the communicable diseases. There is now a preventive vaccine for it, but the virus still manages to afflict a large number of the unprotected each year. The disease and rash can be mild, or severe with a heavy cough. Your body needs vitamins to help fight and recover from it.

Beta-carotene, 10,000 IU (reduce dose for child) one to three times daily

Rose hips vitamin C, 500–1,000 mg. A.M. and P.M.

Vitamin E (dry form), 200–400 IU A.M. *or* P.M.

355. Mononucleosis

Commonly contracted by adolescents and young adults, mono (glandular fever), or "the kissing disease" as it is often called, can affect anyone and can deplete the body of massive amounts of nutrients.

Diet is important, and supplements are generally considered essential during the long convalescence.

MVP (see section 246) A.M. and P.M. with food

Extra vitamin C, 1,000 mg. A.M. and P.M. for three months

Potassium, 99 mg. three times daily

B complex, 50 mg. A.M. and P.M.

Zinc, chelated, 15–50 mg. daily

Echinacea, American feverfew, and elderberry extract, 1 dropper twice daily for one to three months

356. Mumps

A vaccine for mumps exists, but the disease is still quite common and just as nutritionally debilitating. The virus can spread through the patient's entire system, involving not only the salivary glands but the testicles or ovaries, the pancreas, the nervous system, and sometimes even the heart.

Beta-carotene, 10,000 IU (reduce dose for children) one to three times daily for five days, then stop for two

Rose hips vitamin C, 500–1,000 mg. twice daily

Vitamin E, 200–400 IU (dry form) daily

357. Osteoporosis

Osteoporosis is a progressive decrease in bone density that weakens and makes bones more likely to fracture. Up until the age of about thirty—with adequate nutrition, calcium, and vitamin D 4000 IU—our bones increase in density. After age thirty, bones decrease in density—especially if the body is not able to absorb the needed nutrients. And because estrogen is the main female hormone that helps regulate the incorporation of calcium into bone, osteoporosis occurs most frequently in postmenopausal women.

FACTORS THAT INCREASE A WOMAN'S RISK OF OSTEOPOROSIS

- Family history of osteoporosis
- Thin build
- Smoking
- Drinking alcohol
- Early menopause
- No pregnancies
- Insufficient calcium in diet
- Lack of weight-bearing exercise
- Overactive thyroid
- Excessive caffeine intake
- Excessive intake of carbonated beverages that contain phosphorus (which in high amounts can deplete calcium from the body)

Be aware that only weight-bearing exercises (walking, stair climbing, jogging, tennis) increase bone density. Swimming, for instance, does not.

Suggested Supplements

Vitamin C with bioflavonoids, 1,000 mg.

Vitamin D, 400 IU

Vitamin E, 400–800 IU (dry form)

Vitamin K, 100–200 mcg.

Vitamin B12, 500 mcg. sublingual form

Boron, 1–3 mg. (sodium borate)

Soy isoflavone complex (with 10 mg. daidzein and genistein)

Calcium, 1,200–1,500 mg. (See section 55 for good dietary sources of calcium.)

358. PMS (Premenstrual Syndrome)

For two to ten days before the onset of menstruation, millions of women are affected by a wide range of physical discomforts and mood disorders—from bloating, depression, and insomnia to severe pains, uncontrolled rages, crying spells, and even suicidal depression. This is known as PMS, premenstrual syndrome.

FOODS AND BEVERAGES TO AVOID

- Salt and salty foods (see section 427)
- Licorice (it stimulates the production of aldosterone, which causes further retention of sodium and water)
- Cold foods and beverages (these adversely affect abdominal circulation and worsen cramping)

- Caffeine in all forms (see section 371). Caffeine increases the craving for sugar, wastes B vitamins, washes out potassium and zinc, and increases hydrochloric acid (HCl) secretions, which can cause abdominal irritation.
- Astringent dark teas (tannin binds important minerals and prevents absorption in the digestive tract)
- Alcohol (adversely affects blood sugar, depletes magnesium levels, and can interfere with proper liver function, which can aggravate PMS)
- Spinach, beet greens, and other oxalate-containing vegetables (oxalates make minerals nonassimilable, difficult to be properly absorbed)

FOODS AND BEVERAGES TO INCREASE

- Strawberries, watermelon (eat seeds), artichokes, asparagus, parsley, and watercress (these are natural diuretics)
- Raw sunflower seeds, dates, figs, peaches, bananas, potatoes, peanuts, and tomatoes (rich in potassium)
- Try dong quai and black cohosh, herbs that can improve circulation, regulate liver function, and help remove excess water from the system.

Suggested Supplements

Vitamin B6, 50–300 mg. daily (work up from 50 mg. gradually)

MVP (see section 246)

Magnesium (500 mg.) and calcium (250 mg.) daily (Yes, with PMS it is twice as much magnesium as calcium, because a magnesium deficiency causes many of the PMS symptoms.)

Vitamin E (dry form), 100–400 IU daily

Pantothenic acid (vitamin B5), 1,000 mg. (1 g.) daily

Evening primrose oil, 500 mg., one to three times daily
CBD, 50 mg. daily

And exercise! Aside from the fact that this will improve abdominal circulation, perspiration helps remove excess fluids.

Brisk walking for thirty minutes twice daily and/or swimming is highly recommended.

359. Prostate Problems: BPH (Benign Prostatic Hyperplasia or Benign Prostatic Hypertrophy)

It is common for the prostate gland to become enlarged as a man ages. It's a condition known as BPH (benign prostatic hyperplasia or benign prostatic hypertrophy). Most men over the age of forty-five experience some amount of prosate enlargement. This enlargement is usually harmless, but it often results in problems urinating. In fact, many men are unaware of the condition until this happens.

BPH can cause problems that over time may lead to serious bladder and kidney damage. Caught early, there is less chance of this happening and of developing prostate cancer, which is why it is important for men to have prostate examinations on a regular basis and be proactive in protecting the prostate.

PROTECTING THE PROSTATE

- Eat at least three servings of cruciferous vegetables weekly.
- Minimize your intake of sugars, processed foods, and unsaturated fats.
- Get your omega-3 fatty acids from fish.
- Avoid flaxseed oil supplements (ALA in these may increase cancer risk).

- Maximize your intake of phytonutrients (see section 106).
- Include antioxidants and lycopene-rich foods in your diet (see section 107).
- Incorporate the herbs saw palmetto, nettle, and pygeum into your diet.
- Avoid tobacco.
- Limit your intake of caffeine.
- Be sure you're getting enough zinc, vitamin D, and selenium.
- Stay active.
- Watch your weight.

Suggested Supplements

MVP (see section 246)

Combination saw palmetto, pygeum, selenium, stinging nettle, beta-sitosterol, zinc, and lycopene tablet, twice daily.

360. RLS (Restless Legs Syndrome)

Characterized by strong urges to move the legs, this condition is usually accompanied by uncomfortable sensations in the legs such as cramping, tingling, burning, and pain. RLS discomfort worsens when lying down, especially when trying to fall asleep, but also during other forms of inactivity, including just sitting. If leg twitching or jerking also occurs, periodic limb movements during sleep (PLMS) may be the cause. Massage and walking alleviate the discomfort, and eliminating caffeine can definitely help.

RLS can begin at any age, but becomes more severe in middle to old age. An iron deficiency can contribute to RLS. If a blood test that measures ferritin levels reveals this, an iron supplement (ferrous sulfate) can help. If levels are normal, a supplement of 5-HTP, 100–200 mg., taken about twenty minutes before retiring can provide relief.

Suggested Supplements

MVP (see section 246)
Folic acid
Vitamin E

CAUTION: *Antihistamines found in many cold, allergy, and over-the-counter sleeping pills can worsen RLS.*

361. Sinusitis

Sinusitis is an inflammation of the sinuses (the hollow chambers in the bones around the nose). Caused by an allergy—or a bacterial, viral, or fungal infection—it can be either a short-lived or an ongoing condition characterized by pain below the eyes and over the cheeks, headache, and toothache.

MVP (see section 246) A.M. and P.M. with food
Coenzyme-Q10, 60 mg. one to three times daily
MSM, 1,000 mg. one to three times daily
Zinc, 15 mg. one to two times daily
Garlic, 500 mg. daily
Echinacea as directed on label

CAUTION: *Forceful nose blowing, overuse of decongestants, and irritant fumes and sidestream smoke can often worsen symptoms.*

362. Shingles

Shingles (herpes zoster) is caused by a virus much like the one that causes chicken pox. But where chicken pox causes a general skin eruption, shingles usually erupts along a nerve path. Differences aside, the nutritional deficit caused by both diseases is high.

Beta-carotene, 10,000 IU daily

Vitamin B complex, 50 mg. A.M. and P.M.

Rose hips vitamin C with bioflavonoids, 1,000–2,000 mg. A.M. and P.M.

Vitamin D, 5000 IU DAILY

Lysine, 1,000 mg. twice daily between meals on an empty stomach

363. Tonsillitis

An inflammation of the tonsils that can afflict any age group, though it is more common in children. Good nutrition and supplements have been effective in preventing it as well as recovering from it.

MVP (see section 246) A.M. and P.M. with food

Beta-carotene, 10,000 IU (reduce dose for children) one to three times daily

Extra vitamin C complex, 1,000 mg. A.M. and P.M.

Vitamin E (dry form), 200–400 IU daily

3 *acidophilus* caps or 1–2 tbsp. three times daily

Water, 6–8 glasses daily

364. Ulcers

There are two types of peptic ulcer, one in the stomach and the other in the duodenum, usually associated with excessive acidity in the stomach juices (see section 9). For both of these conditions, supplements have been found helpful.

Beta-carotene, 10,000 IU daily

Vitamin B complex, 100 mg. A.M. and P.M.

MSM with vitamin C complex, 1,000 mg., 1 tablet three times daily

L-glutamine, 5 grams, one to two times daily

Aloe vera gel, 1–3 capsules or 1–3 tbsp. liquid daily

365. Venereal Disease

Syphilis and gonorrhea are still among the most widespread venereal diseases, and though sulfa drugs, penicillin, tetracycline, erythromycin, and newer antibiotics are the most effective treatments for them, these remedies cause almost as much need for supplements as the diseases themselves.

MVP (see section 246)

3 *acidophilus* capsules or 1–2 tbsp. liquid three times daily

Extra vitamin C, 1,000 mg. A.M. and P.M.

Vitamin K, 100 mcg. daily if on an extended antibiotic program

Genital herpes, America's number one venereal disease of the 1980s, has unfortunately made it into the twenty-first century. Like herpes simplex type I, which causes cold sores (see section 298); type II herpes, which causes genital infection, also seems to respond well to lysine-rich foods. As a preventive, it wouldn't be a bad idea to increase your intake of cottage cheese, flounder, tuna fish, peanuts, raw chickpeas (garbanzos), and soybeans. Valtrex and Famuir are drugs that—at this writing—seem to be effective in blocking herpes replication, but the final results are not yet in. Meanwhile, I'd suggest a preventive supplement of lysine, 500 mg. daily (with water or juice—no protein) and vitamin C, 1,000 mg. A.M. and P.M. If you already have the virus: lysine, 3 g. (3,000 mg.) three times daily—in divided doses—between meals.

CAUTION: *If you have symptoms of herpes virus simplex I or II, avoid supplementation of arginine and arginine-rich foods (see section 85).*

DID YOU KNOW?

- Broccoli may help protect you against COPD.
- Ordinary table salt can eventually weaken bones.
- Over-the-counter sleeping pills and antihistamines can worsen RLS.

---

366. Any Questions About Chapter XIV?

What are "prostaglandins," and are they good or bad? I've been told to take an aspirin a day to block their formation to help prevent a heart attack. But then I read recently that these substances can lower blood pressure. If so, why block them? I'm very confused.

Your confusion is understandable. Prostaglandins are hormone-like substances that constantly regulate every cell in the body in many complex interactions. Some prostaglandins, when made in excess, play a role in promoting heart disease, inflammation, and pain. Aspirin blocks these "bad" prostaglandins, which is a good thing. Unfortunately, aspirin also blocks the formation of "good" prostaglandins, and in the process suppresses the immune system.

You see, while bad prostaglandins can make blood more likely to aggregate and cause a stroke or heart attack, good prostaglandins lower blood pressure, inhibit blood aggregation—as well as the production of cholesterol—and reduce inflammation reactions. In other words, "good" prostaglandins provide the same heart benefits that aspirin does—without the stomach-upsetting side effects. The problem is that we have to make sure the good prostaglandins outweigh the bad. Hydrogenated oils, a diet high in refined carbohydrates and sugar, viral illnesses, and excessive adrenal hormones secreted in response to stress can create more bad prostaglandins and a deficiency of good ones, most of which are made from omega-3 oils. (See section 100 and Anti-Inflammatory Supplements listed at the end of this section.)

My father is on the mend after his stroke, but he'd like to speed up the process. Any supplement suggestions?

Ginkgo biloba and DMAE have both been found to help improve mental function and memory by boosting blood circulation to brain cells. I'd recommend your dad take an MVP (see section 246) with breakfast and dinner, along with a ginkgo biloba, 60 mg. combination capsule (one that contains club moss, vinpocetine, phosphatidyl-serine and choline, bacopa, and DMAE) three times daily.

I get cystitis a lot. Are there supplements that can help prevent a recurrence?

Because cystitis is an inflammatory condition of the bladder, usually caused by some type of bacteria, supplements that produce an antibacterial effect and make the urine more acid have been found to provide relief and may help to prevent a recurrence.

Cranberry juice helps to keep problem bacteria from clinging to the wall of the urinary tract. (Cranberry also contains compounds called *anthocyanosides*, which are natural antibiotics.) If you find the juice too tart, you can get the benefit—without added sugar—by taking 1 to 2 cranberry concentrate capsules one to three times a day. Drink at least 6–8 glasses of water daily, and avoid caffeine, refined carbohydrates, and alcohol. Increase the natural diuretics in your diet (parsley, celery, asparagus, watercress, cilantro) and decrease citrus fruits, which produce alkaline urine that can encourage bacterial growth. Along with an MVP (see section 246), you might need a potassium supplement of 95 mg. daily to replenish the potassium lost when you lose fluid.

What are beta-1,3-glucans? And how do they help the immune system?

Beta-1,3-glucans are polysaccharides (complex sugar molecules), most commonly derived from baker's yeast but also extracted from the bran of oats and barley and mushrooms such as reishi and shiitaki. They have been found to improve the immune system by enhancing the ability of macrophages in the body to fight off invading bacteria, fungi, viruses, and parasites. And the great thing about them is that while they make the immune system work better, they don't make it overactive, which could be harmful to people with autoimmune diseases.

Is it true that senior women vegetarians have an increased risk of osteoporosis?

Apparently so. To foster bone mineral density, premenopausal and postmenopausal women's diets should contain adequate amounts of protein (15 to 20 percent of daily calories). Meat, poultry, eggs, and cheese are sources of complete, protective protein; vegetable protein sources are not. But combining amino acids from nonanimal sources in proper proportion to one another can diminish this risk—and making the grain quinoa (see section 90) a staple in your vegetarian diet can eliminate it.

What is prediabetes—and what are its symptoms?

Prediabetes, which often causes no symptoms, is a condition that doctors have been given new guidelines for diagnosing. It is serious because even before full-scale diabetes occurs it can cause damage to the heart and circulatory system. The latest guidelines lower the acceptable level of blood glucose to 100 mg. a deciliter from 110, enabling doctors to recognize prediabetics and work with them to prevent the condition from getting worse.

I've read about a supplement called hydroxyapatite for osteoporosis. What is it?

It's hard to pronounce, but it is an effective calcium supplement—and one of the few that is well absorbed by the body. It contains calcium that is identical to the calcium found in our bones, along with other minerals essential for strong bones, including magnesium, fluoride, sodium, and potassium.

Several supplements containing hydroxyapatite are available. Be sure to look for one that provides at least 1,000 mg. of calcium. You can make up the other 200–500 mg. with food. (See section 55.) If you're a vegetarian, calcium citrate is also highly absorbable by the body.

I have arthritis and have heard that glucosamine can help ease my joint pain. I'm reluctant to use it because I'm not quite sure what it is and if there are contraindications or side effects. What should I be looking for to get optimal benefits?

Here's a quick crash course on glucosamine that should tell you what you want to know. Glucosamine is a natural constituent of cartilage that stimulates the production of connective tissue in the body. It's used for joint pain, connective tissue repair, tendon and ligament health, and to treat symptoms of osteoarthritis and rheumatoid arthritis. (Although these two conditions are very different, they are both characterized by the destruction of connective tissue, cartilage. When cartilage wears down, it leaves bone endings exposed, causing pain, stiffness, and swelling of the joints.)

As we age we're unable to make enough glucosamine. As a result, the cartilage can't retain water and act as a shock absorber. Glucosamine relieves pain by helping to restore lost cartilage. It works best with two other supplements: chondroitin, which is also found in cartilage; and pregnenolone, a natural hormone.

Misleading label claims have occurred with glucosamine and chondroitin sulfate products. Check to see that potassium chloride (as opposed to sodium chloride) has been used as a stabilizer. You don't need more sodium in your diet (see section 428).

As for side effects, in rare instances glucosamine may cause nausea or heartburn. This can be alleviated by taking the supplement with meals. Some research has suggested that glucosamine might affect insulin resistance, which could contribute to diabetes, but there is little evidence that this is the case. If you're concerned, a 200 mcg. dose of chromium picolinate daily (which also helps burn fat and reduce cholesterol and triglycerides) can prevent it.

Supplements are available in capsules, powder, and liquids. I recommend glucosamine HCl (40 percent more potent than regular glucosamine), one to three 500 mg. tablets daily. If you're taking aspirin or other analgesics, it may take a longer period of time to see and feel glucosamine's benefits.

I've been told that inflammation is the root of most chronic diseases—not just arthritis and asthma. If this is true, what diseases are they, and what supplements would you recommend?

It's true and the current findings are eye-openers. It appears that chronic low-grade inflammation may be the underlying cause of coronary heart disease, Alzheimer's, certain cancers, and even obesity and diabetes. Research by Dr. Paul Ridker of Harvard Medical School, using a particularly sensitive blood test on C-reactive protein (CRP), a blood protein that promotes as well as reflects inflammation levels throughout the body, has shown that elevated inflammation levels quadruple the risk of heart attack. That high blood levels of CRP have been found in a variety of chronic conditions has resulted in what's being called an "inflammation syndrome." Jack Challem, author of *The Inflammation Syndrome*, cites the inflammation present in obesity and diabetes that may appear throughout the body as setting the stage for inflamed blood vessels and an increased risk of heart disease.

Inflammation is a sign that your body's pro- and anti-inflammatory responses are unbalanced. But there are anti-inflammatory supplements that can even the nutritional playing field.

ANTI-INFLAMMATORY SUPPLEMENTS

GLA (gamma linolenic acid): Derived from linoleic acid, also known as omega-6 fatty acid, GLA is the precursor for important prostaglandins that can help suppress inflammation. GLA, primarily found in borage oil, black currant seed oil, and evening primrose oil, can also be produced in the body from omega-6 fatty acids. Unfortunately, although omega-6 is readily available in the American diet, many of the oils containing it are hydrogenated, which can inhibit the conversion of omega-6 to GLA.

EPA (eicosapentaenoic acid): A precursor for the production of anti-inflammatory agents in the body. Although

EPA, an omega-3 fatty acid, can be produced in the body from the conversion of alpha-linolenic acid (see section 49), it can also be obtained directly by eating certain kinds of cold-water fish, such as salmon, mackerel, and sardines (see sections 100 and 102).

Oleic acid: The chief omega-9 fatty acid in olive oil, oleic acid is anti-inflammatory and enhances the activity of EPA.

Vitamin E: Vitamin E (see section 48), along with other antioxidants (see sections 106–130), destroys free radicals, which can stimulate inflammation.

Omega-3 Fatty Acids: Among the best anti-inflammatory supplements (see section 100), omega-3 fatty acids fight the harmful effects of prostaglandins, which lower immunity. Infants whose formulas are fortified with omega-3 fatty acids (plentiful in breast milk) develop natural immunities more quickly.

CBD and curcumin: 50 mg. of each can be taken daily as anti-inflammatory supplements

I have Lyme disease, and my doctor has me on an extended regimen of antibiotics. Are there supplements you can recommend for speeding up my recovery and minimizing the health toll this disease might have already taken on my body?

Yes, there are. While antibiotics have been proven the most effective for this tick-borne disease, natural supplements to boost the immune system used in combination with prescribed medicines can be quite effective in treating symptoms and mitigating damage to your body (see section 459). Caution: Before taking any supplements while under treatment for Lyme disease, consult with your physician or licensed healthcare provider to prevent any interactions that might undermine your treatment. That said, I'd suggest increasing antioxidant-rich foods in your diet (see chapter VII) and a regimen that includes a good vitamin-mineral supplement (see section 246), along with vitamin C, 500 mg.; coenzyme-Q10; and 1–3 omega-3 EPA/DHA fish oil capsules twice daily.

XV

DRUGS AND YOU

367. How Vitamins and Minerals Affect Your Moods

The first scientifically documented discovery to relate mental illness to diet occurred when it was found that pellagra (with its depression, diarrhea, and dementia) could be cured with niacin. After that, it was shown that supplementation with the whole B complex produced greater benefits than niacin alone.

Evidence of biochemical causes for mental disturbances continues to mount. Experiments have shown that symptoms of mental illness can be switched off and on by altering vitamin levels in the body.

Dr. R. Shulman, reporting in the *British Journal of Psychiatry,* found that forty-eight out of fifty-nine psychiatric patients had folic-acid deficiencies. Other research has shown that the majority of the mentally and emotionally ill are deficient in one or more of the B-complex vitamins or vitamin C. And even average happy people have been found to become depressed and experience other symptoms of emotional disturbance when made niacin or folic-acid deficient.

368. Proactively Combat Depression, Anxiety, and Stress with Nutrients

Before running to the pharmacy to fill a prescription for an antidepressant or antianxiety drug, give your brain and body a fighting chance to ward off—or alleviate—the symptoms of those disorders (e.g., feelings of panic, heart palpitations, sleeplessness, obsessive thoughts, and overwhelming sadness) with nutrient supplements that may be able to combat those symptoms naturally—without unwanted side effects!

Vitamin B1 (thiamin)	Above-average amounts can help alleviate depression and anxiety attacks.
Vitamin B6 (pyridoxine)	Aids in the proper production of natural antidepressants such as dopamine and norepinephrine.
Pantothenic acid	A natural tension-reliever.
Vitamin C (ascorbic acid)	Essential for combating stress.
Vitamin B12 (cobalamin)	Helps relieve irritability, improve concentration, increase energy, and maintain a healthy nervous system.
Choline	Sends nerve impulses to brain and produces a soothing effect.

Vitamin E (dry form) (alpha-tocopherol)	Aids brain cells in getting needed oxygen.
Folic acid (folacin)	Deficiencies have been found to be contributing factors in mental illness.
Zinc	Promotes mental alertness and aids in proper brain function.
Omega-3 fatty acids (EPA & DHA)	Boost levels of the brain's feel-good chemical, serotonin.
Magnesium	The antistress mineral, necessary for proper nerve functioning.
Manganese	Helps reduce nervous irritability.
Niacin	Vital to the proper function of the nervous system.
Calcium	Alleviates tension, irritability, and promotes relaxation.
Tyrosine	Helps increase the rate at which brain neurons produce the antidepressants dopamine and norepinephrine.
Tryptophan	Works with vitamin B6, niacin, and magnesium to synthesize the brain chemical serotonin, a natural tranquilizer.
5-HTP	Enhances activity of serotonin much like Prozac (without side effects); alleviates depression and functions as a sleep aid.

L-theanine	Focuses the brain and decreases anxiety by inhibiting neuron excitation; a free amino acid found almost exclusively in tea plants.
SAM-e (S-adenosylmehionine)	Works as a natural alternative to tricyclic antidepressants.
Phosphatidylserine (PS)	A premier brain lipid. Enhances mental performance, suppresses stress and helps fight depressive symptoms.
Phenylalanine	Necessary for the brain's release of the antidepressants dopamine and norepinephrine.

369. Other Drugs Can Add to Your Problem

Alcohol is a nerve depressant. If you take tranquilizers and a drink, the combination of the two can cause a severe depression—or even death.

If you take a sedative with an antihistamine (such as any found in over-the-counter cold preparations), you might find yourself experiencing tremors and mental confusion.

Oral contraceptives deplete the body of B6, B12, folic acid, and vitamin C. If you're on the pill and depressed, it is not surprising. Your need for B6, necessary for normal tryptophan metabolism, is fifty to a hundred times a non-pill-user's requirement.

370. It's Not All in Your Mind

The following list is not all-inclusive, but all the drugs mentioned deplete the body—in varying degrees—of

important mood-regulating nutrients. (See section 381.)
So if you're taking medication to get well and feeling
down, there's a good chance that it's not all in your mind!

DRUGS AND MEDICATIONS THAT YOU MIGHT NOT THINK WOULD CAUSE DEPRESSION—BUT CAN

- Adrenocorticoids
- Arthritis medicines
- Amphetamines
- Anticonvulsants
- Antidepressants (yes, that's right)
- Antihistamines
- Antihypertensives
- Antibiotics
- Baclofen
- Barbiturates
- Beta-blockers (Inderal)
- Diuretics
- Fluorides
- Hormones (estrogen, including Premarin, and synthetic progestins such as Provera)
- Indomethacin (Indocin)
- Isoniazid (INH, Nydrazid)
- Laxatives, lubricants
- Meprednisone (Betapar)
- Methotrexate (Mexate)
- Narcotics
- Nitrofurantoin (Furadantin, Macrodantin)
- Oral contraceptives
- Painkillers
- Penicillamine (Cuprimine)
- Penicillin (all forms)
- Phenytoin (Dilantin)

- Potassium supplements
- Procainamide
- Propoxyphene (Darvon)
- Pyrimethamine (Daraprim)
- Sleeping Pills
- Systemic corticosteroids (prednisone, cortisone, etc.)
- Tagamet
- Tetracyclines
- Tranquilizers (Halcion, Librium, Rostroil, Xanax, etc.)
- Trimethobenzamide (Tigan)

371. The Caffeine Connection

There are no doubts about it, caffeine is a powerful drug. That's right, *drug*. Chances are you're not just enjoying your daily coffees or colas, you're addicted to them.

Caffeine acts directly upon the central nervous system. It brings about an almost immediate sense of clearer thought and lessens fatigue. It also stimulates the release of stored sugar from the liver, which accounts for the "lift" coffee, cola, and chocolate (the caffeine big three) give. But these benefits may be far outweighed by the side effects:

- The release of stored sugar places heavy stress on the endocrine system. (Eventually, adrenal exhaustion can occur, resulting in hypoglycemia.)
- Heavy coffee drinkers often develop nervousness or become jittery.
- Daily intake adds up over a year, and a lot of caffeine accumulates in the body's fat tissue—and is not easily eliminated.
- Coffee-drinking housewives demonstrated symptoms typical of drug withdrawal when switched to a decaffeinated beverage.

- Dr. John Minton, professor of surgery at Ohio State University and specialist in cancer oncology, has found that excessive intake of methylxanthines (active chemicals in caffeine) can cause benign breast disease and prostate problems.
- Caffeine can rob the body of B vitamins, especially inositol, as well as vitamin C, zinc, potassium, and other minerals.
- Coffee increases the acidity in your gastrointestinal tract and can cause rectal itching.
- Many doctors consider caffeine a culprit in hypertensive heart disease.
- The British medical journal *Lancet* reported a strong relationship between coffee consumption and cancer of the bladder and the lower urinary tract.
- People who drink five cups of coffee daily have a 50 percent greater chance of having heart attacks than non–coffee drinkers.
- The *Journal of the American Medical Association* reports a disease called caffeinism, with symptoms of appetite loss, weight loss, irritability, insomnia, feelings of flushing, chills, and sometimes a low fever.
- Caffeine has been shown to interfere with DNA replication.
- Extremely high doses of caffeine (seven or more cups of coffee daily) can produce sensory disturbances, including hallucinations.
- Caffeine can cause mood swings and depression.
- The Center for Science in the Public Interest advises pregnant women to stay away from caffeine, since studies have shown that the amount contained in about four cups of coffee per day causes birth defects in test animals.

- High doses of caffeine will cause laboratory animals to go into convulsions and then die.
- Caffeine is a strong diuretic and can cause dehydration.
- Caffeine can cause stiffness in your neck, jaw, hands, and legs.
- Caffeine can cause coldness in the extremities because it constricts blood vessels.
- Can dangerously increase heart rate and blood pressure when taken with decongestants or pulmonary bronchodilators such as the inhalers Proventil, Ventolin, Bronkaid, and Primatine.
- Women who drink more than one cup of coffee a day are half as likely to get pregnant as those who don't drink coffee.
- Women who drink more than two cups a day are nearly five times less likely to get pregnant as non–coffee drinkers.
- Caffeine can be highly toxic (the lethal dose is estimated to be around 10 g.). New research shows that one quart of coffee consumed in three hours can destroy much of the body's thiamin.

372. You're Getting More Than You Think

The real eye-opener about caffeine is how much there is in foods and beverages that's consumed unknowingly—by adults and children. In fact, a study done by *Consumer Reports* of twenty-five products likely to be consumed by children showed that some sodas, ice creams, and snacks pack a major caffeine jolt. Although not a lot of research has been done with children and caffeine, the concensus among doctors and nutritionists is that exceeding 100 mg.

a day can cause anxiety, tension, and sleeplessness; higher amounts can lead to nausea, vomiting, cramps, and diarrhea. The following table shows the amount of caffeine (in mg.) consumed in specific beverages, drugs, and snacks:

BEVERAGE:	12-OUNCE CAN OR BOTTLE
Coca-Cola	64.7 mg.
Dr Pepper	60.9 mg.
Mountain Dew	54.7 mg.
Diet Dr Pepper	54.2 mg.
Tab	49.4 mg.
Pepsi-Cola	43.1 mg.
RC Cola	33.7 mg.
Diet RC Cola	33.0 mg.
Diet-Rite	0.0 mg.

Beverages: Per 8-Ounce Serving

Starbucks Coffee Frappuccino	83.0 mg.
AMP energy drink	74.0 mg.
Red Bull energy drink	80.0 mg.
Red Fusion	80.0 mg.
Rockstar energy drink	80.0 mg.
SoBe Essential Energy	48.0 mg.
Sunkist orange soda	24.0 mg.

Coffee: Per 5-Ounce Serving

Instant	40–108 mg.
Percolated	64–124 mg.
Dripolated	110–150 mg.
Light coffee-grain blend	12–35 mg.
Decaffeinated	2–5 mg.
Instant decaffeinated	2 mg.

Tea: Per 5-Ounce Serving

Black 5-minute brew	20–50 mg.

Black 1-minute brew	9–33 mg.
Green 5-minute brew	35 mg.
Instant	12–28 mg.
Iced	22–36 mg.
Decaffeinated	10–41 mg.
Cocoa	13.0 mg.

Chocolate

Milk chocolate, 1 oz.	6.0 mg.
Dark semisweet chocolate, 1 oz.	20.0 mg.

DRUGS	PER PILL
Actamin Super	65.4 mg.
Alka-Seltzer Morning Relief Tablets	65.0 mg.
Anacin (also available without caffeine)	32.0 mg.
Aspirin-Free Excedrin Caplets	65.0 mg.
Bayer Select Maximum Strength Headache Pain Relief	65.4 mg.
B.C. Headache Powder	65.0 mg.
Cafergot	100.0 mg.
Darvon Compound 65 Puvules	40.0 mg.
Dexatrim (also available without caffeine)	200.0 mg
Dexatrim Results	40.0 mg.
Dristan Capsules	16.0 mg.
Excedrin	65.0 mg.
(Excedrin P.M. has no caffeine, but does have an antihistamine.)	
Fiorinal	130.0 mg.
Midol	32.4 mg.
No-Doz	100.0 mg.
Norgesic Forte	60.0 mg.

Norphadrine Forte	60.0 mg.
Soma CMPD	32.0 mg.
Triaminicin	30.0 mg.
Vanquish	33.0 mg.

SNACKS

Dannon Natural Flavors Low-Fat Coffee-Flavored Yogurt (6 oz.)	36 mg.
Starbucks Coffee Java Chip Ice Cream (½ cup)	28 mg.
Haagen-Dazs Coffee Ice Cream (½ cup)	24 mg.
M&M's Milk Chocolate Candies (½ cup)	16 mg.
Hershey's Syrup, Chocolate (2 tbsp.)	5 mg.

373. Caffeine Alternatives

Decaffeinated coffee is *not* the best solution to the caffeine problem. Trichlorethylene, which was first used to remove caffeine, was found to cause a high incidence of cancer in test animals. Though the manufacturers have switched to methylene chloride, which is safer, it, too, introduces the same carbon-to-chloride bond in the body that is characteristic of so many toxic insecticides.

Regular tea is not the answer either, since that has nearly as much caffeine. But herb teas can be quite invigorating, and most natural-food stores have a wide variety to choose from. Then, too, ginseng can give you a real lift, much like the one you get from caffeine, without the side effects.

Colas, diet or regular, have become as popular as coffee for those who enjoy the caffeine boost. Try substituting club soda or mineral water, or even a flavored soda if you must. You won't get the caffeine lift, but you'll be doing your body a big favor.

374. What Alcohol Does to Your Body

Alcohol is the most widely used drug in our society, and because it is so available, most people don't think of it as a drug. But it is, and if misused it can cause a lot of damage to your body.

- Alcohol is not a stimulant, but actually a sedative-depressant of the central nervous system.
- It is capable of rupturing veins.
- It does not warm you up, but causes you to feel colder by increasing perspiration and body heat loss.
- It destroys brain cells by causing the withdrawal of necessary water from them.
- It can deplete the body of vitamins B1, B2, B6, B12, folic acid, vitamin C, vitamin K, zinc, magnesium, and potassium.
- Four drinks a day are capable of causing organ damage.
- It can hamper the liver's ability to process fat.

375. What You Drink and When You Drink It

Just because the alcohol content varies in different beverages, don't be fooled. It is true that beer has only about 4 percent alcohol, wine about 12 percent, and whiskey up to 50 percent; but a can of beer, a glass of wine, and a shot of whiskey all have virtually the identical inebriation potential. In other words, 4 cans of beer can get you just as tipsy as 4 shots of tequila.

Surprisingly, what you drink doesn't matter nearly as much as *when* you drink it. Dr. John D. Palmer, of the University of Massachusetts, reports that the length of time alcohol remains in circulation in your blood varies throughout the day. Which means, of course, the more time the alcohol spends in your blood, the more time it has to act on your brain cells. Between 2 A.M. and noon are the most vulnerable hours, while late afternoon to early evening are the least. A cocktail at dinner will be burned away 25 percent faster than a Bloody Mary at breakfast, and the last drink of a party, consumed after midnight, is metabolized relatively more slowly than the ones that preceded it, producing a more lasting rise in blood alcohol.

376. Vitamins to Decrease Your Taste for Alcohol

Research at the University of Texas has shown that if alcoholic mice are fed nutritious, vitamin-enriched diets, they quickly lose their interest in alcohol. This seems to hold true for people, since heavy drinkers have been able to break the habit—and even lose interest—with the right diet and proper nutritional supplements. Vitamins A, D, E, C, and all the B vitamins—especially B12, B6, and B1—along with calcium and magnesium, choline, inositol, niacin, and a very high-protein diet have brought about the best results. Dr. H. L. Newbold, of New York, who has worked with alcoholics, recommends building up to 5 glutamine capsules (200 mg.)—not glutamic acid—three times a day to control drinking, and working with a good nutritionally oriented doctor for the best all-around regimen (see section 462).

Recently, the ancient Chinese herb kudzu (see section 204), which has been used as an antidote for hangovers, is being used to help break alcohol addiction. This is not really surprising since Asian herbalists have used a tea brewed from the kudzu root to treat alcoholism for the past two thousand years. Kudzu contains two phytochemicals, daidzin and daidzein, which help reduce blood alcohol levels. It is available as a supplement in 500 mg. capsules. For best results, take 1 three times daily, before or after drinking alcohol.

377. The Lowdown on Marijuana and Hashish

Marijuana and hashish come from the hemp plant *Cannabis sativa*. The marijuana consists of the chopped leaves and stems of the plant, while the hashish is formed from the resin scraped from the flowering tops.

Both of these drugs can be either smoked or eaten. If smoked, the effects usually last from one to three hours. If eaten, they can last from four to ten hours, though it takes longer for the user to feel them.

Unlike other illicit drugs, marijuana and hashish have the unusual property of "reverse tolerance," meaning that seasoned users need less of the drug to get high than first-timers. Essentially, these drugs act as intoxicants, relaxants, tranquilizers, appetite stimulants, and mild hallucinogenics, though effects vary with the individual.

The smoking of one joint can cause a rise in blood pressure, an increased heartbeat, a lowering of body temperature and vitamin C levels in the blood. It has been found, too, that smoking marijuana during pregnancy can cause low birth weight in newborns and increase the risk of lung cancer.

CAUTION: *Toxic psychosis can occur if Cannabis is eaten and the user hasn't been able to judge the amount ingested.*

SUPPLEMENTS AND FOODS THAT CAN HELP USERS

Increase your intake of citrus fruits and green leafy vegetables. (Those "munchies" usually give you more than your share of refined sugars and carbohydrates, meaning that you've deprived yourself of necessary B vitamins.)

Vitamin C, 1,000 mg. A.M. and P.M.

Vitamin E, 100–400 IU one to three times daily to protect your lungs

378. Cocaine Costs a Lot More Than You Think—in More Ways Than One

Cocaine is a vasoconstrictor, a stimulant of the central nervous system, and potentiates the effects of nerve stimulation. Applied externally, it blocks nerve impulses and produces a numbing sensation.

What users get—no matter how much they pay—is rarely more than 60 percent pure cocaine. The rest is the "cut," which is used by dealers to dilute or enhance the drug for more profit. Some cuts are relatively harmless: lactose, dextrose, inositol (a B vitamin), and mannitol. Other nondrug cuts, such as cornstarch, talcum powder, and flour, can be dangerous because they are basically insoluble in blood and can clot up in the body. *Benzocaine,* which is pharmacologically active, can also cause blood clots and serious complications when used as a cut for cocaine.

Because the drug is absorbed rapidly through the mucous membranes, nasal inhalation is the most popular form of taking cocaine, though it is also often applied locally under the tongue and eyelids, and on the genital region. It can also be injected intravenously or smoked in a process called "freebasing," or as crack, which is cocaine, baking soda, and water distilled into an instantly smokable "rock."

The short-lived effects of coke (about a half hour) are usually euphoria, feelings of psychic energy, and self-confidence, but then more of the drug is necessary to recapture the high. Dependence is intense.

Aside from causing nosebleeds, rapid heartbeat, cold sweats, appetite loss, and in some cases the feeling that gnats or bugs are crawling on you, cocaine can cause convulsions, vomiting, anaphylactic shock, and death. Its toxicity is unpredictable. Even small doses with the wrong cut or taken by susceptible individuals can be lethal.

Supplements and Foods to Help Users

MVP (see section 246)

Chelated calcium (500 mg.) and magnesium (250 mg.) tablets, twice daily—one at bedtime

A kava capsule may be taken at bedtime for restless sleep.

Vitamin C, 1,000 mg.; vitamin E, 200–400 IU; and vitamin B complex, 100 mg., all one to three times daily

379. Help for Coming Down or Kicking the Cocaine Habit

Tyrosine, an amino acid that's usually found in meat and wheat (see section 89), has been found to alleviate the depression, fatigue, and irritability that make quitting cocaine so difficult. At Fair Oaks Hospital in Summit, New Jersey, addicts took the amino acid in their orange juice for twelve days. They also took vitamin C, the B vitamins (thiamin, niacin, and riboflavin), and tyrosine hydroxylase, the enzyme that helps the body use tyrosine. The results were remarkably effective. One St. John's wort complex tablet taken in the morning is also effective in alleviating depression.

380. Whether Rx or Over-the-Counter, There Are Alternatives to Drugs

Americans consume more than 1.5 million pounds of mood-altering drugs and well over 4 million pounds of antibiotics a year. Are all these drugs necessary? Probably not; but when people pay for a visit to their doctor, they expect to walk away with a prescription.

But there are alternatives, which orthomolecular physicians and nutritionally minded individuals are trying before resorting to drugs.

The late Dr. Robert C. Atkins, author of *Dr. Atkins' New Diet Revolution,* had patients try pantothenic acid and about 2,000 mg. of inositol as sleep-inducers, instead of Seconal, Nembutal, Butisol, or other barbiturate sleeping pills. He also had success using B15 to control blood sugar, and B13 (orotic acid) to lower high blood pressure.

So before you pop that next pill, you might want to consider some natural alternatives.

DRUG	NATURAL ALTERNATIVES
Antacids	Deglycyrrhizinated licorice extract (DGL), papaya, lukewarm herbal teas such as fenugreek, slippery elm, comfrey, and meadowsweet (no lemon), MSM (methylsulfonylmethane).
Antibiotics and Antihistamines	Garlic, vitamin C, and (yep, it's true) chicken soup have amazing antibiotic and antihistamine properties. Other fine infection fighters

and histamine-hinderers are vitamin A, zinc, selenium, grapefruit-seed extract, echinacea, pantothenic acid, quercetin, and green tea.

Antidepressants Goji extract capsule and CBD 50 mg. can be taken daily, plus jujube seed extract complex, with calcium and magnesium; vitamins B1, B6, and B12, tyrosine and phenylalanine (do not take in conjunction with MAO inhibitors).

Antidiarrhetics Rice, bananas, and *Lactobacillus acidophilus* yogurt for diarrhea caused by antibiotics.

Antihypertensives Omega-3 fatty acids, magnesium, calcium; cruciferous vegetables (broccoli, cabbage, kale), celery; vitamin C, potassium (not for anyone with a kidney disorder); dong quai, Siberian ginseng.

Antinauseants Vitamins B1 and B6 can help alleviate nausea due to motion or morning sickness; gingerroot capsules; Niacin, bioflavonoids, and standardized ginkgo biloba can help in the treatment of dizziness and queasiness due to diseases of the inner ear.

Cholesterol-lowering drugs	Niacin (see section 33), the "no-flush" formula; vitamin C, magnesium, calcium, copper, vitamin E; psyllium (1–2 tsp. daily) and water; N-acetyl cysteine, green tea, PCOs or proanthocyanidins (grape-seed extract, cayenne, curry; guggul. CBD 50 mg. daily
Decongestants	Vitamins A and C; quercetin, echinacea, goldenseal, and bayberry herbal teas; potassium.
Diuretics	Alfalfa, asparagus, celery, dandelion leaves, and vitamin B6 can work as natural diuretics.
Laxatives	Vitamin C, vitamins B1, B2, B6, and B12, potassium, magnesium, *acidophilus*, alfalfa, hawthorn berry, gotu kola, skullcap, bran, and water.
Tranquilizers (sedatives, relaxants, etc.)	Valerian, melatonin, choline, CBD 50 mg., niacin, vitamins B1, B6, B12, calcium, and magnesium; manganese, zinc, pantothenic acid, and inositol; Dual action St. John's wort complex; phenylalanine and tyrosine.

CAUTION: *If you are already on a medication, do not go off it suddenly to switch to a natural alternative. Work with* *an experienced, nutritionally oriented professional (see section 462) so you can adjust dosages properly while you wean yourself from drugs.*

381. The Great Medicine Rip-Off

More than ever before, Americans are gulping down drugs. What most people don't realize is that a lot of these medications—prescription as well as over-the-counter— are taking as much as they're giving, at least nutritionally. All too often the drugs either stop the absorption of nutrients or interfere with the cells' ability to use them.

A recent study showed that ingredients found in common over-the-counter cold, pain, and allergy remedies actually lowered the blood level of vitamin A. Since vitamin A protects and strengthens the mucous membranes lining the nose, throat, and lungs, a deficiency could give bacteria a cozy home to multiply in, prolonging the illness the drug was meant to alleviate.

Aspirin, the household wonder drug, the most common ingredient in pain relievers, cold and sinus remedies, is a vitamin C thief. Even a small amount can *triple* the excretion rate of vitamin C from the body. It can also lead to a deficiency of folic acid and vitamin B, which could cause anemia as well as digestive disturbances.

Corticosteroids (cortisone, prednisone), used for easing arthritis pain, skin problems, blood and eye disorders, and asthma, have been found to be related to lowered zinc levels.

According to a study that appeared in the *Postgraduate Medical Journal,* a significant number of people who take barbiturates have low calcium levels.

Laxatives and antacids, taken by millions, have been found to disturb the body's calcium and phosphorus metabolism.

And any laxative taken to excess can deplete large amounts of potassium as well as vitamins A, D, E, and K.

Diuretics, commonly prescribed for high blood pressure, and antibiotics are also potassium thieves.

According to Dr. Stephen Holt, chairman of the New York Department of Integrative Medicine, "Pharmaceuticals remain an underestimated cause of nutritional depletion."

The following is a list of commonly prescribed drugs that can induce nutrient deficiencies and the nutrients they deplete. Look it over before you take your next medicine.

THIEVING DRUG	NUTRIENTS DEPLETED
Alcohol (including alcohol-containing cough syrups, elixirs, and OTC medications such as Nyquil)	Vitamins A, B1, B2, biotin, choline, niacin, vitamin B15, folic acid, and magnesium
Ammonium Chloride (e.g., Ambenyl, expectorant, Triaminicol, decongestant cough syrup, P.V. Tussin syrup)	Vitamin C
Antacids (e.g., Maalox, Mylanta, Di-Gel liquid)	Calcium, phosphate, copper, iron, magnesium, potassium, zinc, protein
Antibiotics (e.g., Amoxil, Ceclor, Keflex, Augmentin, PenVee K)	B complex; vitamins C, K, *acidophilus*
Anticoagulants (e.g., Coumadin, dicumarol, Panwarfin)	Vitamins A and K
Anticonvulsants (e.g., phenobarbital, phenytoin)	Biotin, copper

Antihistamines (e.g., Chlor-Trimeton, Pyrabenzamine)	Vitamin C
Aspirin (and remember, APC drugs contain aspirin)	Vitamins A, B complex, C; calcium, potassium
Barbiturates (e.g., pheno-barbital, Seconal, Nembutal, Butisol, Tuinal)	Vitamins A, D, folic acid, and C
Beta-blockers (e.g., Inderal, Lopressor, Sectral)	Coenzyme-Q10
Caffeine (present in all APC medicines)	B1, inositol and biotin; potassium, zinc; can also inhibit calcium and iron assimilation; Vitamin K and niacin
Chemotherapy drugs	Most nutrients
Cholesterol-lowering drugs (e.g., Cholestid, Questran, Locholest, Lipitor, Lescol, Lovastatin, Mevacor, Crestor, Zocor)	Vitamins A, D, E, K, B12, beta-carotene, folic acid, iron, and fat Coenzyme-Q10
Clofibrate (Atromid-s)	Vitamin K
Colchicine (Colbenemid)	B12, A, and potassium
Corticosteroids (e.g., cortisone, hydrocortisone)	Calcium, vitamin D, potassium, selenium, zinc
Diethylstilbestrol (DES)	Vitamin B6
Diuretics (e.g., Diuril, Hydrodiuril, SER-AP-ES, Lasix, Hydrocholorthiazide [HCTZ])	B complex, potassium, magnesium, zinc and coenzyme-Q10
Estrogen replacement (e.g., Premarin, Menest, conjugated estrogens)	Vitamin B6

Fluorides	Vitamin C
Glutethimide (Doriden)	Folic acid
Gout medications (e.g., Zyloprim)	Beta-carotene, vitamin B12, sodium, potassium
Isoniazid (INH, Nydrazid)	Vitamin B6
Kanamycin (Kantrex)	Vitamins K and B12
Laxatives, lubricant (e.g., castor oil, mineral oil)	Vitamins A, D, E, K, calcium and phosphorus
Meprednisone (Betapar)	Vitamins B6, C, zinc, and potassium
Methotrexate (Mexate)	Folic acid
Nitrofurantoin (e.g., Furadantin, Macrodantin)	Folic acid
NSAIDs (e.g., Anaprox, Dolobid, Indocin)	Vitamins B1, C, and folic acid
Oral contraceptives	Folic acid, vitamins C, B2, B6, B12, and E
Penicillamine (Cuprimine)	Vitamin B6
Penicillin (in all its forms)	Vitamins B6, niacin, and K
Phenylbutazone (e.g., Azolid, Butazolidin)	Folic acid
Phenytoin (Dilantin)	Vitamin B12, D, folic acid, and calcium
Prednisone (e.g., Meticorten, Prednisolone, Orasone)	Vitamins B6, D, C, zinc, and potassium
Propantheline (Pro-Banthine)	Vitamin K
Proton pump inhibitors (e.g., Prevacid, Prilosec)	Vitamin B12, protein
Pyrimethamine (Daraprim)	Folic acid
Quinolones (e.g., Cipro, Noroxin)	Iron and zinc

Statins (e.g., Zocor, Lipitor, Pravachol)	Coenzyme-Q10
Sulfonamides, systemic (e.g., Bactrim, Gantanol, Tantrisin, Septra)	Folic acid, vitamins K, and B12
Sulfonamides and topical steroids (e.g., Aerosporin, Cortisporin, Neosporin, Polysporin)	Vitamins K, B12, and folic acid
Tetracyclines (e.g., Achromycin-V, Sumycin, Tetracyn)	Vitamin K, calcium, magnesium, and iron
Tobacco	Vitamins C, B1, and folic acid; calcium
Tranquilizers (e.g., Clorazil, Haldol, Moban, Loxitane)	Vitamin B2, coenzyme-Q10
Tricyclic antidepressants (e.g., Elavil, Tofranil, Norpramin)	Vitamin B2, coenzyme-Q10
Trifluoperazine (Stelazine)	Vitamin B12
Triamterene (Dyrenium)	Folic acid
Tuberculosis drugs	Vitamins B6, D, E, niacin, and calcium
Ulcer medications (e.g., Tagamet, Pepcid, Axid, Zantac)	Vitamin D, B12, folic acid, and zinc

382. Multivitamin Drug Interactions

The following drugs interact with multivitamins:
    Anisindione, moderate interaction
    Bortezomib, moderate interaction
    Caffeine, major interaction

Cholestyramine, moderate interaction
Colesevelam, moderate interaction
Colestipol, moderate interaction
Dicumarol, moderate interaction
Fluorouracil, major interaction
Orlistat, minor interaction
Sevelamer, moderate interaction
Warfarin, moderate interaction

383. Individual Vitamin-Drug Interactions

Biotin: antibiotics, anticonvulsants
Folate: alcohol, anticonvulsants (phenobarbital, phenytoin), 5-fluoracil, metformin, methotrexate, oral contraceptives, primidone, sulfaalzaine, trimethoprine, triamterene
Niacin: alcohol, isoniazid
Riboflavin: alcohol, barbiturates, phenothiazides, thiazide diuretics, tricyclic antidepressants
Vitamin A: cholestyramine, mineral oil
Vitamin B6: alcohol, anticonvulsants, corticosteroids, cycloserine, hydralazine, isoniazid, levodopa, oral contraceptives, penicillamine
Vitamin C: corticosteroids
Vitamin D: anticonvulsants, antipsychotics, corticosteroids, mineral oil, rifampin
Vitamin E: mineral oil, warfarin
Vitamin K: antibiotics, anticonvulsants, mineral oil, warfarin

384. Supplements and Drug Interactions

Antibiotics, antihypertensives, osteoporosis drugs, thyroid drugs, diuretics, and heart drugs are the types of drugs most likely to cause adverse interactions. The following supplements also have interactions with some drugs, listed below. The severity may vary, so consult your doctor if you take these drugs and supplements.

1. Coenzyme-Q10: blood thinners, cancer drugs, antihypertensives
2. DHEA: estrogen drugs, cancer drugs, blood thinners, antidepressants, tuberculosis vaccines
3. Fish oil: cancer drugs, antihypertensives
4. Garlic: birth control pills, HIV/AIDS drugs, immunosuppressants, tuberculosis treatment drugs
5. Ginger: antihypertensives, blood thinners, diabetes and immune suppressant drugs
6. Gingko biloba: anti-anxiety drugs, anticoagulants, antidepressants, diabetes and immune suppressant drugs.
7. Ginseng: blood thinners, antihypertensive and diabetes drugs
8. Green tea extract: cancer and heart drugs, amphetamines, antipsychotics, asthma drugs
9. Melatonin: anticoagulants, antihypertensives, diabetic drugs
10. St. John's wort: anti-anxiety drugs, anticoagulants, antihypertensives, birth control pills, cholesterol lowering drugs, heartburn drugs (PPI), immunosuppressants, antidepressants, blood thinners.
11. Valerian: anti-anxiety drugs
12. Vitamin C: blood thinners, cancer drugs, HIV/AID drugs, estrogen
13. Vitmain D: antihypertensives, cholesterol lowering drugs
14. Vitamin E: cancer drugs, immunosuppressants, blood thinners

385. Drug Effects on Mineral Metabolism

1. Diuretics (thiazides and corticosteroids) deplete potassium.
2. Laxatives, cortisol, desoxycorticosterone, and aldosterone can deplete potassium and can cause sodium retention, which leads to higher blood pressure.
3. Sulfonylureas and lithium (Rx) impair uptake or release of iodine by the thyroid.
4. Oral contraceptives decrease blood levels of zinc and copper.
5. Certain antibiotics (e.g., tetracycline) decrease iron absorption.

386. Drug Effects on Vitamin Absorption and Metabolism

1. Ethyl alcohol impairs thiamin utilization.
2. Isoniazid interferes with niacin and vitamin B6 metabolism.
3. Ethyl alcohol and oral contraceptives inhibit folate utilization.
4. Phenytoin, phenobarbital, primidone, phenothiazines can cause folate deficiency.
5. Anticoagulants can cause vitamin D deficiency.
6. Aminosalicylic acid, slow-release potassium iodide, colchicine, trifluoperazine, metformin, ethyl alcohol, and oral contraceptives interfere with absorption of vitamin B12.
7. Protein pump inhibitors deplete vitamin B12, vitamin C, iron, calcium, and magnesium.

387. Drugs That Deplete Nutrients

1. Ace inhibitors (e.g., Lotensin and Vasotec) deplete zinc and sodium.

2. Antibiotics (penicillin, sulfonamide, erythromycin) deplete calcium, magnesium, potassium, vitamin K, and probiotics.

3. Benzodiazepines (e.g., Valium, Xanax) deplete melatonin.

4. Beta-blockers (e.g., Inderal, Lopressor) deplete coenzyme-Q10 and melatonin.

5. Birth control pills (e.g., Ovral, Demulen) depletes folate; vitamins B1, B2, B6, B12, and C; zinc; selenium; and trace minerals.

6. Bronchodilators (e.g., albuterol, Serevent) depletes potassium.

7. Calcium channel blockers (e.g., Cardizem, Norvasc) deplete potassium.

8. Diabetes drugs (e.g., Glucophage, Avandia) deplete vitamin B6, folate, vitamin B12, coenzyme-Q10, sodium, zinc, magnesium, and potassium.

9. Estrogen (e.g., Premarin, Prempro) depletes vitamin B6.

10. NSAIDs (e.g., ibuprofen, naproxen) deplete folate, iron, and vitamin C.

11. Potassium sparing diuretics (e.g., Aldactone, Dyrenium) deplete folate, vitamin C, iron, and zinc.

12. SSRIs (e.g., Prozac, Paxil) deplete sodium, melatonin, and folate.

13. Statins (e.g., Mevacor, Zocor) deplete coenzyme-Q10.

14. Thiazide diuretics (e.g., hydrochlorothiazide) deplete magnesium, coenzyme-Q10, potassium, sodium, zinc, thiamin, and vitamins B6 and C.

15. Thyroid drugs (e.g., Synthroid) deplete calcium.

388. When Good Foods Are Bad for You

Foods—even those that are normally good for you—can interfere with how medicines are absorbed by the body. If a food is decreasing your medication's effectiveness, it means your body is metabolizing less of it, allowing more to circulate in the bloodstream and increasing the chance of side effects. And if a food is increasing your drug's effect, you're getting a larger dose than intended. Either way, it's a prescription for trouble.

DON'T EAT THAT (Foods)	IF YOU'RE TAKING THIS (Medications)
Milk (dairy products with calcium)	Tetracycline (and any antibiotics labeled "cyclines") as well as Cipro, Levaquin, and iron supplements. Also, if taking laxatives containing bisacodyl (e.g., Correctol and Dulcolax), the milk might make those laxatives work "too well."
Grapefruit or grapefruit juice	Cholesterol-lowering drugs (statins such as Zocor, Lipitor, and Mevacor), many heart medications, calcium channel blockers (e.g., Plendil, Sular, and Procardia), immune system drugs (e.g., Sandimmune and Neoral), some allergy

	medicines (e.g., Allegra), antibiotics (the "mycins"), hormone replacement drugs
Dark green vegetables, asparagus, red leaf lettuce	Blood thinners e.g., Coumadin)
High-fiber foods	Acetaminophen
Bran or oatmeal	Heart medication digoxin
Aged cheeses, avocado, tofu, soy products (foods containing tyromines)	Monoamine inhibitors (MAO) and antidepressant drugs

PERSONAL ADVICE: *Before taking any medication, don't forget to ask your doctor or pharmacist if there are any interactions with foods. Also, to minimize stomach upset and maximize effectiveness of most drugs, it's best to take them with a full glass of water.*

CAUTION: *Do not take medicines with hot drinks (heat can destroy the drug's effectiveness), and avoid taking supplements and medicines at the same times (certain vitamins and minerals can interact with many drugs). Also, don't mix medications in food or take capsules apart unless instructed to do so.*

DID YOU KNOW?

- Alcohol can lower testosterone levels for up to twenty-four hours afterward.
- One cup of Haagen-Dazs coffee ice cream has more caffeine than a can of Coke.
- There are calories in coffee.

---

389. Any Questions About Chapter XV?

I know that coffee can give you the jitters, but I've switched to drinking decaffeinated and still find myself getting moody and uptight. Can such a small amount of caffeine do this?

Caffeine isn't the only substance in coffee that has an effect on behavior. There is, though not yet identified, another substance in both regular and decaffeinated coffee (but not in tea) that blocks the normal activity of brain opiates (endorphins), which act as painkillers and mood elevators.

Some prescription medications that I take are specifically labeled "Do not drink alcoholic beverages while taking this medication." If there is no label, does that mean it's safe to have a drink while on them?

Only if you think that Russian roulette is safe. Alcohol can interact adversely with almost all drugs. In fact, any drug that's available in time-release or spansule form can become dangerous if taken in conjunction with alcohol. The coating that's supposed to allow the drug to be released slowly over an extended time period (usually eight to twelve hours) can dissolve rapidly in alcohol and give you an uncomfortable and potentially toxic dose of the medication. My advice is get well first, then celebrate afterward.

As the producer of a daily television show, I live in Stress City. I eat sporadically, so I'd like to know if there are some foods that would be better for me than others.

There are. Whether it's a power breakfast or an on-the-set lunch, go for the complex carbohydrates instead of the protein. In other words, take the pasta, rice, or cereal instead of the steak and eggs. Complex carbohydrates help boost your brain levels of the chemical *serotonin,* making you calmer and less stressed—but no less alert.

Every once in a while I find myself depressed when there's really nothing in my life to be depressed about. I'm a twenty-nine-year-old male, happily married, and I don't know why I go into these depressions. Could there be a dietary reason?

Absolutely! Especially if you're consoling yourself with sugar-rich foods. Sugar, be it in refined carbohydrates, alcohol, or whatever, can deplete your body of B vitamins, especially vitamin B1, which can bring on depression. Amino acids (see sections 82 and 89) such as tyrosine and phenylalanine can all be used as antidepressants. Check with your doctor, but I'd recommend 500–2,000 mg. (2 g.) of a combination of these amino acids, taken at bedtime or in the morning, with water or juice (no protein). Also, you might want to try 50 mg. CBD daily.

I take Tagamet for my acid indigestion. I was told that while I was taking it I should not eat aged cheddar cheese or other tyramine-rich foods. Could you tell me why—and also what foods contain tyramine?

Foods that are high in the amino acid tyramine can cause severe headaches and temporarily raise your blood pressure when eaten while using Tagamet (cimetidine). Any type of protein such as meat, fish, or a dairy product that has been sitting around for too long will start to form tyramines. To be safe, don't eat leftovers more than a few days old, and check freshness dates when you buy fish, meat, and dairy products. Any type of aged, pickled, or fermented product such as aged cheeses, wines, and pickles may contain tyramines.

FOODS HIGH IN TYRAMINE

Aged cheeses

Raisins

Aged dairy products; sour cream

Avocado

Beef and chicken liver

Dried and pickled fish

Flavor enhancers such as hydrolyzed vegetable protein

Sausages, pepperoni, salami, bologna

Soy products such as tofu, miso, soy sauce, teriyaki sauce

Wine, beer, liqueurs, champagne

Yeast

Tyramine may also interfere with the sympathomimetic drugs used in many asthama inhalers, including albuterol, salmeterol, and epinephrine. Parents of asthmatic children using sympathomimetic drugs need to be extra careful of tyramine-containing foods. An inhaler dose that follows a bologna sandwich has the potential for causing a serious interaction.

XVI

LOSING IT—DIETS BY THE POUND

390. Top 2020 Diets

- Nutrisystem
- Noom
- WW (formerly Weight Watchers)
- Diet to Go
- Jenny Craig
- Freshology
- WonderSlim
- South Beach Diet
- Medifast
- Mediterranean Diet
- DASH Diet
- Flexitarian Diet
- Mayo Clinic Diet
- Volumetrics
- TLC Diet
- Nordic Diet

- Ornish Diet
- Vegetarian Diet

391. The Atkins Diet

This diet ignores calorie content and focuses primarily on carbohydrate restriction; but unlike other low-carbohydrate programs, the late Dr. Atkins's weight-loss program calls for almost *no* carbohydrates (at least for the first two weeks, where you're limited to just 20 carbohydrates a day). By doing this, the body begins to throw off ketones (tiny carbon fragments that are by-products of incompletely burned fat) in amounts sufficient to account for substantial weight loss. According to Dr. Atkins, because carbohydrates are the first fuel your body burns for energy, if none are taken in then the body will draw upon stored fat for fuel, and as ketones are excreted, hunger as well as weight will disappear.

The pros and cons are many, especially since the diet encourages high fat consumption. Although a report in the *New England Journal of Medicine* found that the diet did not cause the expected deterioration in blood cholesterol levels (bad cholesterol did rise slightly, but there was an off-setting improvement in good cholesterol and triglycerides), the Atkins diet did have a high dropout rate, and, as with other diets, most of the lost weight was regained within a year or two. If you are on this diet, I would suggest following the MVP program outlined in section 246, and taking an additional 1,000 mg. vitamin C with bioflavonoids if you've cut out citrus fruit. Also at least 50 mg. B complex with morning and evening meal, 1 g. potassium divided over three meals, and 400–800 mcg. folic acid daily.

What would be even better would be to burn fat and cut your carb intake naturally with the following supplements:

banaba leaf extract: 16–48 mg. daily; gymnema sylvestre (reduces the urge to eat sugars), two 200 mg. capsules daily; and MSM (methylsulfonylmethane), two 1,000 mg. tablets daily.

392. The Zone Diet

The "zone" is an expression often used by athletes to describe a near-euphoric state where the body and mind work at peak efficiency. In *Mastering the Zone,* Barry Sears, PhD, presents a dietary approach to reaching this state by tightly controlling portions of protein, carbohydrates, and fat in an equal number of "blocks" at every meal. Three "blocks" for women, four for men (1 protein block = 7 g. protein; 1 carbohydrate block = 9 g. carbohydrates; 1 fat block = 1.5 g. of fat). Essentially, the zone diet obtains 30 percent of calories from protein, 40 percent from carbo-hydrates, and the remaining 30 percent from fat. Sears believes that getting 55–60 percent of your daily calories from carbohydrates, which is what the Food Guide Pyra-mid recommends, is too much. His diet restricts foods with a high glycemic index (see section 414), but not just refined carbs. Sears also advises avoiding carrots, bananas, brown rice, and whole-grain breads—which I don't agree with.

Essential fatty acids are necessary for reaching the "zone," which is good. Gamma-linolenic acid (GLA), of the omega-6 fatty acids, is, according to Sears, the most important. But too much GLA—through supplements or foods—can negate zone benefits unless the GLA is prop-erly balanced with enough eicosapentaenoic acid (EPA), which can be tricky to figure out.

The diet advocates healthy foods, but rigid quanti-ties at prescribed times—even if you're not hungry. Whether you're successful at reaching the "zone" or not, I suggest covering your nutritional bases with an MVP (see section 246).

393. Weight Watchers

This is a long-term regimen that advocates three meals a day with measured portions of protein, carbohydrates, and fat.

Though the program is nutritionally well-rounded, most Weight Watchers that I've met agree that supplements have helped them keep up their energy levels while their calorie intake goes down. The MVP in section 246 should fill the bill.

394. Jenny Craig

This is a reduced-calorie diet (around 1,200 calories a day) focused on balanced nutrition (60 percent carbs, 20 percent protein, 20 percent fats), with prepackaged meals to control portion size. This is fine for short-term weight loss, but it falls short of helping dieters learn how to handle food selection and portion control in the long run. Also, the program does not emphasize exercise, which is key to keeping lost weight off and staying in good health.

Although this diet is nutritionally acceptable, the MVP in section 246 is recommended for retaining maximum energy output while restricting caloric intake.

395. Liquid Protein Diets

These diets have been found to be dangerous and potentially lethal. In fact, the Food and Drug Administration has a ruling that all protein supplements (liquid or powder) used in reducing diets must carry the following label:

Warning—Very low-calorie protein diets (below 800

calories per day) may cause serious illness or death. Do not use for weight reduction without medical supervision. Use with particular care if you are taking medication. Not for use by infants, children, or pregnant or nursing women.

Radical diets such as these can cause disastrous effects on the body, not the least of which are abnormal heart function and severe deficiencies in vital minerals due to extremely rapid weight loss. I couldn't in good conscience offer supplement suggestions, since I firmly believe that these diets should not be undertaken without strict medical supervision.

396. The South Beach Diet

Not totally unlike the Atkins diet, Dr. Arthur Agatston's South Beach diet advocates an overall cut in carbs and teaches you to rely on low glycemic index carbs (see section 414) for those that you do eat. It allows ample portions of protein and good fats, relying on the low glycemic carbs to provide blood sugar control and hunger satisfaction. Chicken, turkey, and fish are recommended, along with nuts and low-fat cheeses and yogurt.

The strictest part of the South Beach diet is meant to last for two weeks, where there can be significant weight loss. At this point, your cravings for sweets and starches are supposed to have vanished. Of course if they don't, staying on this—or any—diet won't exactly be "a day at the beach." Covering your nutritional bases can help you stick to it by keeping your spirits up while you keep your weight down. (See section 246 for an MVP.)

397. Zen Macrobiotic Diet

Contrary to popular belief, this diet is not connected with the Zen buddhists, but is the creation of a Japanese man named George Ohsawa. Though it has gained many adherents, it is nutritionally dangerous when strictly followed.

There are ten stages to the diet, and milk is prohibited. You start by giving up dessert and eating nothing but grains, preferably brown rice. The diet, based on the Oriental yin-yang philosophy, restricts fluid intake, which is dangerous, as is the lack of nutrients provided in meals consisting of nothing but brown rice. Followers believe that if your thoughts are right you can produce vitamins, minerals, and proteins within your own body, and actually change one element to another.

Just in case your thoughts aren't always right, it would be advisable if you are on this diet, or any strict vegetarian diet, to take supplements. A high-potency vegetarian multi-vitamin-mineral tablet twice daily along with a good B complex with folic acid is recommended. Also vitamin B12, 100 mcg. one to three times a day.

398. The Cookie Diet

This diet is the creation of Dr. Sanford Siegal. Although no clinical studies have been done on it, its appeal is obvious. The no-no on other diets—the cookie—becomes the yes-yes of this one. Eat six prepackaged cookies a day (*which will set you back about $56 each week*), plus one "real" meal (skinless chicken and steamed vegetables), and you can lose ten pounds a month. No magic involved, the cookies (allegedly containing special amino acids that curb hunger, also contain a plant fiber that acts as a bulking agent, along with a mixture of protein and sugar) essentially put you on an 800–1,000 calorie a day diet so, of course, you'll lose weight. Although Dr. Siegal says his product is nutritionally sound, I doubt it. In fact, he might have his doubts, too, because when you order his cookie six-packs, you also get a seven-day supply of multivitamins to "take care of any deficiencies that might arise."

Dieter beware: Diets below 1,000 calories a day do not lead to long-lasting weight loss and they can result in heart palpitations, weakened kidney functions, potassium deficiencies, and other health problems. But if your weakness for cookies entices you to try this one, be sure the multivitamin you're taking has the nutrients you might be missing. Check out my MVP (see section 246).

399. Kelp, Lecithin, Vinegar, B6 Diet

This low-profile, word-of-mouth diet has been around for more than three decades and is still popular. The basic components of the diet can be obtained in one tablet that contains kelp, lecithin, apple cider vinegar, and vitamin B6. There are two potencies available: single strength and double strength. (With the single strength you take 2 tablets with each meal, and with the double strength you take 1.)

As with any diet that cuts down caloric intake, an MVP with breakfast and dinner is recommended. Also a B complex and 500 mg. vitamin C twice daily.

400. DASH Diet

This diet is heart healthy, nutritionally sound, and is rich in fruits, veggies, whole grains, lean protein, and low-fat dairy. Other benefits of the DASH diet include that it is low in saturated fats and sodium and can prevent high blood pressure.

401. Mediterranean Diet

This diet is low in red meat, sugar, and saturated fats, as well as being high in produce, nuts, and other healthy foods. One of its key secrets is that it is rich in olive oil, which helps in weight loss. Eating this diet is heart and brain healthy. It can also decrease one's risk of developing cancer and diabetes. Yet another benefit of this way of eating is that it is rich in resveratrol, found in red wine, which seems to be important in slowing the aging process.

402. Flexitarian Diet

This diet is very flexible, heart healthy, and all vegetarian, which promotes longevity. It is also one of the few diets that emphasizes home cooking.

This diet makes you feel full, and nothing is off-limits. It is high in fruits and vegetables.

403. TLC Diet

This low-fat, heart-healthy diet is government endorsed. It is rich in vegetables, fruits, beans, cereals, pastas, and lean meats. It is rich in sea foods, organic produce, and glycemic foods.

404. Nordic Diet

This diet is high in fruits, vegetables, and whole grains.

405. Ornish Diet

This popular diet is low in fat, animal protein, and refined carbohydrates.

406. Vegeterian Diet

This heart-healthy, lacto-ovo diet contains no meat or fish.

407. Fertility Diet

With this diet, women can increase their chances of getting pregnant faster. It contains good fats, whole grains, and plant proteins. It is low in carbohydrates and recommends eating full-fat dairy products.

408. Asian Diet

This filling diet is rich in fruits, vegetables, seeds, and whole grains such as brown rice, millet, and buckwheat. It also is rich in soy, fish, and shellfish. It does require you to drink at least six glasses of clean water or tea daily, but also allows the drinking of sake, wine, and beer in moderation.

409. Dr Weil's Anti-Inflammatory Diet

In this diet 20–30 percent of the calories you take in are from protein, 30 percent are from fats, and the remaining 40–50 percent are from carbohydrates. It is also high in omega-3 fatty acids.

410. Nutritarian Diet

This diet is rich in salads, such as those made from kale, collards, and mustard greens. It also has reduced animal protein.

411. Vegan Diet

This filling, rich diet is high in fiber foods and environmentally friendly. It is also high in fruits, vegetables, leafy greens, whole grains, nuts, seeds, and legumes.

412. The Engine 2 Diet

This environmentally friendly diet increases lean muscle mass, as well as energizing your body. There is no calorie counting and no vegetable oils in this program.

413. Biggest Loser Diet

There are no foods that are off-limits in this diet. It consists of four servings of fruits and vegetables daily, three servings of whole grains daily, and 200 calories of desserts are allowed. Analyzing this diet we find 23 percent of the calories taken in are from fats, 30 percent from protein, and 45 percent from carbohydrates.

414. All Carbohydrates Are Not Equal: Look Yours Up on the Glycemic Index

All carbohydrates are not equal when it comes to their ranking on a scale known as the glycemic index, a calculation based on how fast and how high blood glucose is elevated after a particular food is eaten. Foods with a high glycemic index are carbohydrate-rich (high in sugar and starch), and allow glucose to enter the bloodstream quickly. There's nothing wrong with glucose (it's the fuel used by every cell in the body), but to process it, the pancreas has to produce insulin. The more high-glycemic foods you eat, the harder your pancreas has to work. And if it has to work too hard too often, it can wear down and diabetes can result.

Additionally, high-glycemic refined carbohydrates cause a surge in blood sugar and, consequently, insulin; insulin then turns all the extra glucose into fat. This is why low-fat and no-fat foods are still making so many Americans fat.

The glycemic index ranks foods on how each 50 g.

serving affects blood sugar levels two to three hours after eating. Generally foods ranking between 1 and the low 60s only minimally affect blood sugar levels and are therefore preferable. Foods ranking betweeen the low 60s and high 80s are considered moderate and should be eaten in moderation, and foods ranked 90 and above are higher and should be used sparingly. But the glycemic index itself doesn't take portion size into account. (A 50 g. portion of carrots is about seven carrots, which adds up to much more than most people would eat at one sitting—which is why they have a higher GI than a quarter cup of sugar that also has 50 g. of carbohydrates.) There is another measurement that does take portion size into consideration. It's called the glycemic load (GL). But this can be confusing because glucose response to a particular food can vary from person to person. Additionally, the same type of food can also vary tremendously. Potatoes, for instance, can show different measurements depending on the variety, where they are grown, how they are cultivated, and the way in which they are prepared.

The key to keeping healthy and trim is replacing high-glucose starches with slowly digested high-fiber carbohydrates. (Unfortunately, food labels do not distinguish between the good and bad carbs. But you can if you check the fiber content. Dietary fiber, although carbohydrates, cannot be broken down by the body; it passes right through you without being converted to blood sugar.) To score high nutritionally, look for foods on the low-glycemic index. My simple guideline lists below should point you in the right direction for making the right food choices.

HIGH-GLYCEMIC FOODS (GI ABOVE 85)

- Refined white sugar
- Snack candies, cakes, crackers, and cookies
- Potato chips, pretzels, and related snacks
- White-flour pastas
- Instant rice
- Waffles
- Macaroni and cheese
- Bagels
- Potatoes
- Carbonated soft drinks
- Sweet corn
- Cornflakes
- Cream of wheat
- Watermelon

MODERATE GLYCEMIC INDEX FOODS
(GI between 60 and 85)

- All-bran cereal
- Baked beans
- Kidney beans (canned)
- Popcorn (air popped)
- Oranges and orange juice
- Grapes
- Mangoes
- Pineapple juice
- Pita bread (white)
- Bananas
- Peas
- Low-fat ice cream

LOW-GLYCEMIC FOODS (GI below 60)

- Whole-grain pasta

- Hard beans (soy, mung, kidney, lima, green beans, butter beans, split peas)
- Pearled barley
- Whole wheat breads
- Bran
- High-fiber fruits and vegetables (apples, asparagus, blackberries, broccoli, brussels sprouts, celery, chard, cucumber, grapefruit, peppers, raw peaches and pears)
- Soy milk, skim milk, 2 percent milk
- Peanuts
- Dried dates and figs
- Yogurt (plain)

415. Low-Carb Dieter's Guide to Fruits and Veggies

Just because you're cutting carbs from your diet doesn't mean you need to deprive yourself of fiber-rich, nutrient-packed fruits and vegetables. In fact, I think it's so important to include them, I've put together a top ten list of the most bang-for-the-buck low-carb veggies and fruits to choose from.

FRUITS	VEGETABLES
Strawberries	Dark greens (spinach, collards, chard)
Blueberries	Avocados
Raspberries	Green beans
Blackberries	Tomatoes
Peach	Carrots
Tangerine	Artichokes
Kiwi	Turnip
Papaya	Broccoli

Cherry   Scallions
Cantaloupe   Ginger and garlic

416. Mindell Dieting Tips

- Before starting any diet, check with your physician. If you don't feel that your family doctor understands your dieting needs, contact a bariatrician, who specializes in the field. For the name of one in your area, write to the American Society of Bariatric Physicians (ASBP), 5453 East Evans Place, Denver, Colorado 80222-5234 (Tel: 303-770-2526; Fax: 303-779-4843) or E-mail: infor@asbp.org.

- If you're on a low- or no-carbohydrate diet, keep away from diet sodas. These beverages contain aspartame, which has been found to inhibit your body from converting fat into glucose.

- Be aware that a low-carb claim on a product generally means that the naturally occurring carbohydrates have been replaced with ingredients such as fiber and artificial sweeteners. Not a good trade-off.

- If you're on a diet that allows alcohol, a glass of wine before dinner stimulates the gastric juices and aids in proper digestion.

- If you do have wine, remember that dry white has fewer calories than red.

- If you're eating popcorn as a low-calorie snack, be aware that movie-theater popcorn has twice the calories per cup as "light" microwave—and two and a half times that of air-popped.

- Keep in mind that protein requires your body to expend 25 percent more calories than fat or carbohydrates does just to digest it.

- When a recipe calls for a cup of sour cream, substitute low-fat yogurt and you'll save more than 300 calories.
- Remember that the body's natural response to a decreased food intake is to burn *fewer* calories—which is why diets without exercise don't work in the long run.
- Whatever you're eating, sit down to eat it, and eat it slowly. (You might expend more calories standing than sitting, but you tend to eat more that way, too.) Also, don't read or watch TV until you finish your meal.
- When selecting fruit, remember that all fruits are not equal, that an apple, a banana, or a pear has more calories and carbohydrates than a half cantaloupe, a cup of raw strawberries, or a fresh tangerine.
- When choosing your vegetable, take green beans instead of peas (you save 40 calories on a half-cup serving), spinach instead of mixed vegetables (you save 35 calories), and mashed potatoes—if you must—instead of hash browns (you save 139 calories).
- Carbohydrate watchers, don't underestimate onions; one cup of cooked onions has 18 g. of carbs.
- If you're counting every calorie, realize that 1 tbsp. of lecithin granules contains 50 calories and a lecithin capsule about 8.
- Try a one-day-a-week water fast (the ancient Greeks did it). Limit yourself to cold filtered tap or bottled (not iced) or herb tea with lemon or lime juice. Nothing else. This should pep you up, too.

417. Mindell Vitamin-Balanced Diet to Lose and Live By

I know your mother told it to you, but it is true anyway—breakfast *is* the most important meal of the day. It comes after the longest period of time that you've been without food, and you cannot catch up nutritionally by eating a good lunch or dinner later.

If you're dieting, it is especially important to perk up your energy level at the start of the day.

BREAKFAST

8 oz. of no-sugar almond milk

A flavored low-calorie, low-carbohydrate whey protein powder

4 ice cubes

Mix well in blender for 60 seconds. Calories: approximately 150.

This mixture can be frozen and used as a dessert for dinner or a pick-me-up snack if your calorie quotient allows.

Lunch is a tricky meal. Fast-food restaurants are seductively convenient, and nothing blows a diet faster than "a few french fries" and a "tiny milk shake." If you really want to lose weight, think more along these lines:

LUNCH

A modest portion (3–5 oz.) of water-packed canned or fresh fish, skinless chicken or white meat turkey, a raw vegetable salad (with lemon or vinegar dressing), and a piece of fruit.

OR

A low-cal turkey sandwich (3 oz. turkey, 1 tsp. mayo, 2 slices whole wheat bread, lettuce, thin-slice tomato), small carrot, ½ cup unsweetened applesauce, mixed with ½ cup low-carbohydrate yogurt.

OR

A diet pizza (2 oz. sliced low-fat mozzarella cheese, ½ whole wheat muffin, small sliced tomato, 1 tsp. olive oil with oregano sprinkled on top), ¼ cantaloupe or 1 cup frozen melon balls.

(Vary lunches from day to day.)

Dinner is usually a dieter's downfall, but it doesn't have to be that way:

DINNER

Five nights a week you should have fish (sole, trout, salmon, halibut, etc.) or poultry broiled, boiled, or roasted (remove skin before eating—but leave on for cooking); and two nights a week you can have meat, once again broiled, boiled, or roasted; a cooked vegetable; a large salad (no more than 1 tsp. oil in the dressing); a small boiled or baked potato once or twice a week; and a fresh fruit for dessert. Substituting tofu for meat or poultry is a great way to cut calories and fat.

BEVERAGES

For best results (and improved health) stay away from alcohol—try sparkling mineral water with lemon or lime instead. I make a drink with an instant mix powder containing L-phenylalanine, a natural amino acid that increases my energy. It gives me a feeling of well-being while it helps reduce my appetite; it really gets me fired up!

Also be sure to drink at least six to ten 8-ounce glasses of filtered water daily. (To find out how much water your body needs see section 73.) Herb teas, hot or iced, are recommended alternatives to diet sodas—especially those that contain caffeine (see section 372).

SUPPLEMENTS

MVP (see section 246)

Calcium (500 mg.) or magnesium (250 mg.), 1 twice daily for men, 2 twice daily for women

Chromium picolinate complex, 200 mcg. one to three times daily

Banaba leaf extract, 50 mg., take a half hour before lunch and dinner

418. Supplements for Eating More and Gaining Less

The amino acids arginine and ornithine (see section 88) have been found to stimulate the pituitary gland to continue to produce growth hormone, which can rejuvenate your metabolism. While some hormones encourage the body to store fat, growth hormone acts as a mobilizer of fat, helping you to look trimmer and have more energy as well.

Best of all, you can rejuvenate your metabolism while you sleep because that's when growth hormone is secreted!

Supplements are available as tablets or powder. The time-release-tablet form is most effective and 1,500 mg. of arginine can be taken twice daily. A combination of arginine and ornithine in powder form works best when taken on an empty stomach with water or juice (no protein). For reducing benefits, take 2 g. (2,000 mg.) immediately before retiring.

CAUTION: *Arginine is contraindicated for growing children, persons with schizophrenic conditions, and anyone who has a herpes virus infection. Doses exceeding 20 g. are not recommended.*

419. More Natural Alternatives to Diet Drugs

Because of the dangers of diet drugs, many people are seeking safer alternatives to weight loss. The following is a list of natural alternatives you might want to consider using along with your diet and exercise regimen if you'd like to be in better shape than the shape you're in.

Chitosan: This is an effective fat blocker that enhances weight loss by preventing the absorption of fat. As it passes through the digestive tract it can absorb four to six times its weight in fat, flushing it out of the body before it can be metabolized and stored as excess pounds. Unfortunately, chitosan can also rob you of important fat-soluble vitamins, such as vitamins E, A, D, and K. It should be used only occasionally, and not for more than two weeks at a time. If you take it, you *must* supplement your diet with fat-soluble vitamins and essential fatty acids. Take one to three 250 mg. tablets daily with meals. Be sure to drink 8 ounces of filtered water with each tablet.

CAUTION: *Do not use chitosan if you have an allergy to shellfish. This supplement (or any other fat blocker) should not be used by pregnant or lactating women or by children.*

Coenzyme-Q10 (Co-Q10): This great antioxidant, which also facilitates the production of energy, may make it easier for the body to burn fat for fuel (see section 119).

Conjugated linoleic acid (CLA): A good fat-fighting and powerful cancer-fighting antioxidant that helps reduce the amount of body fat while increasing muscle. Since muscle burns excess calories, the more muscle you have, the less likely you are to become overweight. CLA also helps reduce the appetite by improving the way the body extracts energy from less food (see section 97).

DHAP: This is a combination of pyruvate and its precursor, dihydroxyacetone, and referred to as DHAP. Available as a supplement, it increases athletic stamina and the amount of fat lost during exercise. Even at rest, it helps the body burn fat for fuel. The recommended dosage is 2–5 g.

taken twice daily with meals. It is not recommended for children or pregnant women.

DL-phenylalanine, tyrosine, and 5-HTP: This amino acid combination, soon to be available as a patented formula supplement, has been found to help curb sugar and carbohydrate cravings that are the downfall of binge dieters. (Recommended dosages for individual amino acids can be found in chapter V.)

Gymnema sylvestre: (See section 232.)

Garcinia cambogia: (See section 195.)

Green tea: (See section 198.)

Hydrocitric acid (HCA): This is the active ingredient extracted from the sour Indian fruit garcinia cambogia, which ayurvedic healers have used as a natural appetite suppressant for centuries. Marketed under the tradenames of Citrin and Citrimax, as well as HCA, it is non-habit-forming. Some studies suggest it can reduce caloric intake by as much as 10 percent. For best results, take three 500–750 mg. capsules daily, half an hour before meals—in conjunction with a sensible diet and exercise regimen.

L-carnitine: This vitaminlike nutrient can help increase physical stamina and promote weight loss. (It can also lower high blood cholesterol while raising levels of good HDL cholesterol.) I suggest 1–3 capsules (250–500 mg. strength) taken half an hour before meals.

Licorice flavonoid oil (LFO): Derived from the common licorice plant, this natural flavonoid oil essentially gives the metabolism a fat-burning boost. By inhibiting the action of genes involved in the synthesis of fat while increasing the activity of enzymes involved in its breakdown, it has been found to not only lower weight and body fat percentage, but LDL cholesterol as well.

Pyruvate: Can increase stamina and help you burn fat for fuel—even *without* exercise. Pyruvate is naturally found in the body as a by-product of normal metabolism; it triggers the release of adenosine triphosphate (ATP), the fuel that runs the body. It also helps lower cholesterol and blood pressure. Pyruvate enthusiasts report that doses as low as 5 g. daily have produced good results. There are few side effects, except for occasional stomach upset, but it is not recommended for pregnant women or children.

White Tea: An extract of white tea—the least processed version of the tea plant used to make green and black tea—has been found to effectively inhibit the production of new adipocytes (fat cells) while stimulating fat mobilization from existing mature fat cells. Containing more of the ingredients thought to be active on human cells, such as methylxanthines (like caffeine) and epigallocatechin-3-gallate (EGCG), white tea may be a safe natural source of slimming substances.

Avenca: Avenca promotes weight loss, fights free radicals, lowers blood sugar, and reduces cholesterol and blood pressure.

Research has shown that Avenca inhibits pancreatic lipase, so that the fats in the diet are not broken down and absorbed, but pass through the digestive process and are eliminated. It has the ability to inhibit alpha-amylase and alpha-glucoside. These two digestive enzymes break down starches and sugars the same way lipase breaks down fats in animals. Take 500 mg fifteen minutes before one or two meals.

DID YOU KNOW?

- A medium popcorn and soda at a cineplex can be the equivalent of eating three McDonald's Quarter Pounders with twelve pats of butter!
- Eating the same amount of calories, but different proportions of fat, protein, and carbohydrates, can result in *different amounts of weight loss.*
- Having a weakness for sweets could be caused by low potassium levels.

---

420. Any Questions About Chapter XVI?

I know that no more than 30 percent of my daily calories should come from fat. But I'm not good at figuring out percentages. I read labels, but I'm still confused. Is there an easy way to determine how much I'm getting?

Just remember that 1 g. of fat equals about 9 calories. Therefore, to keep your fat intake below 30 percent daily, when you check food labels be sure that for every 100 calories there are no more than 3 grams of fat.

What is fucoxanthin and how safe is it to use as a diet aid?

Fucoxanthin is a carotenoid derived from brown seaweed that has been shown in animal studies to promote fat burning within fat cells, particularly those around the abdominal area. Its effacacy in humans, though, has not been fully documented. As for its safety, seaweed contains high amounts of iodine, so a potential side effect could be changes in thyroid function due to iodine excess, resulting in goiters. As a diet aid, it would not be my first choice.

What is a set point? And what does it have to do with losing weight?

The set point theory is one of the most widely accepted on weight gain and loss. It holds that fatness is caused by the setting of an area in the hypothalamus (part of the brain), sometimes called an appestat, which controls your appetite for food. Needless to say, everyone's appestat is not on the same setting.

Glycerol, which is bound and released according to the fat content of a cell, along with the blood level of insulin, informs the brain of the body's fat reserves and sets your appestat accordingly. Unfortunately, external influences—such as the aroma and taste of delectable food—can *raise* your appestat.

But you can reset your set point by exercising regularly. In other words, you'll reduce your appetite by lowering the point at which you feel full.

To reset for weight loss, the minimum requirement is half an hour of aerobic exercise three times a week. A simple and effective way to do this is by walking 2 miles in half an hour three times a week (or 1 mile in 15 minutes six times a week.)

I've heard that you're likely to be more successful dieting in warm weather. Is this true?

If this were completely true, dieters would be moving to Florida and Southern California in droves. What has been purported by Susan Perry and Jim Dawson in *The Secrets Our Body Clocks Reveal* (Rawson Associates) is that we are genetically disposed to have extra fat layers in fall and winter. Therefore, when days start getting longer in the spring, it's allegedly easier for us to lose weight. The question is, easier than what?

What real dangers are there in liquid dieting—aside from running the risk of gaining the weight back?

Extremely real dangers. Many people who go on very-low-calorie diets (VLCD) do so without proper medical supervision. They are unaware that a VLCD is designed for people who are at least 30 percent over their ideal weight (as determined by a physician—not a fashion model). Once on a VLCD, a dieter must be medically monitored (receiving regular blood tests, electrocardiograms, and blood pressure checks).

Diets such as Slim-Fast, which advocate a shake only for breakfast and lunch and then a "sensible" dinner (4–6 oz. of poultry, fish, or lean meat; ½ baked potato; 3 steamed vegetables; and fruit for dessert) are not dangerous. But if you are less than 30 percent over your ideal weight, and you go on a quick-loss, over-the-counter (OTC) liquid diet, substituting it for *all* meals, you risk losing too much muscle, bone, and lean body mass in proportion to fat—causing possible heart arrhythmia, permanently slowed metabolism, fatigue, and, in extreme cases, even death.

I've replaced virtually all my fatty foods with low-fat and fat-free substitutes and I'm gaining weight. What gives?

Fat-free and low-fat do not mean sugar-free! Nor do they mean no calories. My guess is that you're eating more sugar and processed carbohydrates than you did before.

Can I gain weight if I just chew on fatty things and then spit them out?

You might not gain weight, but you could be doing something more harmful to your body. Merely tasting fatty foods has been found to raise the amount of fat in your blood. A study done at Purdue University showed that people who chewed and spit out full-fat cream cheese on crackers almost doubled their levels of potentially heart-damaging triglycerides!

Which has less fat, something marked "extra-lean" or "low-fat"?

Foods marked "extra-lean" have less than 5 g. total fat, less than 2 g. saturated fat, and less than 95 mg. cholesterol per 100 g. serving. Low-fat foods have 3 g. or less per serving.

Does a cup of coffee without milk or sugar really have calories?

Well, the bad news is that according to the USDA nutrient database, an 8-ounce cup of regular coffee, brewed from grounds does have calories. The good news is there are just 2 of them. In other words, it's virtually calorie-free and considered a zero-calorie beverage.

Can you explain this body mass index (BMI) thing? My old doctor told me I was okay at 5'5" and 150 pounds—and now my new doctor tells me I'm overweight. What's it all about?

Let me first tell you that you're not alone. There are about twenty-nine million Americans who have just discovered that they are overweight. The old male-female height and weight statistics that have been around since the 1950s have been replaced by a new measurement system, created by the National Heart, Lung, and Blood Institute. The BMI (body mass index) is a single number that represents height and weight without regard to age or sex.

To figure out your BMI, you multiply your weight in pounds by 703 and then divide it by your height in inches squared (your weight in kilograms divided by the square of your height in meters). The number you end up with is your BMI.

BMIs of 22–24 are considered healthy. BMIs above 27 are considered dangerously overweight. Your BMI is 25, and anywhere between 25–26 is now considered overweight. But not by everyone. In fact, the National Center for Health Statistics still feels that you're not overweight unless you're above 27. Let me put it this way: If you're exercising, eating properly, and keeping to a low-fat, high-fiber diet—and you're happy with the way you look and feel—relax and go back to your old doctor.

For those of you who would like to know what your BMI is—without doing the math—the following chart from the National Center for Health Statistics should give you a pretty good idea.

BMI—	23	24	25	26	27	28
5'	118	123	128	133	138	143
5'1"	122	127	132	137	143	148
5'1"	130	135	141	146	152	158
5'5"	138	144	150	156	162	168
5'7"	146	153	159	166	172	178
5'9"	155	162	169	176	182	189
5'11"	165	172	179	186	193	200
6'1"	174	182	189	220	204	212
6'3"	184	192	200	208	216	224

XVII

So You Think You Don't Eat Much Sugar and Salt

421. Kinds of Sugars

More than a hundred substances that qualify as sweet can be called sugars. The ones we come in contact with most often are *fructose,* a natural sugar found in fruit and honey; *glucose,* the body's blood sugar and the simplest form of sugar in which a carbohydrate is assimilated; *dextrose,* made from cornstarch and chemically identical to glucose; *lactose,* milk sugar; *maltose,* the sugar formed from the starch by the action of yeast; and *sucrose,* the sugar that is obtained from sugarcane or beets and refined to the product that reaches us as granules.

Brown sugar, which many people assume to be healthier than white sugar, is merely sugar crystals coated with molasses syrup. (In the United States most brown sugar is made by simply spraying refined white sugar with the molasses syrup.) Raw sugar is banned in the United States because it contains contaminants. When it's partially refined and cleaned up, it can be sold as turbinado sugar. *Honey* is a blend of fructose and glucose.

422. Not-So-Sweet Truths About Sugar Substitutes

Sorbitol, mannitol, and *xylitol* are naturally occurring sugar alcohols that are absorbed more slowly into the blood than glucose or sucrose. The biggest misconception about these sweeteners is that they have no calories. The fact is, they have as many calories as sugar—and in some instances, products using them as sweeteners contain *more* calories than they would if made with regular sugar. Don't be fooled. These are not low- or no-calorie sugar substitutes, even though products containing them are often sold in the dietetic section of food markets. Always check labels. Products using these sweeteners must reveal that they are not a reduced-calorie food or be marked not for weight control.

Aspartame (Equal, NutraSweet, Sugar Twin) is a combination of the amino acids phenylalanine and aspartic acid (see sections 82 and 89) and has no calories. Although deemed safe by the FDA, there have been numerous side effects associated with it. Among them: dizziness, headache, increased appetite, nausea, fatigue, mood changes, and cramps. More serious illnesses have also been associated with aspartame, including anxiety attacks, depression, multiple sclerosis, fibromyalgia, blurred vision, lupus, slurred speech, and various cancers.

Acesulfame K (Sunette, Sweet One) is a nonnutritive sweetener that looks like sugar, is derived from acetoacetic acid, has no calories, and is used in many foods and beverages—without consumers being aware of it. Not a good thing, since acesulfame K contains methylene chloride, a potentially dangerous chemical carcinogen. Long-term consumption is reported to cause cancer, depression, liver disease, kidney disease, and mental confusion.

Saccharin (Sweet 'n Low, Necta Sweet, Sweet* 10), a noncaloric petroleum derivative estimated to be seven hundred times sweeter than sugar, and chemically similar to acesulfame K, saccharin is absorbed but not modified by the body and is excreted unchanged in the urine. At one time the only artificial sweetener in the US, it was banned as a carcinogen for fourteen years, based on flawed studies, but the FDA removed it from the list of suspected carcinogens in 2000.

Sucralose (Splenda) is up to six hundred times sweeter than regular sugar and, like saccharin, has no calories. But because there is a trace of chlorine in Splenda, which is not safe for humans, there have been concerns about its safety—especially for long-term use.

Neotame is one of the most intense sweeteners approved by the FDA. It would take 8,000 tsp. of sugar to equal the sweetening power of 1 tsp. of neotame. Although it has the same amino acids as aspartame, it is metabolized differently, is not a source of phenylalanine, is safe for people with phenylketonuria, and does not require a warning label.

Stevia is an herb that has been safely used medicinally and as a sweetener in South America for centuries. Two hundred times sweeter than sugar, it has no calories, is suitable for diabetics, and has immunity-boosting properties. Sounds great? Well, it is. But (*and here's the catch*) despite the fact that all three of the FDA-approved herb-based sweeteners—Truvia, PureVia, and Sweet Leaf—are made with a stevia leaf extract (rebiana, aka Reb A), stevia itself has still *not* been approved by the FDA as a food additive! Fortunately, stevia is widely available as a dietery supplement and can be obtained as a powder or liquid at health-food stores. It's my pick for a safe, no calorie sugar substitute. (Chose the green or brown liquids or powders, because the clear and white versions are highly refined.)

CAUTION: *If you have diabetes or hypoglycemia, be sure to check with your doctor or a nutritionally oriented dietician before adding any products containing alternative sweeteners to your diet.*

423. Naturally Sweet Sweetening Alternatives

If you have a sweet tooth and want a healthier choice than refined sugar or artificial sweeteners, one that won't adversely affect your health or your body's blood sugar, take your pick from the list below. They're all natural and available in most health-food stores. Now that's sweet!

Agave Nectar: Made from the juice of the agave cactus, this nectar is not only sweeter than refined sugar, it won't create a "sugar rush" and is less disturbing to the body's blood sugar levels than white sugar.

Barley malt: Available as a powder or syrup, it can be substituted one to one for sugar, although it is half as sweet.

Brown rice sugar: Minimally refined from malted brown rice and enzymes, this tasty sugar has a semisweet butterscotch flavor.

Date sugar: It's granulated, tastes like dates, and can be used as a direct substitute for sugar.

Honey: Sweeter than sugar, raw honey has added benefits—small amounts of enzymes, minerals, and vitamins.

Maple sugar: This is dehydrated maple syrup, but twice as sweet as white sugar and much less refined.

Sucanat: This is essentially evaporated organic cane juice made through a mechanical rather than chemical process, thereby retaining many of sugarcane's inherent vitamins and minerals.

Vegetable glycerin: A very sweet odorless, colorless syrupy liquid derived from coconut and palm oils that does not contain sucrose, making it a great choice for Candida sufferers.

424. Dangers of Too Much Sugar

The big problem with sugar is that we eat too much of it (over 154 pounds) and often don't even know it. All carbohydrate sweeteners qualify as sugar, even though they may be called by other names; and when sucrose is the number three ingredient on a box of cereal, corn syrup number five, and honey number seven, you don't realize it, but you're eating something that is 50 percent sugar!

The consumer today is hooked on sugar right from the start. Baby formulas are often sweetened with sugar, as are many baby foods (check labels). Because sugar also acts as a preservative and retains and absorbs moisture, it's often in products we never think of as containing it, products such as salt, peanut butter, canned vegetables, bouillon cubes, and more. Would you believe that the ketchup you put on your hamburger has just less than 8 percent more sugar than ice cream? That cream substitute for coffee is 65 percent sugar compared to 51 percent for a chocolate bar?

The fact is, we're eating too much sugar for our health. It is beyond argument that sugar is a prime factor in tooth decay. Also, one-third of our population is overweight, and obesity increases the possibility of heart disease, diabetes, hypertension, gallstones, back problems, and arthritis. Not that sugar alone is the cause, but its presence in foods induces you to eat more, and if you cut your calorie count without cutting your sugar intake, you'll lose nutrients faster than pounds. Sugar is also the villain where hypoglycemia is concerned, and, though there have been arguments pro and con, directly or indirectly sugar is a factor in diabetes and heart disease.

LABEL ALERT: *"Sugar-free" on a label usually means that artificial sweeteners—which are worse for you than real sugar—or fruit juices have been added. Check those ingredients.*

425. How Sweet It Is

Hidden sugars are where you least expect them. (Would you believe that Canada Dry tonic water has approximately 18¼ teaspoons of sugar in a 12-oz. serving?) If you want to be a sugar detective, my advice is to check labels. Look for sucrose substitutes such as corn syrup or corn sugar, and watch out for words ending in -*ose*, which indicates the presence of sugar. A sugar by any name is still a sugar. And remember that not even medicines are immune from added sweeteners! Pseudoephedrine, a decongestant in some cold and flu medicines, can be high in sugar. Read the label for sure. When in doubt about the sugar or artificial sweetener content of any medication, over-the-counter or prescription, ask your pharmacist.

MEDICINES	SUGAR PER TABLESPOON
Alternagel liquid	2,000 mg.
Basaljel extra-strength liquid	375 mg.
Gaviscon liquid	1,500 mg.
Gaviscon-2 tablets	2,400 mg.
Maalox plus tablets	575 mg.
Mylanta liquid	2,000 mg.
Riopan Plus chew tablets	610 mg.

(When in doubt about sugar or saccharin content of any medication—ask your pharmacist.)

426. Dangers of Too Much Salt

Taking things with a grain of salt is all well and good, but eating things with it might be a different story. The normal intake of sodium chloride (table salt) is 6 to 18 g. daily, but the American Heart Association recommends an intake of no more than 3 g. (3,000 mg.) daily. An intake of more than 14 g. is considered excessive. And too many of us are being excessive. The average American consumes about 15 pounds (a bowling ball) of salt each year!

According to the Center for Science in the Public Interest (CSPI), a hefty 77 percent of the sodium intake of the average American is from sodium added to processed foods. CSPI also asserts that manufacturers add unnecessary amounts of salt to products, an assertion based on comparisons of products that are similar but have enormously different amounts of sodium. For example: Contadina tomato paste has about three times the salt as Hunt's tomato paste; Burger King french fries about three times the amount of salt as McDonald's.

Too much salt can cause hypertension (high blood pressure), which increases the chances of heart disease, and has recently been cited as one of the causes for migraine headaches. It causes abnormal fluid retention, which can result in dizziness and swelling of the legs. Also it may cause potassium to be lost in the urine and interfere with the proper utilization of protein foods. In addition, recent studies have linked excess sodium in the diet and low potassium-to-sodium ratios as high risk factors for colorectal cancer—particularly in men.

427. High-Salt Traps

Just because you stay away from pretzels and snack foods and don't pour on the table salt doesn't mean you're not getting more salt than you should. Salt traps are as hidden from view as sugar ones.

If you want to keep your salt intake down:

- Hold back on beer. (There's 25 mg. sodium in every 12 oz.)
- Avoid the use of baking soda, monosodium glutamate (MSG, Accent), and baking powder in food preparation.
- Stay away from laxatives, most of which contain sodium.
- Do not drink or cook with water treated by a home water softener; it adds sodium to the water.
- Look for the words *salt*, *sodium*, or the chemical symbol *Na* when reading food labels.
- Watch out for tomato juice. It's low in calories, but very high in sodium.
- Don't eat cured meat such as ham, bacon, corned beef, frankfurters, sausage; shellfish; any canned or frozen meat, poultry, or fish to which sodium has been added.
- When dining out, ask for an inside cut of meat, or chops or steaks without added salt.
- Watch out for diet sodas—the calories might be low, but in many the sodium content is still *high*!
- Be aware that 2 slices of most processed breads (even if "lite" or whole wheat) contain approximately 230 mg. of salt.

428. How Salty Is It?

APPROXIMATE SODIUM CONTENTS OF COMMON FOODS

Item	*Amount*	*Salt (mg.)*
Pickle, dill	1 large	1,928
Frozen turkey three-course dinner (Swanson)	1 (17 oz.)	1,735
Soy sauce	1 tbsp.	1,320
Pancakes (Hungry Jack Complete)	3 pancakes 4 in. each	1,150
Chicken noodle soup (Campbell's)	10 oz.	1,050
Tomato soup (Campbell's)	10 oz.	950
Green beans, canned (Del Monte)	1 cup	925
Cheese, pasteurized, processed American (Kraft)	2 oz.	890
Baked red kidney beans (B&M)	1 cup	810
Pizza, frozen (Celeste)	4 oz.	656
V8 vegetable juice	6 oz.	654
Danish cinnamon rolls w/raisins (Pillsbury)	1 serving	630
Bologna (Oscar Mayer)	2 slices	450
Tuna, in oil	3 oz.	430
Frankfurter, beef (Oscar Mayer)	1	425

DID YOU KNOW?

- Sorbitols, mannitols, and hexitols in artificially sweetened "sugarless" gum and candies are metabolized as carbohydrates, *only more slowly*!
- Water softeners can unhealthily increase your daily salt intake.
- Bread and breakfast cereals are two of the top sources of sodium in the diet.

---

429. Any Questions About Chapter XVII?

Isn't it true that in very hot weather you need salt supplements, especially if you do exercise and perspire heavily?

No! This is not only a myth, but one that could result in dangerous consequences. The truth is that salt tablets have a dehydrating effect, and are never indicated. When you exercise, your body uses mechanisms to conserve salt—and since the average American eats somewhere around sixty or more times the salt than is needed by the body, salt depletion is highly unlikely. In fact, too much salt under those conditions can contribute to heat exhaustion and heat stroke. (In the very, *very* rare case where a salt deficiency might occur, replacement should be administered with a 0.1 percent solution of salt administered in drinking water—and a doctor should be consulted.)

I've been told that eating a candy bar before running is not good for you. I don't understand why a quick energy fix would be bad. Can you explain?

Eating sugar or drinking a sugar drink within a half hour before exercise has been shown to stimulate the release of insulin, causing a drop in blood sugar (and, therefore, needed energy). Research done at the Human Performance Lab at Ball State University in Muncie, Indiana, found that once exercise starts, the insulin response is inhibited, which is why athletes can then drink beverages, such as Gatorade, that contain sugar in a glucose form that won't cause bloating.

Does sugarless chewing gum really help prevent cavities?

The claim for sugarless gum is that it doesn't *promote* cavities. There is no claim that it actually has a prophylactic effect. In fact, sugarless gum, or candy, that contains sorbitol or mannitol can increase your chances of tooth decay!

No, sorbitol and mannitol don't actually promote cavities, but both of them nourish and increase the type of bacteria in your mouth—namely, *Streptococcus mutans*—that do. According to Dr. Paul Keyes, founder of the International Dental Health Foundation, *Streptococcus mutans* have the mechanism to stick to teeth but will remain harmless until you eat something containing sugar or sucrose, with which they then quickly combine to cause decay. Because the sorbitol and mannitol have swelled the ranks of these bacteria, there are more of them available to use passing sugars to attack your teeth.

Rinsing your mouth with water within fifteen minutes after eating or drinking anything containing sucrose is the best preventive.

I've switched from Splenda to Truvia as a no-cal sweetener because it's been advertised as all natural. But I see it also contains erythritol. Can you tell me what erythritol is and if it's safe?

Erythritol is a polyol (sugar alcohol) that has been declared safe by the FDA for more than a decade. It is virtually calorie-free (0.2 calories per gram as opposed to sorbitol's 2.6 calories per gram) and found naturally in fruits like pears, melons, and grapes. It's expensive to produce commercially, which is why it's usually blended with other sweeteners in most products. But unlike other polyols (e.g., sorbitol, mannitol, xylitol), erythritol is digested almost entirely in the large intestine and 90 percent is excreted virtually unchanged, which is why it is lower in calories and less likely to cause diarrhea. It is also safe for people with diabetes, can be used in baking, doesn't contribute to tooth decay, and has no aftertaste. Personally, I am not a fan of artificial sweeteners (see section 422), but if I were, then erythritol alone or blended would be my choice.

Do some types of salt have less sodium than others?

They do. When it comes to how much sodium you get, size matters. The larger the salt crystals, the less actual salt—and therefore sodium—you'll get per teaspoon. Kosher salt, for example, with its large grains, has almost half the sodium per teaspoon as regular salt. Larger crystals affect how your taste buds perceive their flavor, meaning you could use less and get the same taste effect. Sea salts may also provide more flavor bang while using less because of their mineral content.

XVIII

STAYING BEAUTIFUL—STAYING HANDSOME

430. Vitamins for Healthy Skin

What you look like on the outside depends a lot on what you do for yourself on the inside. And as far as your skin is concerned, vitamins and proper nutrition are essential.

Topical cosmetic creams may promise the same age-defying results as expensive wrinkle-filling injections, but to quote Dr. Marsha Gordon, vice president of dermatology at Mount Sinai School of Medicine, "If creams could accomplish the same thing as a medical procedure, they would be drugs and not cosmetics."

To look your best, make sure that you drink 8 glasses of water daily (herbal teas can count for a few of them) and keep your milk and yogurt consumption restricted to the nonfat variety. Keep away from chocolates, nuts, dried fruits, fried foods, cola drinks, coffee, alcohol, cigarettes, and excessive salt. Also, do not use sugar. Small amounts of honey will sweeten just as well, and you'll look better for it.

A good start toward healthy, glowing skin is a daily soy-food protein drink. It can be taken in place of any meal, but it makes an especially good breakfast.

PROTEIN DRINK

2 tbsp. whey protein powder
2 tbsp. lecithin granules
1½ cups almond milk
2 tbsp. fresh or frozen fruit, or 1 banana
3–4 ice cubes
Mix in blender at high speed for one minute.

SUPPLEMENTS

Take with meals unless otherwise indicated.

• An all-natural, high-potency multivitamin and amino acid–chelated mineral complex (containing vitamin A, beta-carotene or carotenoids, vitamins B1, B2, B3, B5, B6, B12, biotin, choline, folic acid, inositol, vitamin C, vitamin D, vitamin E, boron, calcium, chromium, copper, magnesium, manganese, selenium, vanadium, and zinc)—1 twice daily, A.M. and P.M.

Essential for skin tone and nerve health.

• A broad-spectrum antioxidant formula (containing alpha- and beta-carotene, lutein, lycopene, vitamin C, vitamin E, selenium, ginkgo biloba, coenzyme-Q10, bilberry, L-glutathione, soy isoflavones [genistein and daidzein], grape-seed extract, and green tea extract)—1 twice daily, A.M. and P.M.

Helps replenish antioxidants that protect skin and keep it healthy and young-looking.

If your multivitamin-mineral complex and antioxidant formula do not contain the following supplements, add them separately to your daily intake:

- RNA/DNA complex—Stimulates formation of new cells; helps improve texture of skin.
- Superoxide dismutase (SOD) time-release and wild yam, 300 mg.—Aids in growth and repair of tissues and helps to maintain soft, pliant skin.
- Beta-carotene, 10,000 IU—Helps protect skin from free radical damage.
- Vitamin C with bioflavonoids, 500 mg.—Aids in preventing breakage of capillaries; promotes healing of wounds, bruises, and scar tissue.
- Vitamin E, dry form, 400 IU—Improves circulation in tiny face capillaries. Aids in replacing cells on the skin's outer layer.
- Vitamin B complex with pantothenic acid, 50 mg.—Helps in cell building and aids in wound healing.
- MSM (methylsulfonylmethane), 1,000 mg.—Promotes the formation of collagen, which helps produce new skin.
- Essential fatty acids, 1,000 mg. Flaxseed oil is a fine source of moisture-replenishing omega-3 fatty acids.
- L-cysteine, 1 g. daily (taken between meals with juice or water)—Helps maintain supple, young-looking skin.
- Zinc, 15–50 mg.—Aids in growth and repair of badly blemished skin.
- Astaxanthin, 5 mg.—a skin healthy supplement.

431. Vitamins for Healthy Hair

Shampoos and conditioners are not enough. In fact, hair isn't made up of living cells, so vitamins in shampoos, conditioners, and treatments, though they may change your hair's appearance, don't make any difference to its actual health. To make sure that you're giving your crowning glory its due, you have to be aware that nutrition plays a very important role in having terrific, shiny hair. Unlike the skin, hair cannot repair itself; but you *can* get new, healthier hair to grow.

The first thing to do is examine your diet. Does it include fish, wheat germ, yeast, and soybeans? It should. The vitamins and minerals that these foods supply are what your hair needs, along with frequent scalp massage, a good pH-balanced, protein-enriched shampoo, and supplements.

SUPPLEMENTS

Take with meals unless otherwise indicated.

- An all-natural, high-potency multivitamin and amino acid–chelated mineral complex (see section 430 above for optimal supplement contents)—1 twice daily, A.M. and P.M. Essential for general health of hair.
- A broad-spectrum antioxidant formula (see section 430 above for optimal supplement contents)—1 twice daily, A.M. and P.M. Aids in replenishing antioxidants and protecting hair from oxidative damage.

If your multivitamin-mineral complex and antioxidant formula do not contain the following supplements, add them separately to your daily intake:

- Essential fatty acids (flaxseed or any omega-3 fatty acid), 1,000 mg.—Prevents dry, brittle hair; improves texture.
- Silica, 500 mg., 1–3 daily—Aids in forestalling hair loss; helps keep hair shiny.
- Biotin and inositol, 50–100 mg.—Helps prevent hair loss; vital for hair growth.

- Coenzyme-Q10, 60 mg.—Helps improve scalp circulation.
- L-cysteine, 1 g. (Take between meals with juice or water.)—Cysteine is the chief protein constituent of hair, and can help keep tresses looking lustrous.
- MSM (methylsulfonylmethane), 1,000 mg.—Helps promote thicker and shinier hair.
- B complex, 50–100 mg. with pantothenic acid, folic acid, and PABA—Essential for hair growth; can help hair retain natural color.
- Beta-carotene, 10,000 IU—Works with the B vitamins to keep hair shiny.

Keep in mind that it is normal to lose 50–100 hairs a day.

432. Vitamins for Hands and Feet

Your hands take lots of abuse. Detergents strip away natural oils, and water and weather alone can cause chapping. Rubber gloves are a good idea, but if you already have splits in your skin or some sort of dermatitis, they should *not* be put directly on your hands. (A pair of cotton gloves beneath the rubber ones will absorb perspiration and prevent reinfection.) Also, do not use cornstarch in the gloves; it can promote the growth of microorganisms. If you want to use something to absorb the moisture, try plain unscented talcum powder.

As for toenails and fingernails, the best remedy for problems is diet. Gelatin is commonly accepted as the cure for weak nails, but this is a misconception. The nails do need protein, but gelatin is a poor supplier. Not only are two essential amino acids missing, but another amino acid, glycine, is supplied in amounts you do not need. Two supplements that have been shown to produce a marked increase in the thickness of brittle nails are biotin and silicon. As a regimen, I'd suggest taking 2.5 mg. of biotin and 10 mg. of silicon daily. But keep in mind that keratin is the primary protein in nails, so be sure your diet includes enough vitamin C, zinc, B vitamins, and amino acids, particularly cisteine and methionine, for your body to manufacture it.

SUPPLEMENTS

Take with meals unless otherwise indicated.

- An all-natural, high-potency multivitamin and amino acid–chelated mineral complex (see section 430 for optimal supplement contents)—1 twice daily, A.M. and P.M. Promotes health, growth, and strength of nails.
- A broad-spectrum antioxidant formula (see section 430 for optimal supplement contents)—1 twice daily, A.M. and P.M.—Helps protect against free radical damage to tissues.

If your multivitamin-mineral complex and antioxidant formula do not contain the following supplements, add them separately to your daily intake.

- RNA/DNA complex—Stimulates formation of new cells; helps improve skin texture and nail strength.
- B complex, 50–100 mg., with pantothenic acid— Helps build resistance to fungus infections; vital to nail growth.
- Beta-carotene, 10,000 IU—Aids in preventing splitting nails.
- Silica, 500 mg., one to three times daily—Helps prevent white spots and peeling nails.

- Vitamin E, 400 IU succinate dry form—Necessary for proper utilization of vitamin A.
- Zinc, 15–50 mg—Aids in strengthening brittle nails and eliminating white spots.

433. Natural Cosmetics—What Could Be in Them?

Many cosmetics nowadays are advertised as "natural," but looking at the ingredients can cause you to wonder. To be sure of what you're getting, read the label carefully. The following explanation of cosmetic ingredients should make things clearer.

Amyl dimethyl PABA—a sunscreening agent from PABA, a B-complex factor

Annatto—a vegetable color obtained from the seeds of a tropical plant

Avocado oil—a vegetable oil obtained from avocados

Caprylic/capric triglyceride—an emollient obtained from coconut oil

Carrageenan—a natural thickening agent from dried Irish moss

Castor oil—an emollient oil collected from the pressing of castor bean seeds

Cetyl alcohol—a component of vegetable oils

Cetyl palmitate—a component of palm and coconut oils

Citric acid—a natural organic acid found widely in citrus plants

Cocamide DEA—a thickener obtained from coconut oil

Coconut oil—obtained by pressing the kernels of the seeds of the coconut palm

Decyl oleate—obtained from tallow or coconut oil

Diethenolamine—can be an irritant, used to lighten skin

Disodium monolaneth-5-sulfosuccinate—obtained from lanolin and used to improve the texture of hair

Formaldehyde—an irritant

Fragrance—oils obtained from flowers, grasses, roots, and stems that give off a pleasant or agreeable odor

Glyceryl stearate—an organic emulsifier obtained from glycerin

Goat milk whey—protein-rich whey obtained from goat's milk

Hydrogenated castor oil—a waxy material obtained from castor oil

Hydroquinone—may be cancer-causing

Imidzaolidinyl urea—a preservative derived naturally as a product of protein metabolism (hydrolysis)

Lanolin alcohol—a constituent of lanolin that performs as an emollient and emulsifier

Laureth-3—an organic material obtained from coconut and palm oils

Methyl glucoside sesquistearate—an organic emulsifier obtained from a natural simple sugar

Mineral oil—an organic emollient and lubricant

Monoethanolamine—similar use as ammonia

Olive oil—a natural oil obtained from olives

Paraffin—wax to make surfaces shiny

Peanut oil—a vegetable oil obtained from peanuts

Pectin—derived from citrus fruits and apple peel

PEG lanolin—an emollient and emulsifier obtained from lanolin

Petrolatum—petroleum jelly

POE (20) methyl glucoside sesquistearate—an organic emulsifier from a simple natural sugar

Potassium sorbate—obtained from sorbic acid found in the berries of mountain ash

Pthalates—nail polish solvents

Safflower oil-hybrid—a natural emollient obtained from a strain of specially cultivated plants

Sesame oil—oil of pressed sesame seeds

Sodium cetyl sulfate—a detergent and emulsifier obtained from coconut oil

Sodium laureth sulfate—a detergent obtained from coconut oil

Sodium lauryl sulfate—a detergent obtained from coconut oil

Sodium PCA—a naturally occurring humectant found in the skin, where it acts as a natural moisturizer

Sorbic acid—a natural preservative derived from berries of mountain ash

Triclosan—artificial antibacterial and antiviral, not generally recognized as safe

Triethanolamine—PH balancer, can be toxic and cause allergies

Tocopherol—a natural vitamin E

Undecylenamide DEA—a natural preservative derived from castor oil

Water—the universal solvent, and the major constituent of all living material

434. Not-So-Pretty Drugs

Medications are necessary for certain conditions, but doctors often fail to mention their possible side effects. It is a rare physician who puts his patient on the pill and tells her that her face might break out, or that she might suffer hair loss; but many women on oral contraceptives find this out soon enough. In fact, many drugs can be the cause of skin and other cosmetic problems. The following is a list of just a few:

Alfenta	Skin rash, flushing
Codeine	Skin rash, itching, sweating
Coumadin	Skin rash, itching, hives
Darvon	Skin rash, flaking skin, itching
Demerol	Skin rash, flushing, water retention
Doxycycline	Rashes, open sores, teeth discoloration
Fentanyl	Flushing, sweating, allergic reactions
Miltown	Welts, flaking skin, itching
Nembutal	Skin rash
Phenobarbital	Rash, itchy skin, swollen eyelids
Quaalude	Pimples, welts
Talwin	Rash, facial swelling, skin peeling
Tetracycline	Taken during pregnancy and in infancy may cause permanent discoloration of child's teeth
Thorazine	Peeling skin, jaundice, welts, swelling
Tofranil	Rash, itchy skin, jaundice
Tuinal	Can aggravate existing skin condition
Valium	Jaundice, rash, swollen patches

DID YOU KNOW?

- Gelatin is a poor cure for weak nails.
- It is normal to lose 50–100 hairs a day.
- Collagen in antiaging creams cannot be absorbed by the skin.

---

435. Any Questions About Chapter XVIII?

What do you think of jojoba oil as a beauty aid?
Personally, I think it's one of the best. It's available in

a variety of forms—an oil, a cream, a soap, a shampoo—and it works wonders naturally!

For example: As a moisturizer, use a few drops under your makeup. Massage gently into your skin, particularly around the eyes where lines occur. (Be careful to avoid direct contact with the eyes and if any irritation results, discontinue use.) At night, use the oil to soften your skin as you sleep. Just apply a light layer over your face and neck—after they've had a good cleansing, of course.

The oil can also be used to soften skin after showers (all you need is a few drops) and as a luxuriant bath oil (again, just a few drops). For dry, chapped, or recently shaved skin, it should be applied directly.

After shampooing your hair, try rubbing a few drops of the oil into your hair and scalp. (Don't rinse.) Daily use will help even the driest hair return to its natural luster.

My nails just won't grow. I've tried all sorts of vitamins, but they don't work. Where do I go from here?

It's possible that you might have a thyroid problem, so you might want to check with a nutritionally oriented physician. (See section 462.)

In the meanwhile, you could try silica, an organic herb that's also known as horsetail and *Equisetum arvense,* which is changed by the body into readily available calcium—which nourishes nails, skin, hair, bones, and the body's connective tissue.

My hairdresser told me I should look into something called amor crescido. What is it?

A natural nutrient for your hair. Used for centuries by indigenous communities in the Amazon rain forest as a treatment for thinning hair, amor crescido is a plant extract (*Portulaca pilosa*) that is extremely rich in mucilage, vitamins A, B1, B2, and C. It stimulates hair growth and volume by nourishing the scalp with its inherent nutrients. It's available in shampoos and conditioners that usually also contain sea kelp extract, which increases circulation to hair follicles. It may also be helpful in minimizing dandruff and repairing damaged hair.

Do vitamins in cosmetics work?

They do work—but they don't work miracles. The skin's job is to protect against substances entering the body. Vitamins in cosmetics have difficulty entering beyond the skin's top two or three layers. Formulas containing vitamins A, C, and E do have some effect on these layers. For instance, although not absorbed at high levels, a form of vitamin A (tretinoin) can act on the skin cells, stimulate the production of new ones, and in so doing improve the appearance the skin. Vitamins C and E (often included in cosmetics because their antioxidant properties act as natural preservatives) have shown some effect at protecting against the aging effects of free radicals. However, few cosmetics on the market have high enough levels of these vitamins to make any long-term difference and neither one is very well absorbed into the skin. Panthenol, a provitamin form of B5, traps moisture in the top layer of skin, making it feel softer and appear smoother. It also can plump up the skin, making wrinkles less apparent. But antiaging creams with collagen have little effect since the collagen molecules are too big to be absorbed in the skin. For lasting beauty results, let your vitamins work from the inside out.

XIX

STAYING YOUNG, ENERGETIC, AND SEXY

436. Slowing the Aging Process

Aging is caused by the degeneration of cells. Our bodies are made up of millions of these cells, each with a life of somewhere around two years or less. But before a cell dies, it reproduces itself. Why, then, you might wonder, shouldn't we look the same now as we did ten years ago? The reason is that with each successive reproduction, the cell goes through some alteration—basically, deterioration. So as our cells change and deteriorate, we grow old.

The good news is that deteriorating cells can be rejuvenated if provided with substances that directly nourish them—substances such as nucleic acids.

DNA (deoxyribonucleic acid) and RNA (ribonucleic acid) are our nucleic acids. DNA is essentially a chemical boilerplate for new cells. It sends out RNA molecules like a team of well-trained workers to form them. When DNA stops giving the orders to RNA, new cell construction ceases—as does life. But by helping the body stay well supplied with nucleic acids, you can look and feel six to twelve years younger than you actually are.

We need 1½ g. of nucleic acid daily. Though the body can produce its own nucleic acids, they are broken down too quickly into less useful compounds and need to be supplied from external sources if the aging process is to be slowed.

Foods rich in nucleic acids are wheat germ, bran, spinach, asparagus, mushrooms, fish (especially sardines, salmon, and anchovies), chicken liver, oatmeal, onions, and certain types of nutritional yeast that clearly say on the label "rich in RNA and DNA."

Soon after I started eating a diet high in nucleic acids and taking RNA-DNA supplements many years ago, I noticed a dramatic difference in how I looked and felt. I had more energy and my skin looked healthier and more youthful. Many clients and friends experienced similar results. Though a high–nucleic acid diet and RNA-DNA supplementation might not reverse the aging process, I believe it can slow it down.

CAUTION: *Gout and certain forms of arthritis may be aggravated by a diet rich in nucleic acids. If you have these conditions, check with your physician before eating these foods or taking any supplements.*

OTHER ANTIAGING SUPPLEMENTS

SOD (superoxide dismutase) is one of the most popular arrivals in the battle to combat aging. (See section 129). This enzyme fortifies the body against the ravages of free radicals, destructive molecules that speed the aging process by destroying healthy cells as well as attacking collagen ("cement" that holds cells together).

As we age, our bodies produce less SOD, so supplementation—along with a natural diet that restricts free radical formation—can help increase our energetic and productive years. It's important to note, though, that SOD can become inactive very quickly if essential minerals such as zinc, copper, and manganese are not supplied. Supplements of sod should be time-release for better absorption.

Grape-seed extract is also being touted as a potent free-radical fighter and antiaging supplement. It contains *proanthocyanidins,* bioflavonoids that greatly enhance the activity of vitamin C. By helping vitamin C enter cells, grape-seed extract aids in strengthening the cell membranes and protecting the cells from oxidative damage. It can improve circulation, strengthen capillaries, and help protect collagen fibers—necessary for the growth and repair of cells—from damage caused over the years by free radicals. (Proanthocyanidins are also in grape skins, bilberries, cranberries, blackcurrants, and green and black tea.)

As an antiaging supplement, I suggest taking 1–2 grape-seed extract capsules (30–100 mg.) daily.

Coenzyme-Q10, a substance that can be synthesized by the body (although it is also obtained from food) is used by our cells during the process of respiration, and deficiencies are common in the course of normal aging. In fact, studies have shown that reduced levels of coenzyme-Q10, which shares many of vitamin E's antioxidant properties, may directly contribute to aging and that increasing levels can slow the process, as well as:

- reduce the risk of heart attack (aid respiration of the heart muscle; help provide a protective effect against viral-caused heart inflammations; help prevent cardiac arrhythmias; minimize myocardial injury caused

by heart bypass surgery; reduce frequency of angina attacks)
- stimulate the immune system
- aid in the treatment of periodontal disease
- help lower blood pressure
- aid in the prevention of toxicity from drugs used to treat many diseases associated with aging.

As a supplement, I recommend one 100 mg. capsule twice daily with food.

DHEA (dehydroepiandrosterone), a natural hormone that is produced by the adrenal glands and the most abundant steroid hormone in the body, decreases as we age. (Steroids are a class of compounds that help balance emotions and increase the body's ability to handle stress, among other functions.) About the age of forty-five, we produce only *half* of the DHEA we produced at age twenty. By age seventy, production falls to almost nothing. Leading researchers link the decline in hormones such as DHEA with the physical and mental decline of normal aging. Boosting DHEA back to youthful levels may prevent and even reverse many age-related problems. Older people given DHEA have an increased sense of well-being, more energy, an increase in lean body mass, and produce more sex hormone.

DHEA has been found to strengthen the immune system, slow down the production of fats that contribute to obesity, offer postmenopausal women protection against heart disease, reduce fatigue, increase cognitive function, and enhance mood and stress responses.

New research indicates that DHEA may be a promising treatment for osteoporosis and depression, as well as in reducing the symptoms of lupus, an autoimmune disorder for which, at this time, there is no cure. (Anyone with lupus should certainly talk to his or her physician about trying DHEA.)

If you are over forty, have your DHEA level checked by a physician. The usual dose is one 25 mg. tablet daily for women over age forty; one 50 mg. tablet for men over forty. As a supplement, look for "pharmaceutical grade" on the DHEA label—it ensures as pure a product as possible.

An advantage for women in taking DHEA (or DHEA combined with pregnenolone) instead of hormone replacement is that there is apparently no effect on the endometrium—even if the dose is large enough to cause changes in the lining of the vagina. And, with just DHEA alone, there's no need to worry about balancing an estrogen dose with just the right dose of progesterone.

CAUTION: *DHEA is a hormone and can theoretically stimulate the growth of hormone-dependent cancers. If you have a history of prostate or breast cancer, I advise that you not use DHEA. Abdominally obese postmenopausal women are known to be at a higher risk of breast cancer and are advised not to take DHEA supplements unless a blood test indicates a deficiency.*

Pregnenolone, produced in the brain and adrenal cortex from cholesterol, functions as a parent hormone, converting into DHEA, estrogen, testosterone, progesterone, and other hormones.

Touted as a general antiaging supplement for men and women, pregnenolone levels peak in our thirties and then decline. Recent studies suggest that supplements may improve concentration and memory, act as an antidepressant, reduce stress, and help relieve symptoms of rheumatoid arthritis, lupus, and multiple sclerosis.

The usual supplement dose is 5–10 mg. daily.

CAUTION: *Pregnenolone can elevate levels of sex hormones and interact adversely with other medications. It should not be taken by pregnant women. Before taking this hormone, I recommend that you consult with a knowledgeable physician.*

437. Controlling Cortisol—the Stress or Death Hormone

Secreted by the adrenal glands, cortisol is an important part of the body's response to stress. The stress can be physical, environmental, chemical, or psychological (and all of these different sources are cumulative in their effects). Under normal circumstances, cortisol is involved in a variety of functions, from regulating blood pressure to proper glucose metabolism, but during fight-or-flight stress situations, it is secreted in higher than normal levels.

While small increases give you that quick burst of energy for survival, if called upon too often without giving the body a chance to return to being relaxed/normal, prolonged high levels in the bloodstream can create chronic to severe inflammation that eventually causes premature aging and often leads to an earlier death. For this reason, cortisol is frequently referred to as "the death hormone."

Prolonged high levels of cortisol can lead to:
- Higher blood pressure
- Suppression of DHEA
- Osteoporosis
- Loss of muscle tone
- Impaired cognitive function
- Reduced growth hormone, testosterone, and estrogen
- Suppressed thyroid function

- Lowered immunity
- Hyperglycemia
- Increased abdominal fat (associated with elevated cholesterol, heart attacks, and strokes)

FYI: Normally, cortisol levels rise in the morning and drop in the evening. (In night workers, this pattern may be reversed.) If you do not have this fluctuation, you may have overactive adrenal glands and possibly Cushing's syndrome. If you have too little cortisol, you may suffer from chronic fatigue, exhaustion, and Addison's disease.

PERSONAL ADVICE: *Yes, you can reduce stress with nutrition—and without stressing about it. Quick-start your regimen by cutting back on sugar and eating low-glycemic foods (see section 414), put "Rest" on your to-do list, and supplement your diet with the following:*

MVP twice daily with food.

B-Complex, 50 mg. twice daily with food.

Calcium and magnesium, 250 mg., and 125 mg., twice daily. (Last dose can be taken at bedtime.)

5 HTP, DL-phenylalanine, and tyrosine combination taken between meals. (If a combination tablet is unavailable, take separately: HTP, 50 mg.; DL-phenylalanine, 375 mg.; and tyrosine, 500 mg.

Optional: If you are over fifty years of age: DHEA, 25 mg. for women, 50 mg. for men, once daily.

CAUTION: *DHEA is a hormone and can theoretically stimulate the growth of hormone-dependent cancers. If you have a history of prostate or breast cancer, I advise that you not use DHEA. Abdominally obese postmenopausal women are known to be at a higher risk of breast cancer and should* *not take DHEA supplements unless a blood test indicates a deficiency.*

438. Lifesaving Nitric Oxide

It took a Nobel Prize winner—Dr. Louis J. Ignarro—to discover a gas that occurs naturally in the body that may do more than any drug to prevent heart attack and stroke—nitric oxide!

What Nitric Oxide Can Do for You:

- Help prevent blood clots
- Dilate blood vessels
- Regulate blood pressure
- Reduce arterial plaque (the underlying cause of heart disease)
- Lower cholesterol

Beginning in early adulthood, our nitric oxide levels decline as we age. The bad news is that because nitric oxide is a gas, it can't be taken in supplement form. The good news is that taking other supplements can increase the production of nitric oxide.

SUPPLEMENT REGIMEN
L-arginine, 2,000–3,000 mg. twice daily

L-citrulline, 400–600 mg. daily (helps arginine enter cells quickly)

Multivitamin mineral complex (with 200–400 IU natural vitamin E) daily

Vitamin C, 500 mg. twice daily

Plus: Add more dietary fiber to your meals (see section 137), drink eight or more 8-ounce glasses of water a day, and do at least twenty minutes of aerobic exercise three days a week to stimulate cells to keep producing nitric oxide.

439. Basic Keep-Yourself-Young Program

Along with proper diet, a good supplement regimen is important to the success of looking, feeling, and keeping yourself young. (MVP: See section 246.)

If you are over forty years of age add:

Vitamin E succinate 100 IU A.M. and P.M.

Vitamin C, 500 mg. with bioflavonoids A.M. and P.M.

Coenzyme-Q10, 200 mg. daily

SOD, 125 mcg. time-release daily

Ginkgo biloba, 60 mg., 1–3 standardized capsules daily

Cayenne pepper, 500 mg., 1–3 capsules daily

For women: soy isolate complex with 1,000 mg. calcium and 500 mg. magnesium, 1 daily

For men: soy isolate complex with 500 mg. calcium and 150 mg. magnesium, 1 daily

CBD, 25 mg. daily

Astaxanthin, 5 mg. daily

440. High-Pep Energy Regimen

Whether you want to feel good or just look good, exercise, diet, and the right supplements are the tickets to high energy.

If you're not into jogging, can't afford the sneakers, don't play tennis, find yourself reluctant to swim in twenty-below weather, and hate calisthenics, I have the perfect exercise for you—jumping rope.

A jump rope is inexpensive, convenient (you can take it everywhere), and lots of fun to use. And it works! In terms of calories burned, jumping rope can outdo bicycling, tennis, and swimming. An average person of about 150 pounds uses up 720 calories an hour jumping rope (120–140 turns per minute). When you realize that an hour of tennis uses up only 420 calories, you have a better idea of just how good jumping rope can be for you.

For keeping energy high, remember to eat a combination of 2 protein foods (or a protein drink) at each meal; drink at least 6 glasses of water daily (a half hour before or after meals); avoid refined sugar, flour, tobacco, alcohol, tea, coffee, soft drinks, and processed and fried foods.

A good pep-up protein drink:

1 tbsp. whey powder

1 tbsp. lecithin granules

2 tbsp. *acidophilus* (nondairy) liquid

Blend with low-fat or nonfat soy milk, water, or juice, with 3–4 ice cubes, for 1 minute. (Add fresh or frozen fruit if desired. A peeled frozen banana tastes great!)

441. High-Pep Supplements

With breakfast:

MVP (see section 246)

Vitamin E (dry form), 400 IU

Coenzyme-Q10 complex, 100 mg.

Women: soy isolate complex with 1,000 mg. calcium and 500 mg. magnesium

Men: soy isolate complex with 500 mg. calcium and 250 mg. magnesium

With dinner:

MVP (see section 246)

Coenzyme-Q10 complex, 100 mg.

Women: soy isolate complex with 1,000 mg. calcium and 500 mg. magnesium

Men (over 45): saw palmetto, pygeum, zinc, pumpkin seed oil complex, 2 with meals

442. Spicing Up Sex Naturally

Sex-boosting drugs, such as Viagra, Cialis, and Levitra, used for treating erectile dysfunction, work well by increasing blood flow to the penis, but they have potentially serious side effects (including heart failure) and very little—if any—effect on stimulating libido or heightening sexual sensation in men or women.

As Dr. Ray Sahelian points out in his landmark book *Natural Sex Boosters*, sex-enhancing herbs have been used successfully and safely for hundreds of years in numerous countries around the world—increasing desire, strengthening erections, and significantly amplifying genital sensation for men and women.

FOUR SUPPLEMENTS FOR FABULOUS SEX

Ashwagandha: Increases sexual desire and boosts production of nitric oxide, which is known to enhance penile erection and vaginal sensitivity. (May cause drowsiness. Do not drive after taking this herb.)

Suggested dose: 300–500 mg. one to two times daily on an empty stomach

Horny goat weed: Increases libido in both sexes and contains flavonoids that dilate blood vessels to promote firmer erections in men.

Suggested dose: 500–2,000 mg. daily. Start with 500 mg. and increase as needed. (May cause restlessness and insomnia.)

Muira puama: Improves libido while increasing orgasm

intensity, genital sensitivity, and prompting sexual fantasies in men and women.

Suggested dose: 500–1,000 mg. capsules, three consecutive days each week in the A.M. (May cause restlessness and insomnia.)

Tribulus: Promotes firmer erections for men and increases libido for both sexes.

Suggested dose: 500–1,000 mg. daily every other week to minimize the risk of restlessness and increased body temperature.

It's advisable to start with one herb. After a week or two you can combine it with others to heighten the effect, but cut the recommended dose in half to avoid the possibility of side effects, such as restlessness and insomnia.

Remember, vitamins that keep up your energy levels (see section 441) will also do a lot for your sexual performance.

CAUTION: *Before starting this or any new supplement regimen, be sure to check with your physician or a nutritionally oriented doctor, especially if you have a specific physical problem or are taking any medication.*

443. Foods, Herbs, and More Supersupplements for Sexier Sex

Incorporate some of the following into your daily diet and enjoy the results:

Asparagus	Ginseng
Avena sativa	Kava
Avocados	Oysters
Barley	Pine nuts
Brewer's yeast	Quince
Cardamom	Sarsaparilla

Carrots	Shiitake mushrooms
Cinnamon	Soy foods
Coriander	Wheat germ
Fertilized chicken eggs	Whole grains
Ginkgo biloba	Yohimbe (see section 227)

Supplement Regimen

MVP (see section 246)
Vitamin E (dry form), 400 IU daily
Zinc, 15–50 mg. (chelated) daily
Ginkgo biloba complex, 60 mg. twice daily
Women over 40: DHEA 25 mg. daily
Men over 50: DHEA 50 mg. daily
Men: Arginine, 3–6 g. 45 minutes before sex

DID YOU KNOW?

- Soy foods can increase your sex drive.
- A single natural supplement can help people with age-related memory problems regain twelve years of brain power.
- One handful of walnuts daily reduces your risk of developing blood clots.

---

444. Any Questions About Chapter XIX?

I understand that octacosanol can improve a male's sexual performance enormously. What do you feel about this?

I feel that a lot is still going to depend on the male involved. It is true, though, that octacosanol (which is a natural food substance present in very small amounts in many vegetable oils, the levels of alfalfa and wheat, wheat germ, and other foods) has an energy-releasing function, increasing strength and stamina, and in laboratory experiments it seems to improve reproductive disturbances.

If you try it, don't be impatient, it often takes four to six weeks for beneficial effects from octacosanol to be noticed.

Always keep in mind, too, that an energizing diet of raw or lightly cooked foods, rich in B vitamins and amino acids, will contribute to a good sex life.

I'm an active, happily married forty-five-year-old woman, but my sex drive seems to have stalled. What natural love-life enhancers would you recommend?

Along with following my MVP vitamin regimen (see section 246), I'd suggest you increase your diet of soy foods. Soybeans are rich in plant estrogens called isoflavones. They can alleviate some of the symptoms of perimenopause that often interfere with sexual desire. You might also want to have your DHEA levels checked. If they're low, 25 mg. of supplemental DHEA daily could elevate your libido. Additionally, I'd suggest you try the herb damiana, which has the reputation of being a sexual stimulant. Take 1 capsule one to three times daily before meals. Add a little candlelight to the evening, and you may be pleasantly surprised with the results.

I am eighty-two years old and in pretty good health, but hardly the man I used to be. I have difficulty just carrying groceries home these days and often have to ask a neighbor to do my shopping. Is there a safe energizing supplement for someone my age?

There's one that I believe might be tailor-made for you—beta-alanine. It's a non-essential amino acid, found in meat, poultry, and fish, that occurs naturally in the body and is widely used by athletes and bodybuilders to increase muscle mass, strength and aerobic endurance. Researchers in England gave it to a group of older men and women and saw a marked increase in fitness after ninety days, suggesting that beta-alanine could help prevent falls and prolong independent living among your age group.

The test group received just 2.4 g. daily, but the optimal dose is 5 g. daily taken with a high-carbohydrate meal. It may take three to four weeks before you notice any results. You might experience a tingling sensation on the skin for about an hour in the first few weeks directly after taking the supplement, but this will subside after a week or two. If you don't notice any improvement in three months, discontinue use.

What is Spanish fly and is it really a natural aphrodisiac?

Far from it! Spanish fly is actually cantharides made from the outer skeletons of beetles. It causes itching, but not necessarily for sex. In fact, it's a poisonous substance that can be anything *but* a turn-on. It has been linked to convulsions and kidney disorders, and has been reported to make urination virtually impossible, to say nothing of causing men to experience extremely painful erections.

What's legally marketed in this country as Spanish fly is generally nothing more than dried herbs that are no more potent than parsley. I'd advise saving your money for a romantic dinner. As old-fashioned as it sounds, I feel that a candlelight dinner will beat a beetle skeleton as an aphrodisiac every time.

I've been told that there's something called DMG that is an aphrodisiac. Have you heard of it and does it work?

I've heard of it, but I can't vouch for its effectiveness. DMG is dimethylglycine, a derivative of the amino acid glycine, found mostly in seeds and grains. It aids in increasing the supply of oxygen to the bloodstream and body tissues. Those touting it as an aphrodisiac say that the increased oxygen in the tissues enhances your sexual response. (Maybe eating those Wheaties does work.) Anyway, it is available as a supplement, so you might want to give it a try. It might not be your ticket to ecstasy—but it won't hurt.

My father had macular degeneration. I'm a sixty-eight-year-old photographer and very worried about losing my eyesight. Can you recommend any supplements that might lower my risk of inheriting the disease?

Age-related macular degeneration is not necessarily inherited, but, yes, there are vitamins that could lower your risk. Because high blood levels of the amino acid homocysteine have been linked to the disease, supplements of folic acid, B6, and B12—which reduce blood levels of homocysteine—are what you want.

Are there brain nutrients? If so, what are they and what do you recommend for someone who's not old but worried that she's already too forgetful?

Are there brain nutrients? There definitely are. And for anyone who's starting to worry about having too many senior moments—or the possibility of age-related cognitive decline (ARCD), which may begin as early as age forty-five—ensuring that these nutrients are in your diet can make a memorable difference in your life. Among those I've found to be most brain-beneficial are:

Vitamin B6—supplements of 50–75 mg. daily in equal amounts with B1 and B12, which may also help protect your brain from shrinking. (See sections 31, 36 and 37.)

Vitamin E—supplements of 200–400 IU daily. (See section 48.)

Selenium—supplements of 100–200 mcg. daily.

Phosphatidylserine (PS, a phospholipid that already occurs naturally in brain tissue, helping to relay chemical messages from brain cell to brain cell)—supplements of 200 mg. daily can help regain twelve years of brain power.

Ginkgo biloba—supplements of 60 mg. standardized capsules or tablets, one to three times daily.

Dimethyl aminoethanol (DMAE, also found in the brain, and in foods such as sardines and anchovies)—supplements of 1–2 tablets daily. DMAE is available in a combination formula of DMAE, ginkgo biloba, PS, and B vitamins inositol and choline.

Huperzine A—an extract derived from Chinese club moss and found to be a potent memory enhancer. Look for huperzine A (or club moss tea) in formulas designed to enhance mental function.

Vinpocetine—a purified extract of periwinkle (*Vinca minor*) found to be a a powerful cognitive enhancer, facilitating blood flow to the brain, improving short- and long-term mental function.

Wild blueberry extract—deemed "miracle berries" by *Prevention* magazine, this potent antioxidant supplement aids in cerebral circulation and helps support brain and memory function.

XX

SUPPLEMENTS TO BOOST YOUR IMMUNE SYSTEM

Your immune system consists of a complex of cells that process natural chemicals that constantly defend your body against invading pathogens, influenza viruses, toxins, and bacteria. The key to keeping your immune system healthy, so that it can prevent infections and disease, is to eat healthy foods, get enough restful sleep and exercise, and take the right supplements.

445. Foods, Herbs, and Supplements to Keep Your Immune System Working Efficiently

1. Andrographis: This herb controls a terpenoid compound found to have anti-viral effects against respiratory disease-causing viruses.
2. Astragalus: This herb has been used in traditional Chinese medicine. It has been shown in antiviral research that its extract can improve immune-related responses.

3. B-complex vitamins: B6 and B12 are important for a healthy immune response.

4. Vitamin C: This vitamin supports the various immune cell functions and enhances their ability to protect against infection. It also keeps your immune system healthy by clearing out old cells and replacing them with new healthy ones. It is an antioxidant that guards against oxidative stress, which can negatively affect your immune system.

5. Cistanche: This ancient herb is rich in echinacosides, which promote increased development of T cells and natural killer cells.

6. Curcumin: The active ingredient of the herb turmeric, it is one of the strongest antioxidant and anti-inflammatory supplements available. Studies demonstrate that curcumin inhibits the enzyme cycloxygenase-2 (COX-2), which causes inflammation. Curcumin inhibits a nuclear factor protein complex that controls many genes involved in inflammation and blocks the synthesis of nitric oxide. Nitric oxide releases inflammatory factors. Curcumin lowers by 60 percent levels of interleukin-1, which plays a central role in the regulation of inflammation. It reduces the expression of inflammatory makers of astrocytes that support and protect brain neurons.

7. Vitamin D3: This fat-soluble nutrient is really a hormone and is essential to the health and function of your immune system. Vitamin D enhances the pathogen-fighting effects of monocytes and macrophages—white blood cells that are an important part of our immune defense and decreasing inflammation.

8. DHEA (dehydroepiandrosterone): A natural hormone that is produced by the adrenal glands and is the most abundant steroid hormone in your body,

DHEA decreases with age. Supplementing with DHEA to return to youthful levels of the hormone may prevent and even reverse many age-related problems. You will feel an increased sense of well-being, your body will produce more energy and more sex hormones. DHEA supplementation strengthens your immune system, as well as slowing down the production of fats that contribute to obesity. You will notice a reduction in fatigue, increased cognitive function, and enhanced mood and stress response.

9. Echinacea: It has been shown to improve immune health, and may have antiviral effects against several respiratory viruses, including respiratory syncytial virus and rhinoviruses.

10. Elderberry: In test tube studies elderberry extract demonstrated potent antibacterial and antiviral potential, showing success against bacterial pathogens responsible for urinary tract infections as well as strains of influenza viruses. It has been shown to enhance your immune response system.

11. Fish oil: A source of essential fatty acids EPA and DHA, fish oil helps reduce harmful cholesterol and triglyceride levels, which in turn can lower the risk of heart attack and stroke. Fish oil also helps reduce the "stickiness" of blood platelet cells and the amount of fibrin in the blood, which can help prevent clot formation. This supplement also helps prevent arteriosclerosis and reduces inflammation.

12. Garlic: A powerful anti-inflammatory and antiviral, garlic enhances your health by stimulating protective white blood cells like NK cells and macrophages. High-allicin garlic extract, 600–9,000 mg., can be taken daily and is available in an odorless form.

13. Lactoferrin: At doses of 300–1,200 mg. daily, this natural component of mother's milk boosts killer cell activity and can prevent certain viruses from binding to cell membranes and entering the cell, where they replicate.

14. Licorice: The active ingredient in licorice, glycyrrhiza, can protect you against viral infections.

15. Medicinal mushrooms (*reishi, coryceps, lion's mate, maitake, shiitake, and turkey tail*): These mushrooms can promote the maturation and activation of immune system cells such as T cells, natural killer cells, dendrite cells, and macrophages. Lab studies have shown that reishi augments the function of both the innate and adaptive immune system. The innate immune system is your body's first line of defense. It responds rapidly to potentially harmful insults such as viruses, bacteria, and cancer cells. Reishi mushrooms support your body's production of endogenous enzymes such as SOD and glutathione, which support your natural immune defenses against free radical damage.

16. Melatonin: A hormone produced in the pineal gland of your brain. It supports your immune system. High doses over 10 mg. of melatonin taken at bedtime induce a potent immune response. This high dose can facilitate the sleep one often needs to fend off an infection.

17. Propolis: This bioflavonoid produced by bees appears to protect against viruses, especially in the elderly and others with a weak immune system. Dosages of 200–500 mg. can be taken daily.

18. Pu-erh tea: A fermented black tea that has been shown to be a benefit in one's aging immune system,

this tea increases natural killer and T cells, which provide direct antibacterial and antiviral effects. Subjects who supplemented with this tea extract showed improvement in immune status.

19. Selenium: A mineral essential for immune health, selenium functions as an antiviral defense against influenza strains, including H1N1. Dosages of 100–200 mcg. can be taken daily.

20. Whey protein: 2–4 scoops of 1½ tablespoons a day provide a glutathione boost which can ramp up antibody response.

21. White peony root extract: This root has been used in China for more than twelve hundred years to balance the immune system. Its active ingredient and other compounds have been shown to help maintain the balanced responsiveness, sensitivity, and strength of a properly modulated immune system. It produces immune homeostasis—optimal immune health—by limiting production of inflammatory molecules and naturally balancing inflammation, thus suppressing pro-inflammatory cells.

22. Zinc: Zinc has shown a direct effect of inhibiting the ability of certain viruses to latch on to the cells in the back of your throat, where they multiply and can descend into your lungs to potentially cause pneumonia.

XXI

CBD (CANNABIDIOL): THE WONDER SUPPLEMENT OF THE 2020S

CBD is a naturally occurring substance derived from hemp (*Cannabis sativa*). It is a relative of cannabis, but contains none of its psychoactive properties, due to the fact that it contains little or no THC. Its roots are in central Asia, and it is believed to have been first medicinally used around 750 BC. There are more than one hundred cannabinoids in the plant, such as terpenes and CBN. Basically, CBD binds to receptors in your immune system, providing a variety of medicinal benefits. It was patented in 2003 as a neurotransmitter (brain protector) and an antioxidant. Antioxidants are the "good guys" that neutralize the "bad guys" (free radical oxygen molecules) that can speed up the aging process and lead to degenerative diseases.

How does CBD work?
CBD and the other cannabinoids interact with CB1 and CB2 receptors within your endocannabinoid system

to regulate homeostasis (balance). CBD is known for its ability to influence physiological function in your body, such as inducing sleep, improving mood and memory, pain modulation, strengthening immune and cardiovascular function, and improving inflammatory response.

Does CBD have any side effects?

If taken as instructed by a doctor or on the label, there are no known side effects of any consequence. I feel that CBD has side benefits not side effects. If there are untoward effects, it is probably due to the impurities in the oil and substandard manufacturing process. Look for a product that states it is organic (free of pesticides, herbicides, insecticides, and heavy metals such as lead and arsenic).

Is CBD legal and do you need a prescription to obtain it?

CBD extracted from industrial hemp is legal in all fifty states and DC as long as it is grown in accordance with the 2018 Farm Bill and contains less than 0.3 percent by weight of THC. No prescription is required.

What is the dosage?

It is best to start with a smaller amount of CBD and gradually increase to 25–50 mg. daily.

446. History of CBD

In the US hemp and CBD dates back centuries. In 1619 the first general assembly of Virginia established a law requiring farmers to grow hemp: "For hemp also—we do require and enjoin all households of this colony, that have any of those seeds to make trial thereof of the new season." Hemp was even used as a form of currency in tax payments.

Presidents Washington and Jefferson grew hemp on their farms. Benjamin Franklin wrote about hemp in his chronicles and used hemp paper in his publications. The first two drafts of the Declaration of Independence were written on hemp paper, with only the final draft being written on parchment. Betsy Ross even designed a US flag made with hemp.

In 1839, William Brooke O'Shaugnessy, a surgeon, brought cannabis into mainstream medicine after learning of its medicinal benefits in India. By 1850, it had been added to the United States Pharmacopeia, a list of medicines, herbs, and dietary supplements. Later Henry Ford built an automobile of hemp. In 1942, during the hemp prohibition in the US, our government produced a fourteen-minute film entitled *Hemp for Victory*. The idea was to encourage farmers to grow hemp (even though it was illegal) for the war effort, to make products such as military uniforms, parachutes, rope, and sails.

447. Immediate Benefits of CBD

- Nontoxic, not habit forming, and does not create a toxic buildup in your system
- In 2003 the governmental agency the National Institutes of Health patented CBD. The patent states that CBD is neuroprotective and an antioxidant.
- Can relieve discomfort and pain
- Non-psychoactive (no high)
- 100 percent safe and effective
- Can alleviate cancer-related symptoms, such as nausea and vomiting
- Heart healthy and can normalize blood pressure
- Supports positive mental state, including healthy mood and relaxation

- Antipsychotic and may help with schizophrenia
- CBD enhances substance-abuse treatment
- Has been shown to have anti-tumor properties in animals

448. Long-Lasting Benefits When You Use CBD Daily

- Less chronic pain. CBD is able to relieve pain by attaching to the cannabinoid receptors (endocannabinoid system) which naturally occurs in your body.
- Reduces inflammation with the same mechanism as above
- Decreases anxiety such as panic disorder, PTSD, and obsessive compulsion disorder. CBD tells your body to calm down.
- Improves depression, which 300 million people worldwide suffer from
- CBD acts on your brain's receptor for serotonin, a neurotransmitter that regulates mood and social behavior.
- Decreases epileptic seizures. The FDA has approved epidioles (CBD crystal form) to treat two serious kinds of epilepsy in children.
- Antinausea, even from chemotherapy
- Can treat acne, giving you glowing skin
- Decreases the risk of metastatic breast cancer[1]
- Fewer digestive issues. Seventy-four percent of Americans are living with digestive symptoms such as diarrhea, bloating, and abdominal pain.

---

[1] Source: California Pacific Medical Center.

- Better sleep. One out of four Americans develop insomnia every year.
- Can lower blood pressure. The stress- and anxiety-relieving properties can improve blood pressure as well.
- Can lower your risk of type 2 diabetes
- Supports immune system health

XXII

SLAMMING OLD AGE INTO REVERSE

Aging can be defined as deterioration of the physiological function necessary for survival and fertility. Aging is characterized by inflammation, glycation, and mitochondrial decay. Some of the main causes of aging include accumulated cellular damage, caused by free radicals and the shortening of telomeres. Telomeres are structures, located at the ends of chromosomes, that play an important role in cellular division. As we age, telomeres shorten, making cellular division more difficult, which decreases our ability to replace damaged cells.

Smoking tobacco will decrease life expectancy anywhere for three to fifteen years, depending on the amount and length of time a person smokes. Diet can either increase or decrease your longevity as well. Stress, either psychological or physiological, can also be a factor in your longevity. The taking of drugs, prescription or over-the-counter (OTC), is a factor in your life expectancy.

By the year 2050, it is projected that 20 percent of

Americans will be over sixty-five years of age. Today American life expectancy is 78.3 years, yet in Singapore it is over 85 years. We are not dying of old age itself. Most of the reasons for our early demise are inflammatory diseases and conditions such as cancer, dementia, arteriosclerosis, frailty, arthritis, heart disease, stroke, and high blood pressure.

449. Supplements That Support Healthy Aging and Longevity

1. Acetyl-L-carnitine: It supports healthy levels of glutathione, an amino acid molecule utilized by all cells to protect against free radical damage and attacks from foreign compounds.
2. Arginine: It stimulates the release of human growth hormone. It helps metabolize stored body fat and tones up muscle tissue. It also promotes physical and mental alertness.
3. Astragalus: It alleviates fatigue and is an immune system booster.
4. Benfotiamine: It promotes endothelial cell integrity by protecting from the effects of high glucose levels. It also intensifies direct antioxidant capacity and supports DNA function.
5. Black tea: Contains theaflavins and antioxidants, which prevent the damage that can be done by radical oxygen molecules.
6. Carnosine: As we age, proteins in our bodies become irreversibly damaged by glycination reactions, which can lead to alterations of normal cell function. Carnosine is a potent anti-glycination agent, as well as a protector against reactive cytotoxic protein carbonyl species associated with normal aging.

7. Coenzyme-Q10: An antioxidant that your body produces, which declines with aging. It plays an essential role in energy production and protects against cellular damage. It also helps reduce oxidative stress, a condition characterized by an accumulation of free radicals, which accelerate the aging process. This reaction can slow age-related physical decline and improve quality of life in older adults.

8. Collagen: It is an integral component of your skin that helps maintain skin structure. As we age, collagen production slows, causing the acceleration of visible aging.

9. Curcumin: The active ingredient in turmeric, a plant that grows in tropical Asia, its many benefits include:
   o anti-oxidative stress effect
   o anti–joint inflammation
   o liver protection
   o anti-aging effects
   o lipid (fat) lowering effect in obese people
   o stimulates the production of antioxidant enzymes such as SOD, catalase, and glutathione peroxidase

10. Vitamin D3: It increases telomere length. As our cells age, they lose a certain number of base pairs of DNA, known as telomeres, from the end of each chromosome, every time cell division occurs. Telomeres keep our chromosomes intact and functioning to reproduce themselves, the key to healthy aging. Having long telomeres is an indication of a healthy individual. Short telomeres impair the ability of healthy cells to divide and function properly, while longer telomeres are associated with healthy cells and longevity.

11. Gamma tocopherol, NAC, and green tea (EGCG): Help maintain cholesterol levels already within the normal range. They also promote brain health and a

healthy body weight, which benefit immune system function.

12. Lipoic acid: Preserves youthful cellular energy. Helps protect against oxidative stress and reverse the negative effects caused by strokes.

13. Nicotinamide riboside: Promotes youthful cellular production.

14. Pine bark extract: Supports healthy circulation and a healthy inflammation response, as well as helping maintain already healthy glucose levels.

15. Quercetin: Helps your body's cells function optimally. Promotes youthful, healthy cellular function and supports systemic rejuvenation.

16. Resveratrol: A polypeptide-flavonoid family member, it reduces the risk of heart disease and stroke by inhibiting the formation of blood clots. It can also reduce diabetes neuropathy and improve memory. Supports healthy insulin response and helps already healthy glucose levels. Also supports healthy inflammatory response and inhibits oxidation.

450. How to Keep Your Telomeres Healthy and Functional

- Take a polyphenol supplement daily
- Avoid smoking
- Maintain a healthy weight
- Exercise regularly
- Manage your blood sugar
- Maintain a healthy diet
- Maintain a healthy cholesterol
- Check your blood pressure regularly
- Minimize stress
- Have at least 7 to 8 hours of restful sleep per night

451. More Anti-Aging Supplements

1. Crocin: A yellow carotenoid pigment in saffron, it is anti-cancer, anti-inflammatory, anti-anxiety, and anti-diabetic. It is a protectant against mental decline and helps

2. DHEA: Balances emotions, helps handle stress, brings back youthful levels and may prevent and even reverse many age-related problems. It strengthens your immune system and produces more sex hormones.

3. ECGC (green tea): It can slow the aging process by restoring mitochondrial function in cells and acting on pathways involved in aging.

4. Fisetin: A flavonoid compound that can extend life span in animals.

5. Garlic: Powerful antioxidant, anti-inflammatory, and anti-aging agent.

6. Hot chili peppers: Studies suggest these peppers may play a role in the suppression of certain types of cancer.

7. Lipoic acid: A universal antioxidant, lipoic acid helps reverse the negative effects caused by strokes.

8. Lutein: A flavonoid that helps suppress inflammatory cytokines such as Interleukin-1 and tumor necrosis factor-alpha, which are involved in most undesirable consequences of aging.

9. Nicotinamide riboside and nicotinamide "neuroprotective": Both are precursors to nicotinamide adenine dinucleotide (NAD). NAD decreases with age, which can accelerate physical decline and the onset of age-related diseases.

10. PPQ: An antioxidant believed to be a part of the B-complex family. It protects your cells from oxidative damage and supports healthy aging.

11. Pyridoxal-5-phosphate: The active form of vitamin B6, it protects against both lipid and protein glycation reactions. Glycation is the cross-linking of protein and sugar to form nonfunctioning structures, which can lead to alterations of normal cell functions.

12. SAM-e: Promotes the synthesis of chemicals throughout your body that are critical to the vital function of such things as gene expression and DNA repair. According to a 2010 study funded by the National Institute of Mental Health, SAM-e augments existing drug treatments in patients who were resistant to FDA-approved antidepressant drugs. SAM-e is involved in methylation, in which it acts as a methyl donor to support a multitude of chemical reactions such as regulation of gene expression, lipid and mineral metabolism, and membrane structure and fluidity.

13. Sirtuins: A family of proteins that regulate cellular health.

14. Taurine: A brain protector, it strengthens heart function, helps bolster vision, and prevents macular degeneration. It aids in the treatment of anxiety and epilepsy.

15. Theaflavins: Polyphenols formed from the condensation of flavan-3-ols and oolong tea. A powerful antioxidant that may reduce cholesterol and protect your brain.

16. Theanine: It helps protect against mental decline. It has been shown to extend the life span of roundworms by 5 percent.

452. How to Live to Be 100+

- Supplement with vitamin D3.
- Be careful when using pain-relief pills, such as Advil, Motrin, and Aleve. Frequent or excessive use can

raise your risk of heart disease and stroke by 10 percent, according to a 2014 U.S. FDA panel review.

- Sleep eight hours per night. 50 percent of people over sixty-nine have insomnia. Maintain a regular sleep schedule by getting up and going to bed at the same time each day.
- Having a healthy sex life in men was a significant predictor of longevity.
- Married men on average live longer than never married men.
- Drink 3 to 5 cups of coffee per day. A 2015 study showed that those people who drank this much coffee daily had a 15 percent lower risk of premature mortality.
- Eat frozen fruit—it can have higher nutrient counts than fresh.
- Drink green tea. A Japanese study showed that Japanese men who drank 5 or more cups of green tea daily, had a 12 percent decrease in mortality, while women had a 23 percent decrease.
- Do not consume over 25 grams (6 teaspoons) of sugar daily for women, 9 teaspoons for men.
- Eat whole grains such as oatmeal, brown rice, quinoa, barley, and farro. In a 2016 Harvard University research study people who ate whole grains were 20 percent less likely to die prematurely.
- Eat hot chili peppers (active ingredient capsaicin). According to a 2016 analysis of the dietary habits of 16,000 men and women over a twenty-three-year period, it showed a reduced risk of dying by 13 percent.
- If you wish to drink cow's milk, drink organic whole milk. The journal *Circulation* in 2016 showed that those who consumed the most daily fat had a 50

percent lower risk of developing diabetes (which can shorten your life by eight to ten years on average).

- Drink 8 to 10 glasses of clean water daily. This decreases your caloric intake by between 68 and 205 calories per day.

- Eat less and slower. Stop eating when you feel 80 percent full. Cutting back on calories reduces blood pressure, cholesterol, and insulin resistance.

- A 2016 study published in the *Journal of the American Medical Association* found that mortality rates were lower overall for people who eat predominantly veggies and occasionally fish, compared to those who eat no animal products and lacto-ovo vegetarians who eat dairy and eggs.

- Eat a Mediterranean diet: fruits, veggies, olive oil, fish, and nuts.

- Seventh Day Adventists located in Loma Linda, California, have the highest longevity in the US, living eight to ten years longer than average. They do not eat meat, do not drink caffeinated beverages, do not smoke or drink alcohol. They do eat soy-based foods.

- Go nuts! Eating 3½ ounces of walnuts, 8 almonds, and 6 cashews daily can reduce your risk of premature death by 23 percent. Eating a handful of nuts at least five times per week lowers your mortality rate for heart disease by 29 percent, respiratory disease by 24 percent, and cancer by 11 percent.

- Get a pet. Pets can reduce anxiety, lower blood pressure, and even improve the odds of surviving a heart attack.

- Read books, newspapers, and magazines as little as a half hour per day. This amount had a significant survival advantage over non-readers.

- Take the stairs instead of an elevator or escalator if possible. This reduces the risk of dying prematurely by 15 percent.
- Walk briskly at least 10 minutes daily. This benefits your brain, heart, skin, mood, and metabolism. Exaggerate your arm movement when you are walking to help exercise your heart, which is a muscle.

XXIII

FAST FACTS AT A GLANCE

453. Supplements Simplified

So many supplements these days are referred to by letters that nutrition can often seem like an alphabet soup of confusion. I hope this list of commonly used abbreviations simplifies sorting out supplements that might be right for you.

AHAs (alpha-hydroxy acids)—skin exfoliants used to "unglue" old cells and stimulate new cell growth

AKG (alkyglycerol)—disease-fighting compound in shark liver oil

ALA (alpha-linolenic acid)—essential omega-3 fatty acid found in plant sources that needs to be converted by the body to DHA and EPA in order to be made use of

ALC (acetyl-L-carnitine)—slows progression of early-stage Alzheimer's disease; improves cognitive function and memory in older adults

BHAs (beta-hydroxy acids)—skin exfoliants used to "unglue" old cells and stimulate new cell growth

CLA (conjugated linoleic acid)—helps reduce body fat, promote weight loss, enhance muscle tone; protects against many types of cancer

Co-Q10 (coenzyme-Q10)—helps strengthen the heart, reverse gum disease, lower blood pressure

DGL (deglycyrrhizinated licorice)—provides a natural buffer against stomach acid; relieves pain due to excess gas or ulcers; helps reduce pain from arthritis

DHA (docosahexaenoic acid)—essential omega-3 fatty acid that reduces inflammation and can help prevent risk factors associated with chronic diseases such as heart disease, cancer, and arthritis

DHEA (dehydroepiandrosterone)—a natural hormone that strengthens the immune system; may help in treating symptoms of lupus, rheumatoid arthritis, and other autoimmune diseases

DMAE (dimethylaminoethanol)—enhances mental function; acts as a natural alternative to Ritalin in helping children with attention deficit disorder

DNA (deoxyribonucleic acid) and **RNA** (ribonucleic acid)—present in every cell in the body, essential for cell repair and growth; nucleic acids that may slow and even reverse the aging process

EPA (eicosapentaenoic acid)—essential omega-3 fatty acid that works with DHA to reduce inflammation and can help prevent risk factors such as hypertension and high triglycerides associated with heart disease and other chronic conditions

Ev.Ext-33—a patented extract of a unique subspecies of ginger that can reduce pain and inflammation

FOS (fructo-oligosaccharide)—a complex plant sugar; enhances immune function; normalizes blood sugar levels; increases good bacteria in the gut; helps protect against gastrointestinal cancers

GLA (gamma-linolenic acid)—a fatty acid in borage oil used for the treatment of arthritis

HCA (hydrocitric acid)—a natural appetite suppressant

HMB (beta-hydroxy beta-methylbutyrate)—sports supplement; builds muscle, decreases fat

5-HTP (5-hydroxytryptophan)—similar to tryptophan; a natural alternative to Prozac; suppresses appetite; helps alleviate depression and promote restful sleep

IHN (inositol hexanicotinate)—a "no-flush" niacin; helps prevent heart disease by lowering blood triglyceride levels and raising HDL (good cholesterol) levels; may enhance memory

MCP (modified citrus pectin)—a carbohydrate found in plant cell walls; can slow down the spread of cancer

MCTs (medium-chain triglycerides)—saturated fats that are burned rapidly by the body and do not promote weight gain or raise blood cholesterol levels; improve athletic endurance; may help dieters shed pounds

MSM (methylsulfonylmethane)—an organic sulfur; helps reduce allergic symptoms; promotes wound healing; relieves pain and inflammation from arthritis

NAC (n-acetyl cysteine)—increases levels of the body's most abundant antioxidant, glutathione; helps treat ear infections; speed recovery after exercise; protect against cancer-causing chemicals in cigarette smoke

NADH (nicotinamide adenine dinucleotide)—protects against brain aging; helps memory; relieves some symptoms of Alzheimer's and Parkinson's diseases; enhances ability to work out

PC (phosphatidylcholine)—supports liver function; helps to reverse liver damage; aids in preventing memory loss

PCOs (proanthocyanidins)—antioxidants found in the bark, stems, leaves, and skins of some plants; help protect collagen from free radical damage; promote good circulation; may prevent skin from aging

PS (phosphatidylserine)—helps enhance memory and ability to concentrate

PSK (coriolus versicolor extract)—derived from an edible mushroom; boosts and normalizes immune function; improves effect of cancer therapies

SAM-e (s-adenosyl-L-methione)—works as a natural antidepressant and anti-inflammatory; may alleviate pain associated with osteoarthritis

SOD (superoxide dismutase)—a potent antioxidant that can help slow the aging process

TMG (trimethylglycine)—also known as betain; converts harmful homocysteine into a beneficial amino acid; reduces risk of heart disease; helps prevent certain cancers; helps protect against Alzheimer's disease

454. Assorted Acronyms

Although there are acronyms (*abbreviations formed from using the first or first few letters of a series of words to make them easier to pronounce or remember*) for almost anything these days—especially with the advent of texting—the ones for diseases, health organizations, government agencies, and nutritional therapies abound and too often confound. I've compiled the following list to enable quick recognition of those most commonly used and most often confused.

AI (adequate intake)—established for a nutrient when there is insufficient data to calculate an RDA

AMA (American Medical Association)

AMD (age-related macular degeneration)—diminution of vision, partial blindness

APhA (American Pharmacists Association)

BPH (benign prostatic hypertrophy)—an enlargement of the prostate that causes frequent urination

CAM (complementary and alternative medicine)

COPD (chronic obstructive pulmonary disease)—lung disease that makes it difficult to breathe; chronic bronchitis and emphysema

CRP (C-reactive protein)—a blood level marker for inflammation and a risk factor for cardiovascular disease

DRI (dietary reference intake)—umbrella term for groups of values, including RDAs, AIs, EARs, and ULs

DRIs (dietary reference intakes)—the latest nutrient intake recommendations from the Institute of Medicine

DV (percent daily value)—used on food labels as recommendations for nutrients regardless of age or sex

EAR (estimated average requirement)—the accepted standard level of nutrients that an average person requires

FDA (Food and Drug Administration)

IFIC (International Food Information Council)—provides food safety, nutrition, and eating information for making safe food choices

NAS (National Academy of Sciences)

NIAD (National Institute of Allergy and Infectious Diseases)—conducts research to understand, diagnose, treat, and prevent chronic, immunologic, and allergic diseases

ORAC (oxygen radical absorbance capacity)—a standard measure of antioxidant activity in foods

OSHA (Occupational Safety and Health Administration)

PSA (prostate specific antigen)—a blood marker used to screen for prostate cancer

RDA (recommended dietary allowances)—established by the Food and Nutrition Board, National Academy of Sciences, National Research Council; recommended intake levels for various types of dietary supplements

RDI (reference daily intake)—based on recommended dietary allowances; recommends nutrient levels as the percent daily value (DV)

UL (upper limit)—tolerable upper intake level; maximum level of daily nutrient intake that is likely to pose no risk of adverse side effects

USAN (United States Adopted Names Council)—cosponsored by the American Pharmaceutical Association (APhA), the American Medical Association (AMA), and the United States Pharmacopeia (USP) for the specific purpose of coining suitable, acceptable, nonproprietary names in the drug field

US RDA (United States recommended dietary allowance)

455. Finding Good Fats Fast

There's a lot of confusion about good fats and bad fats, which I hope I've cleared up in chapter VI (see sections 91 through 103.) But if you need to know which are the good-for-you fats fast, here's a healthy short list:

Borage oil—contains GLA (gamma-linolenic acid); helpful in reducing inflammation and pain of arthritis; can strengthen adrenal glands; may help regulate menstrual cycles and reduce PMS

Canola oil—excellent source of monounsaturated fat that can raise levels of good cholesterol and lower risk of heart disease

Evening primrose oil—another essential fatty acid containing GLA; converts into hormonelike compounds helpful in treating PMS symptoms, maintaining healthy skin, reducing cholesterol, and controlling high blood pressure

Flaxseed oil—one of the best sources of omega-3 fatty acids; may block growth of cancerous tumors; reduces inflammation; helps normalize hormone levels

Olive oil—high in monounsaturated fat that can raise levels of good cholesterol; lowers risk of heart disease (Go for the extra-virgin cold-pressed if you're using it in food.)

Pumpkin seed oil—high in omega-3 and omega-6 essential fatty acids; helps digestion, circulation, good for pregnant and lactating women

456. Quick Amino Acid Reference

These building blocks of protein are vital to our health, but they, too, can be confusing when it comes to remembering which is which and what does what. (For an in-depth look at individual amino acids, see chapter V, sections 75 through 90.) For faster reference the following list should help:

Alanine: Enhances immune system; lowers risk of kidney stones; aids in alleviating hypoglycemia

Arginine: Increases sperm count; accelerates wound healing; enhances sexual performance in men; tones muscle tissue

Asparagine: Promotes balance in the central nervous system

Aspartic acid: Enhances immune system; increases stamina and endurance; expels harmful ammonia from the body

Branched chain amino acids (leucine, isoleucine, valine): See aspartic acid

Cysteine: Helps prevent baldness; alleviates psoriasis; improves condition of hair, skin, and nails; promotes fat burning and muscle building (converts into cystine as needed)

Cystine: Aids in preventing side effects from chemotherapy and radiation therapy; reduces accumulation of age spots (converts into cysteine as needed)

Glutamic acid: Helps improve brain function; aids in metabolism of sugars and fats; useful in treatment of children's behavioral disorders, epilepsy, and muscular dystrophy (converts into glutamine as needed)

Glutamine: Helps improve brain function; alleviate fatigue; aid in ulcer healing time; build and maintain muscle; elevate mood; reduce craving for sugar and alcohol (converts to glutamic acid in brain)

Glycine: Necessary for central nervous system function; aids in healing; helps treat stomach hyperacidity; helps prevent seizures (can be converted into serine in the body when needed)

Histidine: Helps alleviate rheumatoid arthritis; alleviates stress; aids in improving libido

Isoleucine: Helps promote tissue repair and may prevent muscle wasting

Leucine: Needed for protein synthesis and a healthy immune system

Lysine: Helps improve concentration; enhances fertility; aids in preventing herpes simplex infection

Methionine: Aids in lowering cholesterol; helps in treatment of schizophrenia and Parkinson's disease; may protect against tumors

Ornithine: Works as a muscle-building hormone; increases potency of arginine

Phenylalanine: Acts as an antidepressant; helps suppress appetite; can function in some forms as a natural painkiller

Proline: Aids in wound healing; helps increase learning ability

Serine: Helps alleviate pain; can act as a natural antipsychotic

Taurine: Helps strengthen heart function; may prevent macular degeneration; aids in digestion of fats and absorption of fat-soluble vitamins

Threonine: Necessary for utilization of protein in diet; may provide symptomatic improvement in some patients with Lou Gehrig's disease, amyotrophic lateral sclerosis (ALS)

Tryptophan: Aids in reducing anxiety; helps induce sleep; may help in control of alcoholism

Tyrosine: Improves sex drive; helps alleviate stress; can act as an appetite suppressant and mood elevator

Valine: Necessary for the proper growth and maintenance of body tissues; deficiencies may cause loss of muscular coordination and hypersensitivity to cold, heat, and pain

457. Herbal Sources of Primary Antioxidant Vitamins and Minerals

Vitamin A and Carotenoids: alfalfa, borage leaves, burdock root, cayenne, capsicum, eyebright, fennel seed, hops, horsetail, kelp, lemongrass, nettle, paprika, parsley, peppermint, raspberry leaf, red clover, rose hips, sage, uva ursi, watercress, yellow dock

Vitamin C: alfalfa, burdock root, cayenne, chickweed, eyebright, fennel seed, fenugreek, hops, horsetail, kelp, peppermint, mullein, nettle, oat straw, paprika, parsley, plantain, raspberry leaf, red clover, rose hips, skullcap, yarrow, yellow dock

Vitamin E: alfalfa, dandelion, dong quai, flaxseed, nettle, oat straw, raspberry leaf, rose hips

Selenium: alfalfa, burdock root, catnip, cayenne, chamomile, chickweed, fennel seed, fenugreek, garlic, ginseng, hawthorn berry, hops, horsetail, lemongrass, milk thistle, nettle, oat straw, parsley, peppermint, raspberry leaf, rose hips, sarsaparilla, uva ursi, yarrow, yellow dock

Zinc: alfalfa, burdock root, cayenne, chamomile, chickweed, dandelion, eyebright, fennel seed, hops, milk thistle, mullein, nettle, parsley, rose hips, sage, sarsaparilla, skullcap, wild yam

458. Drug and Supplement Combinations That Don't Mix

Always keep in mind that some supplements may diminish or dangerously increase the effect of a drug and vice versa. It's something to talk to your healthcare provider about *before* filling a prescription. The following is a quick reference list of some of the most potentially incompatible combinations:

AIDS drugs (St. John's wort)

Alcohol (andro products, beta-carotene, chamomile, DHEA, GBL, kava, valerian)

Anesthetics (kava, St. John's wort, valerian)

Anticoagulants (Angelica root, anise, arnica, asafoetida, borage-seed oil, bromelain, capsium, celery, chamomile, clove, Co-Q10, devil's claw, dong quai, fenugre, feverfew, fish oils, flaxseed oil, garlic, ginger, ginkgo biloba, ginseng, goldenseal, green tea, horse chestnut, licorice root, onion, meadowsweet, papain, parsley, passion flower, poplar, red clover, St. John's wort, turmeric, vitamin E, willow bark)

Antidepressants (Ginkgo biloba, SAM-e [S-adenosylmethionine], St. John's wort)

Aspirin (Willow bark and any of the supplements that interact with anticoagulants)

Cholesterol-lowering drugs (Red yeast rice, beta-sitosterol)

Diabetes drugs (Alpha-lipoic acid, bitter melon, chomium picolinate or polynicotinate, D-pinitol, 4-hydroxy-isoleucine)

Diuretics (Aloe, dandelion root, goldenseal, licorice)

Estrogen (Black cohosh, DHEA, saw palmetto, soy isoflavones)

Heart drugs (Aloe, huperzine A, L-arginine, licorice, St. John's wort)

High blood pressure drugs (Aloe, coleus forskohlii, dandelion root, glycerol, goldenseal, guarana, huperzine A, licorice, St. John's wort)

Immunity-suppressing drugs (Astragalus, echinacea, ginseng, melatonin, St. John's wort, vitamin E, zinc)

Methotrexate (Echinacea, high-dose folic acid)

Monoamine oxidase (MAO) Inhibitors (Country mallow, ephedra, melatonin, SAM-e, St. John's wort, yohimbe)

Phenothiazines (Evening primrose oil)

Phenylpropanolamine (Ephedra, synephrine, yohimbe)

Pseudoephedrine (Ephedra, synephrine, yohimbe)

Seizure disorder drugs (Ginkgo biloba, high-dose folic acid, St. John's wort)

Tamoxifen (St. John's wort)

Thyroid hormone (Calcium, guggulsterones)

Tranquilizers or sedatives (chamomile, 5-HIP, guarana, kava, melatonin, St. John's wort, valerian)

459. Big-Time Immune System Boosters

Because the immune system is the most powerful weapon you have for keeping healthy, being able to quickly recall major nutrients, herbs, and supplements that can strengthen it will not only simplify your life—it can help extend it!

Acidophilus
Ashwangandha
Astragalus
Bayberry
Beta-1,3-glucan
Bioflavonoids
Bovine trachel cartilage
Cat's claw (una de gato)
Chlorella
Coenzyme-Q10
DHEA (dehydroepiandrosterone)
Echinacea
Elderberry
Essential fatty acids
Feverfew (American)
Garlic
Germanium
Ginger
Ginseng
Glutathione
Goldenseal
Grape-seed extract
Gugul
Kelp
L-arnine and L-ornithine
Maitake, shiitake, and reishi mushroom
Manganese
Melatonin
Propolis
PSK (coriolus versicolor extract)
Quercetin
Schizandra
Selenium
Shark cartilage/liver oil
Suma
Vitamin A
Vitamin B complex
Vitamin C
Vitamin E
Whey
Zinc

460. Quick-Reference Cancer Defense Guide

Along with antioxidant vitamins and minerals (see chapter VII), there are many naturally occurring substances in foods that appear to have even more powerful anticancer properties. Among them: beta-carotene, quercetin, indoles and isothiocyanatos (in cruciferous vegetables), and omega-3 fatty acids.

Since your best defense against cancer is a strong nutritional offense—be sure you put the following winning foods in your diet.

CANCER-FIGHTING FOODS TO INCREASE IN DIET

Food	Comments
Carrots	Highest in beta-carotene; more easily absorbed when cooked.
Cantaloupe	Great vitamin A, beta-carotene, and vitamin C source; low-calorie and high- fiber; aids in combating excess sodium.
Cabbage	A cruciferous vegetable; can lower risk of colorectal cancer; just 2 tbsp. cooked daily has been found to help prevent stomach cancer.
Squash	Same as carrots above.
Sweet potatoes	Same as carrots above.
Papaya	Same as cantaloupe.
Spinach	Same as cantaloupe.
Broccoli	A cruciferous vegetable that contains indoles and isothiocyanates (substances that help reduce and prevent certain cancerous tumors); rich in carotenoids.
Brussels sprouts	Same as broccoli and other crucifers.
Bok choy	Same as broccoli and other crucifers.
Cauliflower	Same as broccoli and other crucifers.
Kale	Same as broccoli and other crucifers.
Radish	Same as broccoli and other crucifers.

Horseradish	Same as broccoli and other crucifers.
Rutabaga	Same as broccoli and other crucifers.
Kohlrabi	Same as broccoli and other crucifers.
Celery	Same as broccoli and other crucifers.
Onions	High in quercetin (not destroyed by cooking); can suppress malignant cells before they become tumors.
Tuna	Rich in omega-3 fatty acids; helps immune system to prevent and inhibit spreading cancers. (May help halt metastasis once tumor occurs.)
Salmon	Same as tuna.
Sardines	Same as tuna.
Mackerel	Same as tuna.
Bluefish	Same as tuna.
Wheat bran	Dietary fiber content helps prevent colon cancer. (The National Cancer Institute suggests 35 g. of fiber daily.)
Corn bran	Provides protection against carcinogens.
Rice bran	Same as corn and wheat bran.
Oat bran	Same as corn and wheat bran.
Fruits and vegetables	(See sections 30, 46, 48, and 68.) high in vitamins A, C, E, and selenium (See sections 30, 46, 48, and 68.)
Soybeans and soy-based foods	High in many cancer-fighting phytochemicals (See section 143.)

HIGH-RISK CANCER FOODS TO DECREASE IN DIET

Food	Comments
Bacon	Contains nitrite, an additive that can interact with natural chemicals in our foods and bodies to form nitrosamines, potent cancer-causing substances.
Luncheon meats	Same as bacon above.
Frankfurters	Same as bacon above.
Knockwurst	Same as bacon above.
Smoked fish	Same as bacon above.
Butter, margarine, mayonnaise, oils	It's recommended that no more than 20–30 percent of the calories in your diet come from fat. (Individuals whose diets contain over 40 percent fat, saturated as well as unsaturated, are more likely to develop colon, breast, and prostate cancers.) In these foods, 100 percent of the calories are fat.
Coffee (regular or decaffeinated)	Implicated in bladder and pancreatic cancers.
Liver and high-fat meat	Contaminants accumulate in an animal's liver and fat cells.
Tobacco	Cigarettes, cigars, pipes, chewing tobacco, and snuff have been implicated in the development of cancer of the

mouth, throat, esophagus, pancreas, and bladder as well as the lung. (Smoking—as well as secondhand smoke—also increases the risk of cervical cancer for women.)

Alcohol — Found to cause liver cancer and to contribute to cancers of the mouth, larynx, and esophagus, particularly among smokers.

Food additives, particularly BHA, BHT, Food Dyes Red No. 3, Blue No. 2, Green No. 3, and Citrus Red No. 2; propyl gallate and sodium nitrite — Highly suspect carcinogens.

461. Natural Alternatives to HRT

With researchers continuing to find that hormone replacement therapy (HRT) increases women's risks of breast cancer as well as heart attacks, and can—with long-term use—double the risk of developing Alzheimer's and other cognitive problems, the search for natural alternatives is becoming more and more widespread. Diets that regularly contain estrogenic plant compounds add to estrogen levels in the body. The herbs listed below have been found to help lessen hot flashes, vaginal discomfort, and other symptoms of menopause, as well as reduce the risks of osteoporosis and heart disease.

CAUTION: *Be sure to try new herbs and supplements by themselves first, rather than in combinations, so if there is an adverse reaction you know what is responsible.*

Black cohosh (see section 170)

Chasteberry/chaste tree (a hormone balancer that can help alleviate depression; see section 180)

Chickweed (helps relieve hot flashes)

Damiana (an antidepressant with aphrodisiac properties)

Dandelion (reduces stress on liver when hormones are out of balance)

Dong quai (high in plant estrogens; see section 184)

Evening primrose oil (see section 188)

Fenugreek (see section 191)

Flaxseed (helps reduce vaginal dryness)

Ginkgo biloba (see section 121)

Ginseng (see section 135)

Hawthorn (see section 200)

Licorice (a powerful adrenal stimulant and estrogentic herb; see section 205)

Motherwort (lessens severity and duration of hot flashes; helps relieve vaginal dryness and insomnia)

Passionflower (relieves insomnia; see section 209)

Raspberry (an estrogenic herb that helps tone weakened uterine muscles)

Sage (contains estrogen and has many medicinal properties; reduces excessive sweating)

Sarsaparilla (stimulates testosterone production and revives sex drive)

Saw palmetto (can help in treatment of urinary incontinence; see section 217)

Valerian (see section 224)

Wild yam (a powerful estrogenic herb; see section 226)

XXIV

LOCATING A NUTRITIONALLY ORIENTED DOCTOR

462. How to Go About It

If you want to consult a nutritionally oriented physician—or other alternative health practitioner—but don't know any in your area, the following organizations can help you find one. If you're seeking a board-certified physician you should specify that, as not all nutritional health professionals are MDs.

Organizations that have websites, and most do, can provide you with immediate information about licensing, certification, and the fastest way to access a local practitioner.

It should be understood that no endorsement or other opinion of any practitioner contacted through these services (or such practitioner's diagnoses, treatments, or credentials) is implied or should be inferred.

American Academy of Medical Acupuncture (AAMA)
2512 Artesia Blvd, Ste 200
Redondo Beach, CA 90278
(310) 369-8261
Website: www.medicalacupuncture.org

American Academy of Osteopathy (AAO)
3500 DePauw Blvd., Suite 1080
Indianapolis, IN 46268
(317) 879-1881
Website: www.academyofosteopathy.org

American Association of Naturopathic Physicians
300 New Jersey Ave NW, Suite 900
Washington, DC 20001
Fax (202) 237-8150
Website: www.naturopathic.org

American Chiropractic Association (ACA)
1701 Clarendon Blvd., Suite 200
Arlington, VA 22209
(703) 276-8800
Website: www.acatoday.org

American Holistic Nurses Association
2900 S.W. Plass Court
Topeka, KS 66611-1980
(800) 278-2462 or (785) 234-1712
Website: www.ahna.org

Academy of Integrative Health and Medicine (AIHM)
6919 La Jolla Blvd
La Jolla, CA 92037
Website: www.aihm.org

American Massage Therapy Association
500 Davis Street
Suite 900
Evanston, IL 60201
(877) 905-2700
Website: www.amtamassage.org

Council for Responsible Nutrition
1828 L St. NW Suite 810
Washington, DC 20036-5114
(202) 204-7700
Website: www.crnusa.org

Homeopathic Academy of Naturopathic Physicians
(HANP)
600 West Emma Street
Lafayette, Colorado 80026
Website: www.hanp.net

National Center for Complementary and Integrative
Health (NCCIH)
National Institutes of Health
9000 Rockville Pike
Bethesda, MD 20892
Website: www.nccih.nih.gov

National Health Federation
P.O. Box 688
Monrovia, CA 91017
(626) 357-2181
Website: www.thenhf.com

463. Finding Specialized Nutritional Help

For AIDS	The American Foundation for AIDS Research (AMFAR) 1100 Vermont Ave, NW, Suite 600 Washington, DC 20005 (202) 331-8600 Website: www.amfar.org
For alcoholism	Alcoholics Anonymous (AA) World Services 475 Riverside Drive, 11th floor New York, NY 10115 (212) 870-3400 Website: www.aa.org
For allergies	Asthma & Allergy Foundation of America (AAFA) 1235 South Clark Street, Suite 305 Arlington, VA 20222 (800) 7-ASTHMA Website: www.aafa.org
For Alzheimer's	Alzheimer's Disease and Related Dementia Referral Center (ADEAR) National Institute on Aging Building 31, Room 5C27 31 Center Drive, MSC 2292 Bethesda, MD 20892 Website: www.alzheimers.org
For arthritis	Arthritis Foundation 1355 Peachtree St NE Suite 600 Atlanta, GA 30309 Website: www.arthritis.org

For breast-feeding	La Leche League, Int. Inc. 110 Horizon Drive, Suite 210 Raleigh, NC 27615, USA (800) LALECHE Website: www.llli.org
For cancer	American Cancer Society 250 Williams Street NW Atlanta, GA 303031 (800) 227-2345 Website: www.cancer.org National Cancer Institute 9000 Rockville Pike Bethesda, MD 20892 301-496-4000 (800) 4-CANCER Website: www.cancer.gov
For cardiovascular disorders	American Heart Association P.O. Box 3049 Syracuse, NY 13220-3049 (800) AHA-USA1 Website: www.heart.org National Stroke Association (a division of the American Heart Association) 7272 Greenville Ave. Dallas, TX 75231 (800) AHA-USA-1 Website: www.stroke.org
For chronic fatigue syndrome	Chronic Fatigue and Immune Dysfunction Syndrome Association of America, Inc. P.O. Box 220398

Charlotte, NC 28222-0398
(800) 44-CFIDS or
(800) 442-3437
Website: www.cfids.org

For communicative disorders

American Tinnitus Association
P.O. Box 424049
Washington, DC 20042-4049
(800) 634-8978
Website: www.ata.org

National Stuttering Association
3285-B Richmond Avenue #119
Staten Island, NY 10312
(800) 937-8888
Website: www.westutter.org

For depression

Depression and Bipolar Support Alliance (DBSA)
55 E Jackson Blvd, Suite 490
Chicago, IL 60604
(800) 826-3632
Website: www.dbsalliance.org

For diabetes

American Diabetes Association
2451 Crystal Drive, Suite 900
Arlington, VA 22202
(800) DIABETES
Website: www.diabetes.org

Juvenile Diabetes Research Foundation International
200 Vesey Street, 28th FloorNew York, NY 102811-800-533-3873 or 1-800-533-CURE
Website: www.jdrf.org

For eating disorders	Anorexia Nervosa and Related Eating Disorders, Inc. (ANRED) P.O. Box 5102 Eugene, OR 97405 (847) 831-3438 ANAD Website: www.anred.com
For epilepsy	Epilepsy Foundation 3540 Crain Highway, Suite 675 Bowie, MD 20716 301-459-3700 24/7 Epilepsy & Seizures Helpline: 1-00-332-1000 Website: www.epilepsy.com
For infertility	Infertility Resources for Consumers Online directory of infertility services Website: www.ihr.com/infertility/ Resolve The National Infertility Association 7918 Jones Branch Drive, Suite 300, McLean, VA 22102 703.556.7172 (617) 623-0744 or (617) 643-2424 Website: www.resolve.org
For osteoporosis	NIH Osteoporosis and Related Bone Diseases National Resource Center (800) 624-BONE Website: www.bones.nih.gov
For pets	The American Holistic Veterinary Medical Association (AHVMA)

	American Holistic Veterinary Medical Association PO Box 630, Abingdon, MD 21009 (410) 569-0795 Website: www.altvetma.org
For sleep disorders	American Academy of Sleep Medicine 2510 North Frontage Road Darien, IL 60561 Phone: (630) 737-9700 Website: www.aasm.org California Center for Sleep Disorders (several locations in the San Francisco Bay area) Website: www.sleepsmart.com
For women	National Organization for Women (NOW) 1000 16th Street NW, Suite 700 Washington, DC 20036 (202) 331-0066 Website: www.now.org National Women's Health Network 1413 K Street NW, 4th Floor Washington, D.C. 20005 (202) 682-2640 Website: www.nwhn.org

GLOSSARY

Absorption: the process by which nutrients are passed into the bloodstream.

Acetate: a derivative of acetic acid.

Acetic acid: used as a synthetic flavoring agent, one of the first food additives (vinegar is approximately 4–6 percent acetic acid); it is found naturally in cheese, coffee, grapes, peaches, raspberries, and strawberries; generally recognized as safe (GRAS) when used only in packaging.

Acetone: a colorless solvent for fat, oils, and waxes, which is obtained by fermentation (inhalation can irritate lungs, and large amounts have a narcotic effect).

Acid: a water-soluble substance with sour taste.

Adrenals: the glands, located above each kidney, that manufacture adrenaline.

Alkali: an acid-neutralizing substance (sodium bicarbonate is an alkali used for excess acidity in foods).

Allergen: a substance that causes an allergy.

Alzheimer's disease: a progressively degenerative disease, involved with loss of memory, which new research indicates might be helped with extra choline.

Amino acid chelates: chelated minerals that have been produced by many of the same processes nature uses to chelate minerals in the body; in the digestive tract, nature surrounds the elemental minerals with amino acid, permitting them to be absorbed into the bloodstream.

Amino acids: the organic compounds from which proteins are constructed; there are twenty-three known amino acids, but only nine are indispensable nutrients for man—histidine, isoleucine, leucine, lysine, total S-containing amino acids, total aromatic amino acids, threonine, tryptophan, and valine.

Anorexia: loss of appetite.

Antibiotic: any of various substances that are effective in inhibiting or destroying bacteria.

Anticoagulant: something that delays or prevents blood clotting.

Antigen: any substance not normally present in the body that stimulates the body to produce antibodies.

Antihistamine: a drug used to reduce effects associated with histamine production in allergies and colds.

Antioxidant: a substance that can protect another substance from oxidation; added to foods to keep oxygen from changing the food's color.

Antitoxin: an antibody formed in response to, and capable of neutralizing, a poison of biologic origin.

Assimilation: the process whereby nutrients are used by the body and changed into living tissue.

Ataxia: loss of coordinated movement caused by disease of the nervous system.

ATP: a molecule called adenozine triphosphate, the fuel of life, a nucleotide—building block of nucleic acid—that produces biological energy with B1, B2, B3, and pantothenic acid.

Avidin: a protein in egg white capable of inactivating biotin.

Bacteriophage: a virus that infects bacteria.

Bariatrician: a weight-control doctor.

B cells: white blood cells, made in the bone marrow, which produce antibodies upon instructions from T cells, white blood cells manufactured in the thymus.

BHA: butylated hydroxyanisole; a preservative and antioxidant used in many products; insoluble in water; can be toxic to the kidneys.

BHT: butylated hydroxytoluene; a solid, white crystalline antioxidant used to slow spoilage of many foods; can be more toxic to the kidney than its nearly identical chemical cousin BHA.

Bioflavonoids: usually from orange and lemon rinds, these citrus-flavored compounds needed to maintain healthy blood-vessel walls are widely available in plants, citrus fruits, and rose hips; known as vitamin P complex.

Buffered: an antacid has been added to protect the stomach; helps pill dissolve faster.

Calciferol: a colorless, odorless crystalline material, insoluble in water; soluble in fats; a synthetic form of vitamin D made by irradiating ergosterol with ultraviolet light.

Calcium gluconate: an organic form of calcium.

Capillary: a minute blood vessel, one of many that connect the arteries and veins.

Carcinogen: a cancer-causing substance.

Carotene: an orange-yellow pigment occurring in many plants and capable of being converted into vitamin A in the body.

Casein: the protein in milk that has become the standard by which protein quality is measured.

Catabolism: the metabolic change of nutrients or complex substances into simpler compounds, accompanied by a release of energy.

Catalyst: a substance that modifies, especially increases, the rate of chemical reaction without being consumed or changed in the process.

Chelation: a process by which mineral substances are changed into easily digestible form.

Chronic: of long duration; continuing; constant.

CNS: central nervous system.

Coenzyme: the major, though nonprotein, part of an enzyme; usually a B vitamin.

Collagen: the primary organic constituent of bone, cartilage, and connective tissue (becomes gelatin through boiling).

Congenital: condition existing at birth, not hereditary.

Coumestans: estrogenlike substances (phytoestrogens) made by some plants that may have anticancer effects.

Dehydration: a condition resulting from an excessive loss of water from the body.

Dermatitis: an inflammation of the skin; a rash.

Desiccated: dried; preserved by removing moisture.

Dicalcium phosphate: a filler used in pills, which is derived from purified mineral rocks and is an excellent source of calcium and phosphorus.

Diluents: fillers; inert material added to tablets to increase their bulk in order to make them a practical size for compression.

Diuretic: tending to increase the flow of urine from the body.

DHA: docosahexaenoic acid; a member of the omega-3 family of essential fatty acids; made in the body from alpha-linolenic acid; found mainly in cold-water fish.

DNA: deoxyribonucleic acid; the nucleic acid in chromosomes that is part of the chemical basis for hereditary characteristics.

Endogenous: being produced from within the body.

Enteric coated: a tablet coated so that it dissolves in the intestine, not in the stomach (which is acid).

Enuresis: bed-wetting.

Enzyme: a protein substance found in living cells that brings about chemical changes; necessary for digestion of food.

EPA: eicosapentaenoic acids; members of the omega-3 family of essential fatty acids.

Excipient: any inert substance used as a dilutant or vehicle for a drug.

Exogenous: being derived or developed from external causes.

FDA: Food and Drug Administration.

Fibrin: an insoluble protein that forms the necessary fibrous network in the coagulation of blood.

Free radicals: highly reactive chemical fragments that can produce an irritation of artery walls and start the arteriosclerotic process if vitamin E is not present; generally harmful.

Fructose: a natural sugar occurring in fruits and honey; called fruit sugar; often used as a preservative for foodstuffs and an intravenous nutrient.

Galactosemia: a hereditary disorder in which milk becomes toxic as food.

Gamma oryszanol: a by-product of rice bran that helps increase lean body mass while decreasing fatty tissue.

GLA: gamma-linolenic acid; member of the omega-6 family; made in the body from linoleic acid.

Glucose: blood sugar; a product of the body's assimilation of carbohydrates and a major source of energy.

Glutamic acid: an amino acid present in all complete proteins; usually manufactured from vegetable protein; used as a salt substitute and a flavor-intensifying agent.

Glutamine: an amino acid that constitutes, with glucose, the major nourishment used by the nervous system.

Gluten: a mixture of two proteins—gliadin and glutenin—present in wheat, rye, oats, and barley.

Glycogen: the body's chief storage carbohydrate, primarily in the liver.

GRAS: generally recommended as safe; a list established by Congress to cover substances added to food.

HDL: high-density lipoprotein; carries fats and cholesterol through bloodstream; considered the "good" cholesterol.

Hesperidin: part of the C complex.

Holistic treatment: treatment of the whole person.

Homeostasis: the body's physiological equilibrium.

Hormone: a substance formed in endocrine organs and transported by body fluids to activate other specifically receptive organs.

Humectant: a substance that is used to preserve the moisture content of materials.

Hydrochloric acid: a normally acidic part of the body's gastric juice.

Hydrogenation: a commercial process that solidifies oils (margarines and shortenings) by a chemical process; transfatty acids created by this process can raise cholesterol levels.

Hydrolyzed: put into water-soluble form.

Hydrolyzed protein chelate: water-soluble and chelated for easy assimilation.

Hypervitaminosis: a condition caused by an excessive ingestion of vitamins.

Hypoglycemia: a condition caused by abnormally low blood sugar.

Hypovitaminosis: a deficiency disease owing to an absence of vitamins in the diet.

Ichthyosis: a condition characterized by a scaliness on the outer layer of skin.

Idiopathic: a condition whose causes are not yet known.

Immune: protected against disease.

Insulin: the hormone, secreted by the pancreas, concerned with the metabolism of sugar in the body.

IU: international units.

Lactating: producing milk.

Laxative: a substance that stimulates evacuation of the bowels.

LDL: low-density lipoprotein; the "bad" substance that deposits cholesterol along the artery walls when oxidized.

Lignans: chemicals derived from flaxseeds, pumpkin seeds, cranberries, and whole grains that have phytoestrogenic properties.

Linoleic acid: one of the polyunsaturated fats, a constituent of lecithin; known as vitamin F; primary member of the omega-6 family; indispensable for life, and must be obtained from foods.

Lipid: a fat or fatty substance.

Lipofuscin: age pigment in cells.

Lipoprotein: a carrier of fatty substances (fats, oil, cholesterol); transporter of lipids between intestine, liver, and body cells; characterized by weight (i.e., low-density, high-density, etc.).

Lipotropic: preventing abnormal or excessive accumulation of fat in the liver.

Megavitamin therapy: treatment of illness with massive amounts of vitamins.

Metabolize: to undergo change by physical and chemical processes.

Mucopolysaccharide: thick gelatinous material that is found many places in the body; it glues cells together and lubricates joints.

MUFA: monounsaturated fatty acid.

Nitrites: used as fixatives in cured meats; can combine with natural stomach and food chemicals to cause dangerous cancer-causing agents called nitrosamines.

Omega-3: a family of essential fatty acids generally supplied inadequately in the modern diet; the primary omega-3 is alpha-linolenic acid.

Omega-6: a family of essential fatty acids abundant in the modern diet; the primary omega-6 is linolenic acid.

Orthomolecular: the right molecule used for the right treatment; doctors who practice preventive medicine and use vitamin therapies are known as orthomolecular physicians.

Oxalates: organic chemicals found in certain foods, especially spinach, that can combine with calcium to form calcium oxalate, an insoluble chemical the body cannot use.

PABA: para-aminobenzoic acid; a member of the B complex.

Palmitate: water-solubilized vitamin A.

Phospholipids: a class of fatty compounds found in cell membranes; lecithin is best known.

PKU (phenylketonuria): a hereditary disease caused by the lack of an enzyme needed to convert an essential amino acid (phenylalanine) into a form usable by the body; can cause intellectual disability unless detected early.

Polyphenols: beneficial plant chemicals, classified as antioxidants, found abundantly in skins of grapes and red wine.

Polyunsaturated fats: highly nonsaturated fats from vegetable sources; tend to lower blood cholesterol.

Predigested protein: protein that has been processed for fast assimilation and can go directly into the bloodstream.

Proprioception: the mind's ability to know what the body is doing.

Prostaglandins: hormonelike substances that aid in regulation of the immune system.

Provitamin: a vitamin precursor; a chemical substance necessary to produce a vitamin.

PUFA: polyunsaturated fatty acid.

RNA: the abbreviation used for ribonucleic acid.

Rose hips: a rich source of vitamin C; the nodule underneath the bud of a rose called a hip, in which the plant produces the vitamin C we extract.

Rutin: a substance extracted from buckwheat; part of the C complex.

Saturated fatty acids: usually solid at room temperature; higher proportions found in foods from animal sources; tend to raise blood cholesterol levels.

Sequestrant: a substance that absorbs ions and prevents changes that would affect flavor, texture, and color of food; used for water-softening.

Sirtuins: enzymes that are regulators of aging in virtually all living organisms, allowing cells to survive damage and delay cell death.

Syncope: brief loss of consciousness; fainting.

Synergistic: the action of two or more substances to produce an effect that neither alone could accomplish.

Synthetic: produced artificially.

Systemic: capable of spreading through the entire body.

T cells: white blood cells, manufactured in the thymus, which protect the body from bacteria, viruses, and cancer-causing agents, while controlling the production of B cells, which produce antibodies, and unwanted production of potentially harmful T cells.

Teratological: monstrous or abnormal formations in animals or plants.

Tocopherols: the group of compounds (alpha, beta, delta, episilon, eta, gamma, and zeta) that make vitamin E; obtained through vacuum distillation of edible vegetable oils.

Toxicity: the quality or condition of being poisonous, harmful, or destructive.

Toxin: an organic poison produced in living or dead organisms.

Trans-fatty acids: artificial fatty acids produced by hydrogenation; although unsaturated, act like saturated fats and are unhealthy.

Triglycerides: fatty substances in the blood.

Unsaturated fatty acids: most often liquid at room temperature; primarily found in vegetable fats.

Xerosis: a condition of dryness.

Zein: protein from corn.

Zyme: a fermenting substance.

BIBLIOGRAPHY AND RECOMMENDED READING

I owe a great debt of thanks to the many scientists, doctors, nutritionists, professors, and researchers whose painstaking and all too often unrewarding work in the field of vitamins and nutrition has made this book possible.

The following list is given to show my sincere appreciation and make known the foundation upon which I have built my knowledge. Many of the books are highly technical and confusing for the layman, meant as they are for professionals in the field. But others, which I have marked with an asterisk, I heartily commend to you for further reading and a healthier future.

In addition to these many useful books, you can find up-to-date research and information on PubMed.gov.

*Abrahamson, E. M., and A. W. Pezet. *Body, Mind, and Sugar.* New York: Avon Books, 1977.

*Abravanel, Elliot D., MD, and Elizabeth A. King. *Anti-Craving Weight Loss Diet.* New York: Bantam Books, 1990.

*Adams, Ruth. *The Complete Home Guide to All the Vitamins*. New York: Larchmont Books, 1972.

*Adams, Ruth, and Frank Murray. *Minerals: Kill or Cure*. New York: Larchmont Books, 1976.

*Aguilar, Nona. *Totally Natural Beauty*. New York: Rawson Associates, 1977.

*Airola, Paavo. *Are You Confused?* Phoenix, AZ: Health Plus, 1972.

*———. *How to Get Well*. Phoenix, AZ: Health Plus, 1975.

*———. *Hypoglycemia: A Better Approach*. Phoenix, AZ: Health Plus, 1977.

Amberson, Rosanne. *Raising Your Cat*. New York: Bonanza Books, 1969.

Arnot, Robert, MD. "Carbo Unloading." *Men's Health* (June 1997).

*Atkins, Robert C. *Dr. Atkins' Diet Revolution*. New York: David McKay, 1972.

*———. *Dr. Atkins' New Diet Revolution*. New York: Avon Books, 1997.

*Balch, James F., and Phyllis A. Balch. *Prescription for Nutritional Healing: Second Edition*. Garden City, NY: Avery, 1997.

* Ballentine, Rudolph. *Diet and Nutrition: A Holistic Approach*. Himalayan Institute Press, 2007.

* Berger, Leslie. "Herbs for Hot Flashes: New Attention, Mixed Results." *New York Times*. (August 12, 2003).

Bernstein, Richard K. *The Diabetic Diet*. New York: Little, Brown, and Company, 2005.

Berry, Jan. *The Big Book of Homemade Products for Your Skin, Health and Home*. Salem, Mass: Page Street Publishing, 2019.

*Bicks, Jane R., DVM. *Dr. Jane's 30 Days to a Healthier, Happier Cat: The Complete Guide to Nutrition and Health*. New York: Perigee, 1997.

Bieri, John G. "Fat-Soluble Vitamins in the Eighth Revision of the Recommended Dietary Allowances." *Journal of the American Dietetic Association* 64 (February 1974).

*Boldt, Ethan. "Drug-Supplement Interactions." *Physical mag.com.* (June 2003).

*Bolles, Edmund Blair. *Learning to Live with Chronic Fatigue Syndrome.* New York: Dell Medical Library, 1990.

*Borek, Carmia. *Maximize Your Health-Span with Antioxidants: The Baby Boomer's Guide.* New Canaan, CT: Keats, 1995.

*———. "Aging Gracefully with Antioxidants." *Nutrition Science News* (March 1998).

*Borsaak, Henry. *Vitamins: What They Are and How They Can Benefit You.* New York: Pyramid Books, 1971.

*Bricklin, Mark. *Prevention Magazine's Nutrition Advisor.* Emmaus, PA: Rodale Press, 1993.

Brody, Jane E. *The New York Times Guide to Personal Health.* New York: Times Books, 1982.

———. "In Vitamin Mania, Millions Take a Gamble on Health." *New York Times* (October 26, 1997).

*———. " 'Normal' Blood Pressure: Health Watchdogs Are Resetting the Risk." *New York Times* (August 12, 2003).

Brown, Susan. *Better Bones Better Body.* New York: McGraw-Hill, 2000.

Bruno, Gene, MHS. "Natural Treatments for Varicose Veins." *Natural Products Marketplace* (December 2008).

Bulsiewicz, Will, MD. *Fiber Fueled.* New York, Avery: 2020.

Burton, Benjamin. *Human Nutrition.* 3rd ed. New York: McGraw-Hill, 1976.

*Carper, Jean. *Miracle Cures.* New York: HarperCollins, 1997.

CDC Yellow Book 2019: Health Information for International Travel. (Gary W, Blumenthal, et.al, eds). New York: Oxford University Press, 2019

Chalem, Jack, Burton Berkson, and Melissa Diane Smith. *Syndrome X: The Silent Killer: The New Heart Disease Risk.* New York: John Wiley and Sons, 2000.

Chappell, P. *Emotional Healing with Homeopathy.* Berkeley, CA: North Atlantic Books, 2003.

*Charello-Ebner, Kaylynn. "Superfruits: Harnessing the Exotic." *WholeFoods* (August 2009).

*"Chronic Fatigue Syndrome: A Modern Medical Mystery." *Newsweek* (November 12, 1990).

Cichoke, Anthony J. "Nutritional Libido Boosters." *Health Foods Business* (June 1998).

*Consumer Reports, Editors of. *The Medicine Show.* Mount Vernon, NY: Consumers Union, 1981.

Cooper, Kenneth H., MD. *Overcoming Hypertension.* New York: Bantam Books, 1990.

Cordain, Loren. *The Paleo Diet.* New York: John Wiley, 1992.

Cowley, Geoffrey, and Anne Underwood. "Memory." *Newsweek* (June 15, 1998).

Cumulative Index for Journal of Applied Nutrition. La Habra, CA: International College of Applied Nutrition, 1947–76, 1976.

Dowdle, Hillari. "The Super Simple Guide to Healing Herbs." *Natural Health* (September 2009).

*Dufty, William. *Sugar Blues.* Pennsylvania: Chilton, 1975.

Duyff, Robert Larson. *American Dietetic Association Complete Food and Nutrition Guide.* New York: John Wiley, 2006.

*Ebon, Martin. *Which Vitamins Do You Need?* New York: Bantam Books, 1974.

*Ellin, Abby. "A Few Cookies a Day to Keep the Pounds Away?" *New York Times* (October 22, 2009).

Ellis, Brian. "The Essential Vitamin K." *Nutrition Industry Executive* (April 2009).

Farrar, Jill. "Health & Fitness." *Vogue Australia* (December 1990).

Flynn, Margaret A. "The Cholesterol Controversy." *Journal of the American Pharmacy* NS18 (May 1978).

"Food Facts Talk Back." *Journal of the American Dietetic Association,* 1977.

Forister, Glenn J., D.J. Blessing. *Introduction to Research and Medical Literature for Health Professionals, 5th edition.* Burlington, MA: Jones & Bartlett Learning, 2019

*Foster, Steven, and James A. Duke. *A Field Guide to Medicinal Plants and Herbs of the Eastern and Central US.* Boston, Mass: Houghton Mifflin, 2000.

*Frank, Benjamin S. *No-Aging Diet.* New York: Dial, 1976.

*Fredericks, Carlton. *Eating Right for You.* New York: Grosset and Dunlap, 1972.

*———. *Look Younger/Feel Healthier.* New York: Grosset and Dunlap, 1977.

*———. *Psycho Nutrients.* New York: Grosset and Dunlap, 1975.

Garrard, Judith. *Health Sciences Literature Review Made Easy: The Matrix Method.* Jones & Bartlett Learning. Burlington: MA, 2016.

*Gomez, Joan, and Marvin J. Gerch. *Dictionary of Symptoms.* New York: Stein and Day, 1963.

Goodhart, Robert S., and Maurice E. Shills. *Modern Nutrition in Health and Disease.* 5th ed. Philadelphia: Lea and Febiger, 1973.

*Graedon, Joel. *The People's Pharmacy.* New York: St. Martin's Press, 1976.

*Graedon, Joel and Teresa, PhD. *The People's Guide to Deadly Drug Interactions.* New York: St. Martin's Press, 1995.

*Greenwell, Ivy. "DHEA: Anti-aging Medicine." *Life Extension.* (Collector's Edition, 2003).

*Grieve, Maude. *A Modern Herbal.* New York: Dover Publications, 1971.

*Gropper, Sareen S., and Jack L. Smith. *Advanced Nutrition and Human Metabolism.* Wadsworth Publishing, 2008.

Guidelines for the Eradication of Iron Deficiency Anemia. New York: International Nutritional Anemia Consultative Group (INACG), 1976.

Guidelines for the Eradication of Vitamin-A Deficiency and Xerophthalmia. International Vitamin-A Consultative Group (IVACG).

Guthrie, Catherine. "Red-Hot Omega-3." *Natural Health.* (May 2009).

Hanlon, Toby, EdD. "The Love Affair Is Over." *Prevention.* (May, 2003).

Harper, Alfred E. "Recommended Dietary Allowances: Are They What We Think They Are?" *Journal of the American Dietetic Association* 64 (February 1974).

Head, Anthony. "Diet Watch: Resolutions for the Happy—and Healthy—New Year." *Health News & Views* (January 1998).

Hermann, Mindy. "A Call for Calcium." *Modern Maturity* (March/April 1998).

Hermann, Mindy, MBA, RD, "6 Smart Supplements That Promise Protection for Your Heart Health." *Environmental Nutrition* (December 2008).

Hershoff, A. *Homeopathic Remedies.* New York: Avery, 2000.

Holford, Patrick. *The New Optimum Nutrition Bible.* Crossing Press, 2005.

Holley, Kyndra D. *Keto Happy Hour.* Victory Belt Publishing, February 2018

Holt, S. *A Primer of Natural Therapeutics: A Certification Program for Dietary Supplement Counselors.* Little Falls, NJ: Wellness Publishing, 2008.

Holvey, David, ed. *The Merck Manual.* 12th ed. Rahway, NJ: Merck and Co., 1972.

Howe, Phyllis S. *Basic Nutrition in Health and Disease.* 6th ed. Philadelphia: W. B. Saunders, 1976.

"How Nutritious Are Fast-Food Meals?" *Consumer Reports* (May 1975).

*Hunter, B. T. *The Natural Foods Primer.* New York: Simon and Schuster, 1972.

Ignarro, Louis, Ph.D. *No More Heart Disease: How Nitric Oxide Can Prevent—Even Reverse—Heart Disease.* New York: St. Martin's Press, 2006.

Index of Nutrition Education Materials. Washington, DC: Nutrition Foundation, 1977.

Insel, Paul, R. Elaine Turner, and Don Ross. *Discovering Nutrition, Third Edition.* Sudbury, MA: Jones & Bartlet, 2009.

Janowitz, Dr. Eric. *The Synergy Health Solution: The Ultimate Framework to Unlock Your Health Potential.* (Self-published), June 2020

Jones, Cindy, PhD. "Rosemary's Whole Plant Properties Counter Cancer." *Nutrition Science News* (March 1998).

Journal of Applied Nutrition. International College of Applied Nutrition, La Habra, CA, 1974–76.

Khalssa, Suram, MD. *The Vitamin D Revolution.* New York: McGraw Hill, 2005.

*Kilham, Chris. "Gymnema, The Sugar Destroyer." *Physicalmag.com* (June 2003).

*Kirschmann, John, and Inc. Nutrition Search. *Nutrition Almanac.* New York: McGraw Hill, 2006.

Knowlton, Leslie. "Vitamins: Why They're Vital." *Los Angeles Times* (April 3, 1998).

*Kolata, Gina. "Hormone Studies: What Went Wrong?" *New York Times* (April 22, 2003).

*Kowalsi, Robert E. *The 8-Week Cholesterol Cure.* New York: Harper and Row, 1987.

Kristof, Nicholas D. "Something Scary in the Pantry." *New York Times* (November 8, 2009).

Kvidahl, Melissa. "A Functional Future for Superfruits." *Nutrition Industry Executive* (March 2009).

Levin, Neil E. "Vitamin D Beyond the Basics." *Vitamin Retailer* (February 2009).

Lewin, Renate. "Chronic Fatigue Syndrome: It's Not All in Your Head." *Let's Live,* February 1991.

*Lewis, Randine. *The Infertility Cure: The Ancient Chinese Wellness Program for Getting Pregnant and Having Healthy Babies.* New York: Little, Brown & Company, 2004.

Li, William W., MD. *Eat to Beat Disease.* Grand Central Publishing: New York 2019.

Lin, Judith, and Laura Goldstein. "The New Cholesterol Busters." *Prevention,* May 1998.

*Linde, Shirley. *The Whole Health Catalog.* New York: Rawson Associates, 1977.

"The Losing Formula." *Newsweek* (April 30, 1990).

Maroon, Joseph, MD. "The Simple Supplement That May Prevent Killer Diseases." *Bottom Line* (September 2009).

Martin, Marvin. *Great Vitamin Mystery.* Rosemont, IL: National Dairy Council, 1978.

Masters, Maria. "The Truth About Fiber." *Men's Health* (November 2009).

Mazori, Daniel. "Antibiotic Alternatives." *Natural Health* (December/January 2010).

McCord, Holly, RD. "Ins and 'Oats' of Soluble Fiber." *Prevention* (July 1997).

———. "Revealed: How Tofu Helps Your Ticker." *Prevention* (January 1997).

*McGinnis, Terri. *The Well Cat Book*. New York: Random House-Bookworks, 1975.

*———. *The Well Dog Book*. New York: Random House–Bookworks, 1974.

McNeil, Donald G., Jr. "Sometimes, the Labels Lie." *New York Times* (September 9, 2003).

* Merck; 14th Edition. *The Merck Index: An Encyclopedia of Chemicals, Drugs, and Biologicals*. Whitehouse Station, NJ: Merck & Co., 2006.

**The Merck Manual of Medical Information: Home Edition*. Whitehouse Station, NJ: Merck & Co, 2006.

Miller, Sue. "A Natural Mood Booster." *Newsweek* (May 5, 1997).

*Mindell, Earl. *Earl Mindell's Anti-Aging Bible*. New York: Fireside, 1996.

*———. *Earl Mindell's Diet Bible*. Gloucester, MA: Fair Winds Press, 2002.

*———. *Earl Mindell's New Herb Bible*. New York: Fireside, 2002.

*———. *Earl Mindell's Nutrition & Health for Dogs*. Rocklin, CA: Prima Publishing, 1998.

*———. *Earl Mindell's Secret Remedies*. New York: Fireside, 1997.

*———. *Earl Mindell's Soy Miracle*. New York: Fireside, 1995.

*————. *Earl Mindell's Supplement Bible.* New York: Fireside, 1998.

*————, and Hopkins, Virginia. *Prescription Alternatives 4th Edition.* New York: McGraw Hill, 2009.

*————, *Earl Mindell's The Happiness Effect.* New York: Square One, 2015.

*————, and Bruno, Gene, *What's in Your Blood and Why You Should Care.* New York: Square One, 2019

Mitchell, Helen S. "Recommended Dietary Allowances Up to Date." *Journal of the American Dietetic Association* 64 (February 1974).

National Research Council. *Recommended Dietary Allowances.* 10th ed. Washington, DC: National Academy Press, 1989.

*Newbold, H. L. *Dr. Newbold's Revolutionary New Discovery About Weight Loss.* New York: Rawson Associates, 1977.

*————. *Mega-Nutrients for Your Nerves.* New York: Peter H. Wyden, 1973.

*Null, Gary. *The Natural Organic Beauty Book.* New York: Dell, 1972.

*Null, Gary and Steve. *The Complete Book of Nutrition.* New York: Dell, 1972.

**Nutrition Almanac.* New York: McGraw-Hill, 1973.

Nutrition—Applied Personally. La Habra, CA: International College of Applied Nutrition, 1978.

Nutrition Information Resources for the Whole Family. National Nutrition Education Clearing House, 1978.

Nutrition Labeling: How It Can Work for You. National Nutrition Consortium, American Dietetic Association, 1975.

Nutrition Source Book. Rosemont, IL: National Dairy Council, 1978.

Oppel, Marissa, MS. "Cranberry Effective in Treating UTIs during Pregnancy and Lactation." *HerbalGram 80.* (March 2008).

"Organic Chemicals in Water: A Major Health Concern." *Consumer Reports* 69 (February 1983).

Papadimitriou, Dimitri, PhD. "Bountiful Berries Benefit the Body." *Natural Products Marketplace* (January 2009).

*Papas, Andreas M., PhD. "Vitamin E's Powerful Family of Anitoxidants." *Functional Food & Nutriceuticals.* (August, 2003).

*Passwater, Richard A. *The New Supernutrition.* New York: Pocket Books, 1981.

*Pearson, Durk, and Sandy Shaw. *Life Extension.* New York: Warner Books, 1983.

Pelton, Ross, RPh, PhD. "Drug-Induced Nutritional Deficiencies." *Natural Pharmacy* (June 1998).

Pennington, Jean A. T., PhD, et al. *Bowes and Church's Food Values of Portions Commonly Used.* 17th ed. New York: Lippincott, 1997.

*Pitcairn, Richard H., and Susan Hubble Pitcairn. *Dr. Pitcairn's Complete Guide to Natural Health for Dogs and Cats.* Emmaus, PA: Rodale Press, 1995.

*Pitchford, Paul. *Healing with Whole Foods: Asian Tradition and Modern Nutrition.* Berkeley, CA: North Atlantic Books (3rd Edition), 2002.

*Pommery, Jean. *What to Do Till the Veterinarian Comes.* Radnor, PA: Chilton, 1976.

Price, Weston. *Nutrition and Physical Regeneration.* La Mesa, CA: Price Pottenger Nutrition Foundation, 2008.

*Pritikin, Nathan. *The Pritikin Permanent Weight-Loss Manual.* New York: Grosset & Dunlap, 1981.

*Raines, Ben. "Your Deadly Diet." *Health* (June 2003).

Randolph, John. *The Brain Healthy Book.* New York: WW Norton & Company (December, 2019)

*Rodale, J. I. *The Complete Book of Minerals for Health.* 4th ed. Emmaus, PA: Rodale Books, 1976.

*———. *The Encyclopedia of Common Diseases.* Emmaus, PA: Rodale Press, 1976.

Roman, Mark. "Your Sexual Appetite." *Men's Health* (September 1997).

*Rosenberg, Harold, and A. N. Feldzaman. *Doctor's Book of Vitamin Therapy: Megavitamins for Health.* New York: Putnam's, 1974.

Rosenthal, Joshua, Institute of Integrative Nutrition. "Lowdown on Sweet." *New York Times.* (February 2006).

*Sahelian, Ray, MD. *Natural Sex Boosters: Supplements That Enhance Stamina, Sensation, and Sexuality for Men and Women.* New York: Square One Publishers, 2004.

*Schiffman, Susan S., and Joan Scobey. *The Nutri/System Flavor Set-Point Weight-Loss Cookbook.* Boston: Little, Brown, and Company, 1990.

*Seaman, Barbara. *Women and the Crisis in Sex Hormones.* New York: Rawson Associates, 1977.

*Sears, Barry, PhD. *Mastering the Zone.* New York: Reagan Books/HarperCollins, 1997.

Shaghaghi, Mino. "Deliverance from the Deep." *Psychology Today* (2009).

Shapiro, Laura. "Fat, Fatter: But Who's Counting?" *Newsweek* (June 15, 1998).

*Shute, Wilfrid E., and Harold J. Taub. *Vitamin E for Ailing and Healthy Hearts.* New York: Pyramid Books, 1969.

*Sinopoulus, Artemis P., MD, and Jo Robinson. *The Omega Plan.* New York: HarperCollins, 1998.

*Sizer, Frances, and Ellie Whitney. *Nutrition Concepts and Controversies*. Florence, KY: Brooks Cole, 2007.

*Smith, Lendon, MD. *Feed Yourself Right*. New York: McGraw-Hill, 1983.

*Spock, Benjamin. *Baby and Child Care*. New York: Simon and Schuster, 1976.

Starr, Sara. "Ten Supplements That Promise a Younger Future." *Health Foods Business* (October 1997).

*Steinman, David. *Diet for a Poisoned Planet*. New York: Harmony Brooks, Crown Publishers, 1990.

*Stoff, Jesse A., MD. *Chronic Fatigue Syndrome: The Hidden Epidemic*. New York: Harper and Row, 1988.

*Strogov, Leelila. "NADH." *Physicalmag.com* (June 2003).

The World Almanac 2010. New York: Infobase Publishing, 2010.

Thompson, Trisha. "Eat Your Heart Out?" *Fame* (February 1990).

*Tierra, Michael. *The Way of Herbs*. New York: Washington Square Press, 1983.

"Too Much Sugar." *Consumer Reports* 43 (March 1973).

Underwood, Eric J. *Trace Elements in Human and Animal Nutrition*. 4th ed. New York: Academic Press, 1977.

United Nations, Food and Agriculture Organization. *Calorie Requirements*, 2009.

U.S. Department of Agriculture. *Amino Acid Content of Food Research Report*, 2002.

U.S. Department of Agriculture. *Composition of Foods: Raw, Processed, Prepared*, 2008.

U.S. Department of Agriculture. *Nutritive Value of American Foods*, 2009.

U.S. Department of Health, Education and Welfare. *Consumer Health Education: A Directory*, 1975.

"The U.S. Food and Drug Administration: On Food and Drugs." USFDA.com, 2010.

U.S. President's Council on Physical Fitness and Sports (Oct. 13, 2009).

U.S. Senate. Select Committee on Nutrition and Human Needs. *Diet and Killer Diseases with Press Reaction and Additional Information*. Washington, DC: U.S. Government Printing Office, 1977.

U.S. Senate. Select Committee on Nutrition and Human Needs. *National Nutrition Policy: Nutrition and the Consumer II*. Washington, DC: U.S. Government Printing Office, 1974.

"Vitamin-Mineral Safety, Toxicity and Misuse." *Journal of the American Dietetic Association*, 1978.

*Wade, Carlson, and Theresa Digeronimo. *Symptoms, Ailments, and Their Natural Remedies*. Paramus, NJ: Reward Books, 2000.

Walker, Morton, DPM. "New Information on Calcium." *Health Foods Business* (December 1997).

Wardlaw, Gordon M., and Ann M. Smith. *Contemporary Nutrition, Updated Sixth Edition*. New York: McGraw Hill, 2007.

"Weigh Too Much? How to Figure It Out." *USA Today* (February 2, 1998).

Werbach, Melvyn R., MD. "Cataract: the Antioxidant Enzymes." *Townsend Letter* (May 2009).

Weston, Jessica Jean. *Healing Tonics, Juices, and Smoothies* New York: Skyhorse Publishing, June 2017.

*Whalen, Jeanne. "Beyond the Heart, What Else Can Omega 3s Do?" *Wall Street Journal* (September 15, 2009).

*Whelan, Elizabeth M., PhD, and Fredrick J. Stare, MD. *The 100% Natural, Purely Organic, Cholesterol-Free, Megavitamin, Low-Carbohydrate Nutrition Hoax*. New York: Atheneum, 1983.

Whitney, Eleanor Noss, and Sharon Rady Rolfes. *Understanding Nutrition*. Florence, KY: Wadsworth Publishing, 2007.

Willet, Walter C., MD, and P. J. Skerett. *Eat, Drink, and Be Healthy: The Harvard Medical School Guide to Healthy Living*. Free Press, 2005.

Williams, J.E., OMD. *Prolonging Health*. Newbury, MA: Hampton Roads, 2003.

*Yeager, Seleine; Prevention Health Books, ed. *Doctor's Book of Food Remedies*. New York: St. Martin's, 2000.

*Young, L. A., L. G. Young, M. M. Klein, and D. Beyer. *Recreational Drugs*. New York: Macmillan, 1977.

Zimmerman, Marcia, CN. "Is DHEA an Antidote to Aging?" *Nutrition Science News* (October, 1996).

*Zinczenko, David, and Matt Goulding. *Eat This Not That 2010: The No-Diet Weight Loss Solution*. New York: Rodale, 2009.

Zogheib, Susan, MHS, RD. *The Easy Mediterranean Diet Meal Plan*. Emeryville, CA: Rockridge Press, 2019.

INDEX

NOTE: Page references in **bold** indicate numbered main entries